WILD sauna

EMMA O'KELLY

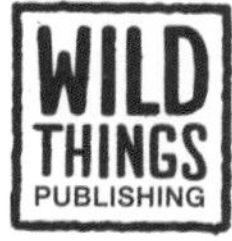

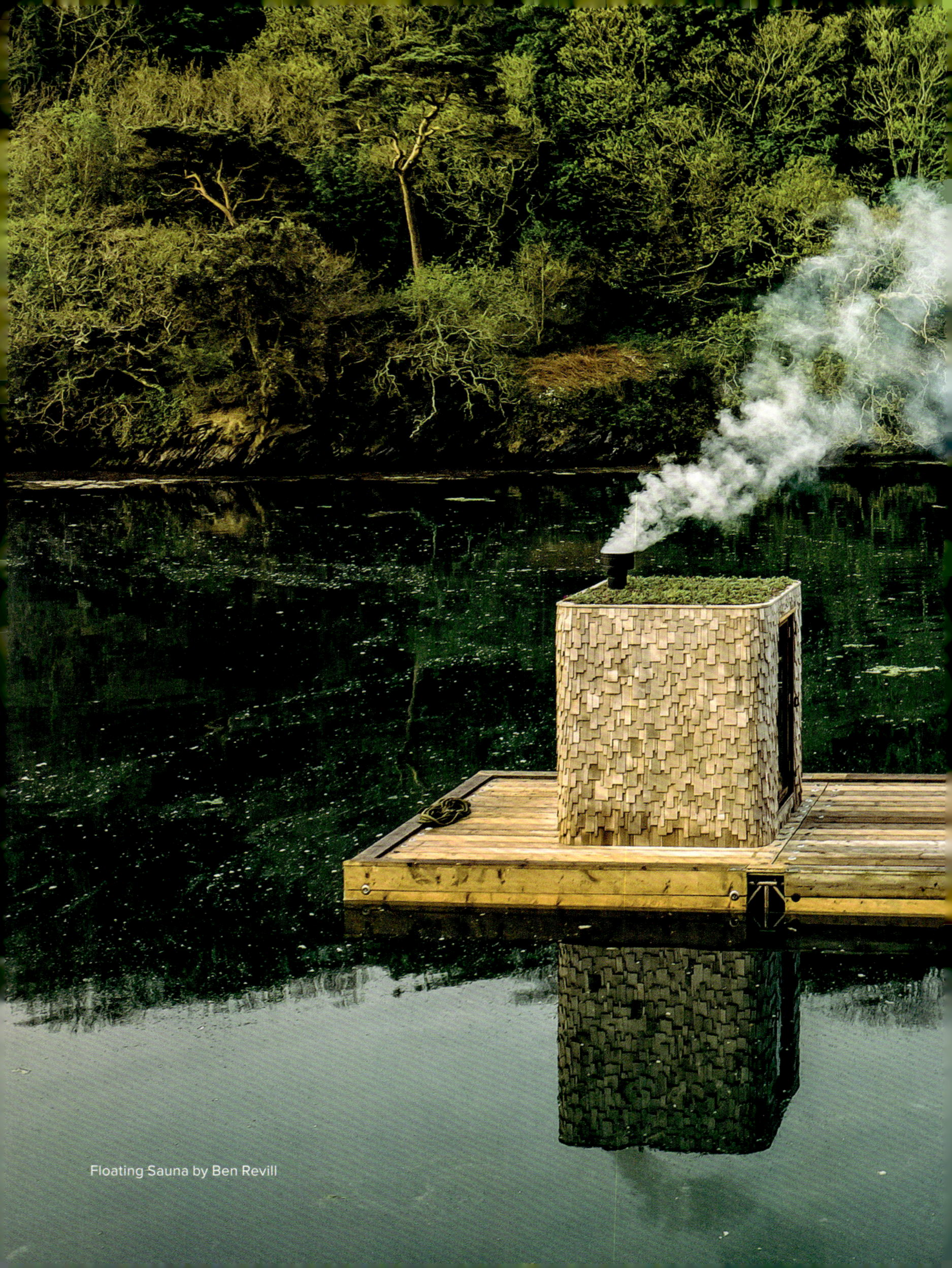
Floating Sauna by Ben Revill

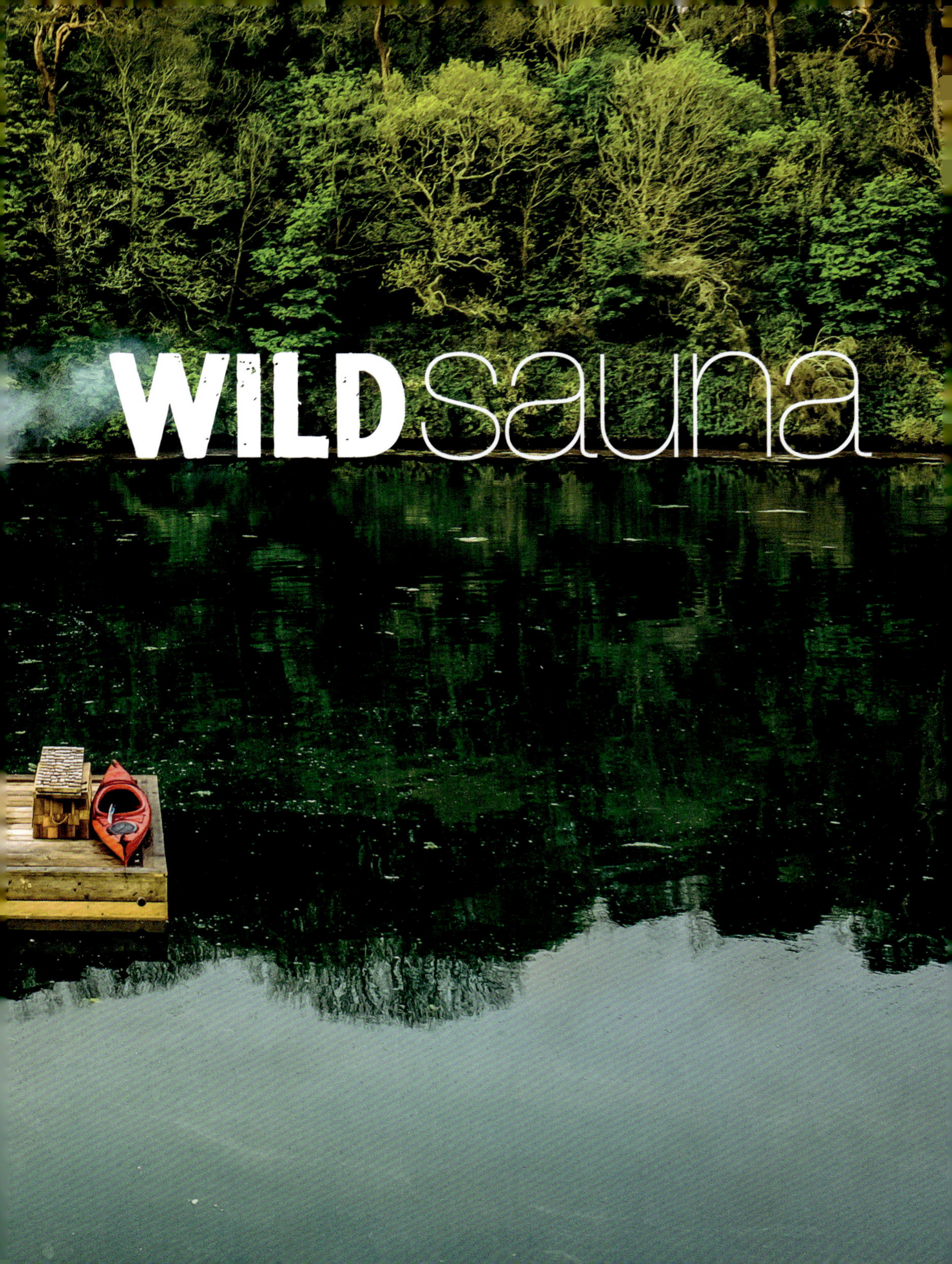
WILD sauna

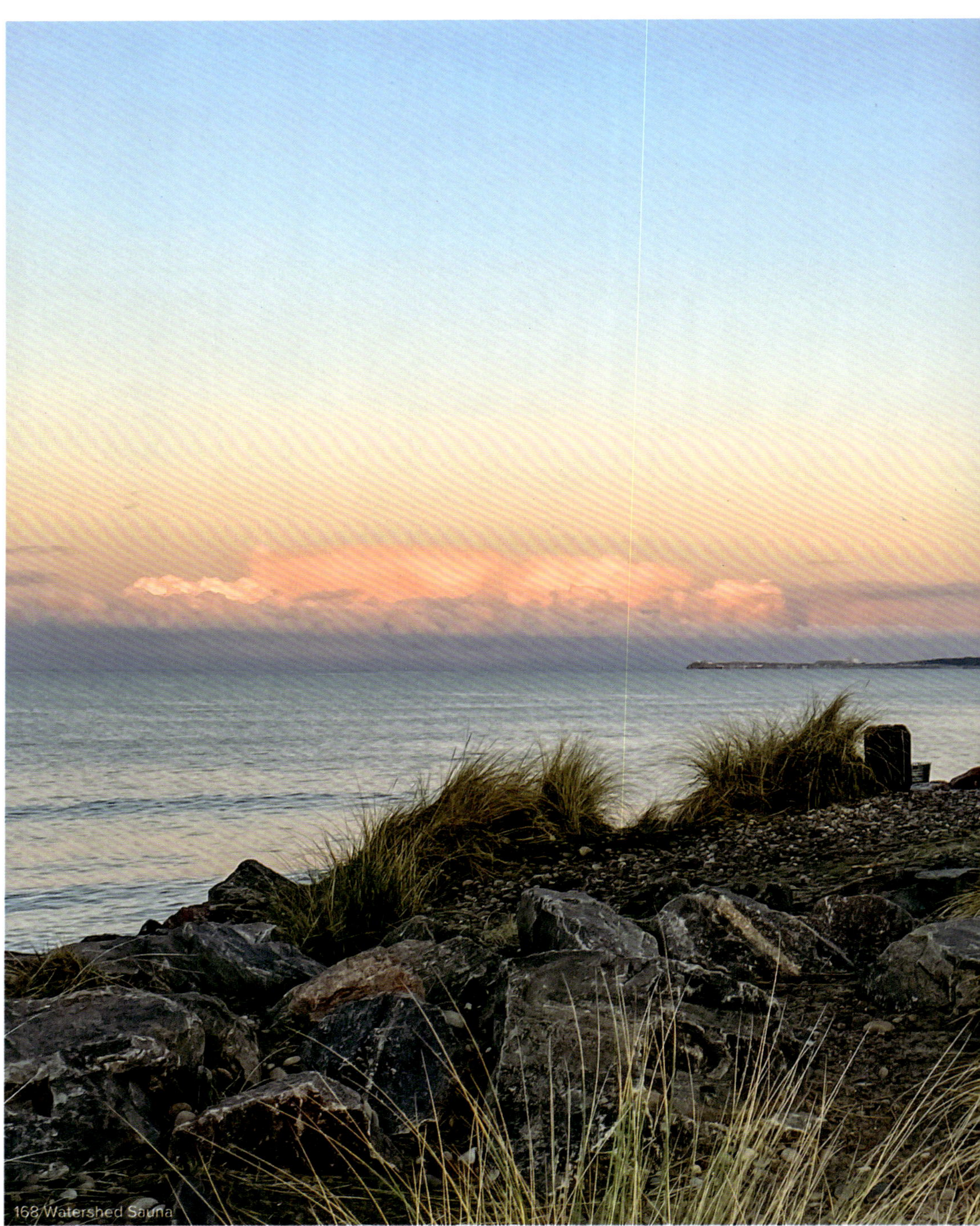
168 Watershed Sauna

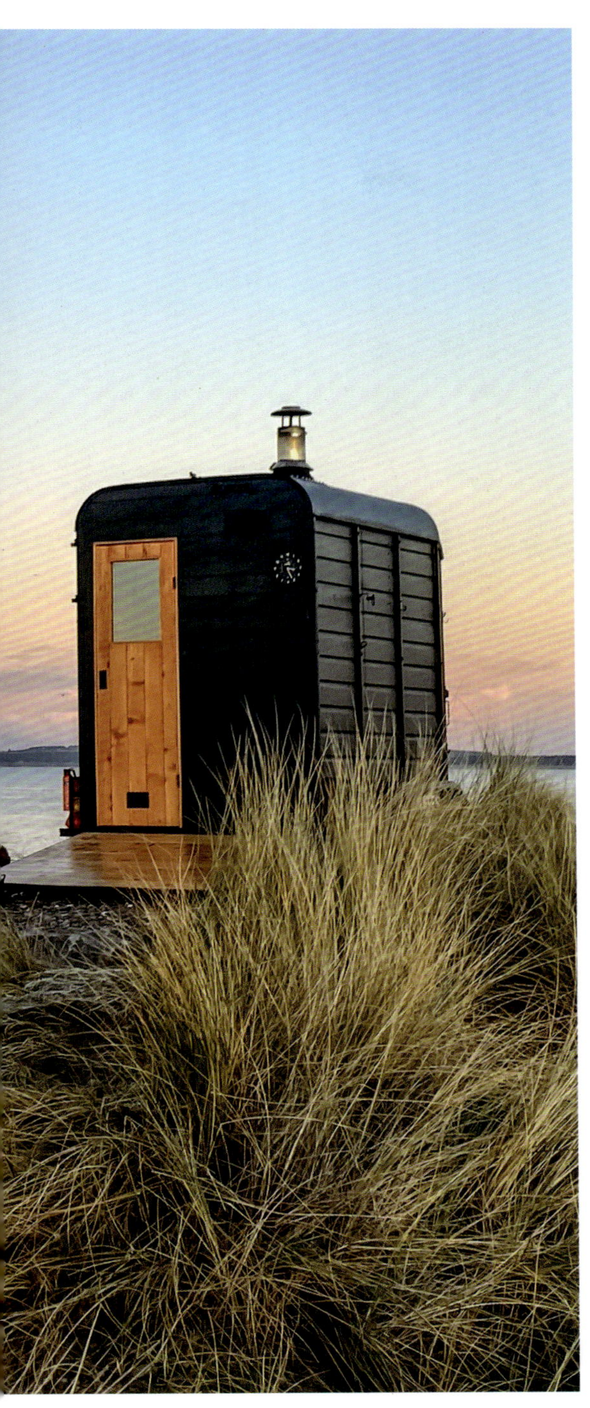

Contents

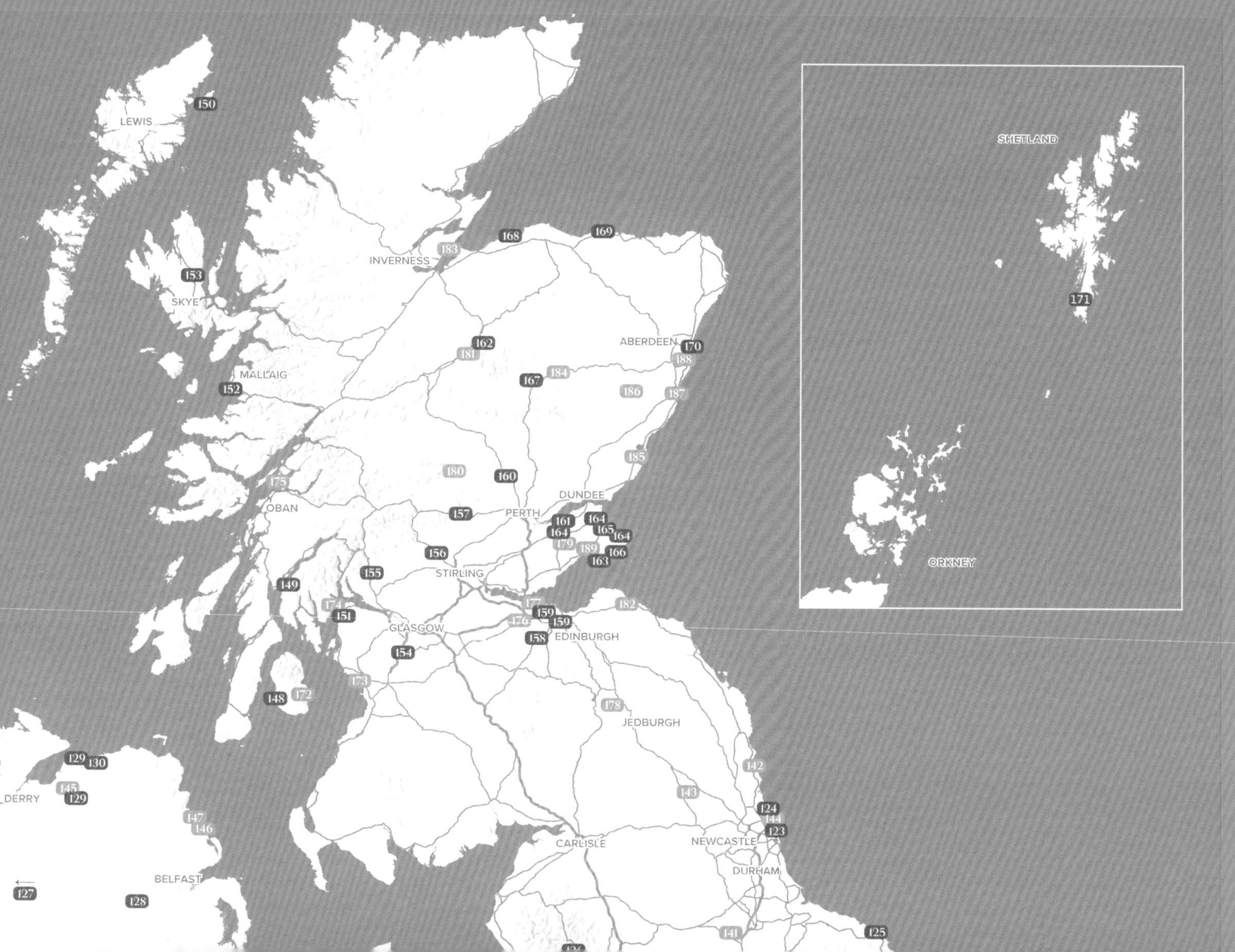
SHETLAND
ORKNEY
LEWIS
SKYE
MALLAIG
INVERNESS
ABERDEEN
OBAN
DUNDEE
PERTH
STIRLING
GLASGOW
EDINBURGH
JEDBURGH
CARLISLE
NEWCASTLE
DURHAM
DERRY
BELFAST
150
153
152
168
169
183
162
181
170
188
167
184
186
187
185
180
160
175
157
161
164
165
166
179
189
163
156
155
149
174
151
177
159
176
158
182
154
173
148
172
178
129
130
145
147
146
142
143
124
144
123
127
128
141
125
171

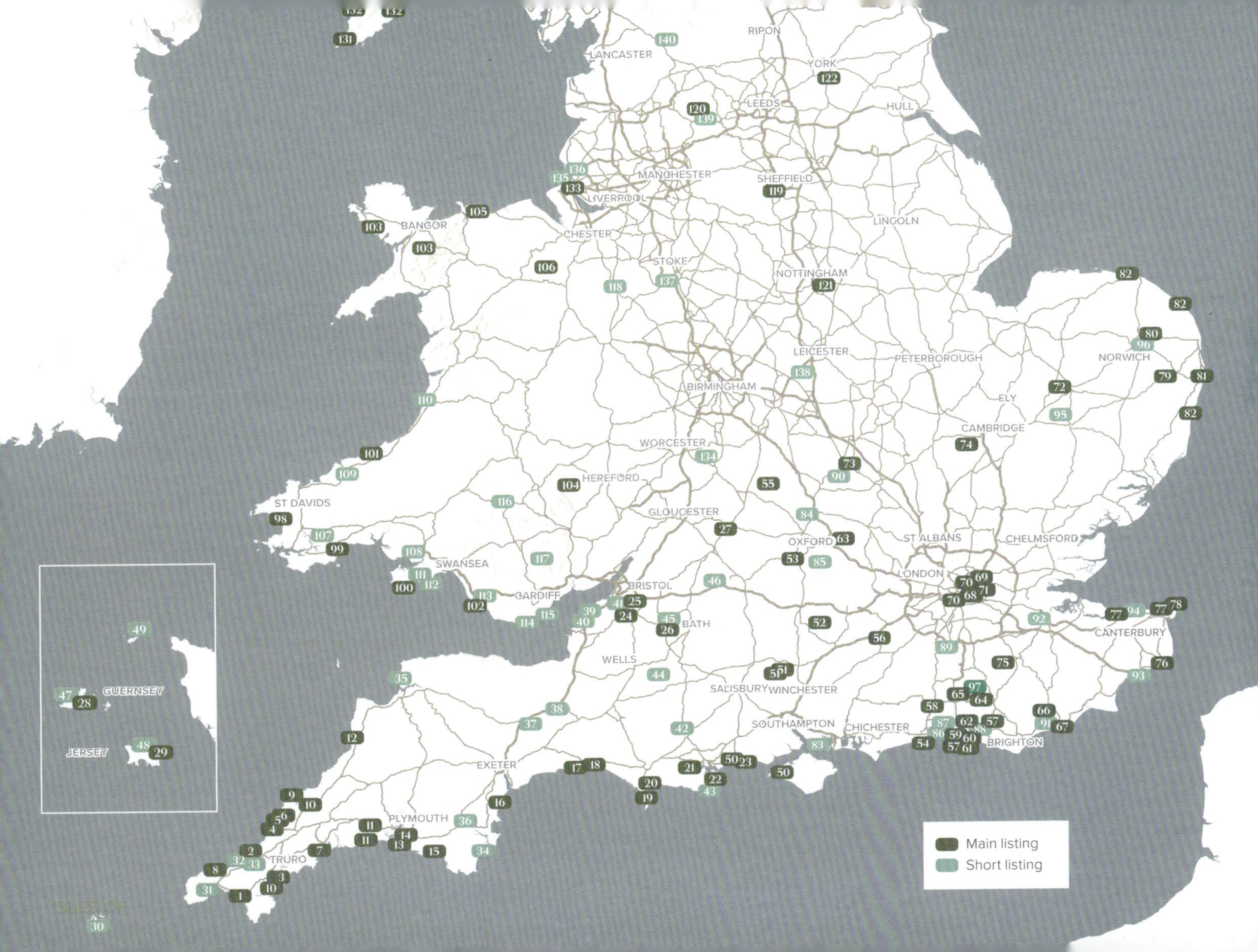
RIPON
LANCASTER
YORK
LEEDS
HULL
MANCHESTER
SHEFFIELD
LIVERPOOL
LINCOLN
BANGOR
CHESTER
STOKE
NOTTINGHAM
LEICESTER
PETERBOROUGH
NORWICH
BIRMINGHAM
ELY
CAMBRIDGE
WORCESTER
HEREFORD
ST DAVIDS
GLOUCESTER
ST ALBANS
CHELMSFORD
OXFORD
SWANSEA
LONDON
BRISTOL
CARDIFF
BATH
CANTERBURY
WELLS
SALISBURY
WINCHESTER
SOUTHAMPTON
CHICHESTER
BRIGHTON
GUERNSEY
JERSEY
EXETER
PLYMOUTH
TRURO
Main listing
Short listing

Foreword

No matter what technology – AI, bots, screens – you put in front of me, I'd still rather pick up a book and lose myself between the pages. So, to be asked to write the preface to *Wild Sauna* is a huge honour, particularly as I devoured Emma's first book *Sauna – The Power of Deep Heat*, from which I learnt so much about this beautiful practice.

I accidentally fell into the sauna world when a mate asked me to buy a sauna so he could get three for the price of two. Since that day, when a wonderful wood-fired Lithuanian sauna came bumping down the lane, my wife Josie and I haven't looked back. Where had this wondrous, transcendent, curative experience been all our lives?

I recently found myself re-reading *Zen and the Art of Motorcycle Maintenance*, a book that I hadn't picked up since my teens, and suddenly my interest in saunas made sense. In 1974, Robert M. Pirsig wrote about the technology monster that 'keeps eating up land and polluting the air and lakes', and it feels to me that sauna operators, aficionados, geeks and recent converts alike see the sauna as a refuge from this monster. The sauna is a place to seek solace, to escape the digital world with its endless pinging and beeping that fills our lives from dawn to bedtime and beyond. It's a last bastion of silence and rebellion against the noise of the 21st century.

And, as Emma's book shows, sauna is so many things: a place to get warm, an expression of freedom, and somewhere to cry, to love, to give birth and even prepare for death. While in the UK we may not have embraced sauna quite that much yet – we still seem stuck on 'it's the new pub' – but we will get there, now that we're starting to understand it.

I've sat in sweat boxes with rebels, punks, super straight naked geeks, grandads, babies, meditating yogis, taxi drivers and builders, and realised that no-one gives a monkey's what you do, or how much money you do or don't have. Instead, you might get a bit of comforting advice or a shoulder to cry (and sweat) on.

So, possibly like you, I want to know more about what it is that makes us want to sit in a box/tent/dome and drip sweat, whether alone or with friends or strangers (even on a hot day, when most people are reaching for a cold flannel). Although I'm making progress, I heartily recommend reading this book to really understand what makes the heart of the sauna tick.

ROB DA BANK

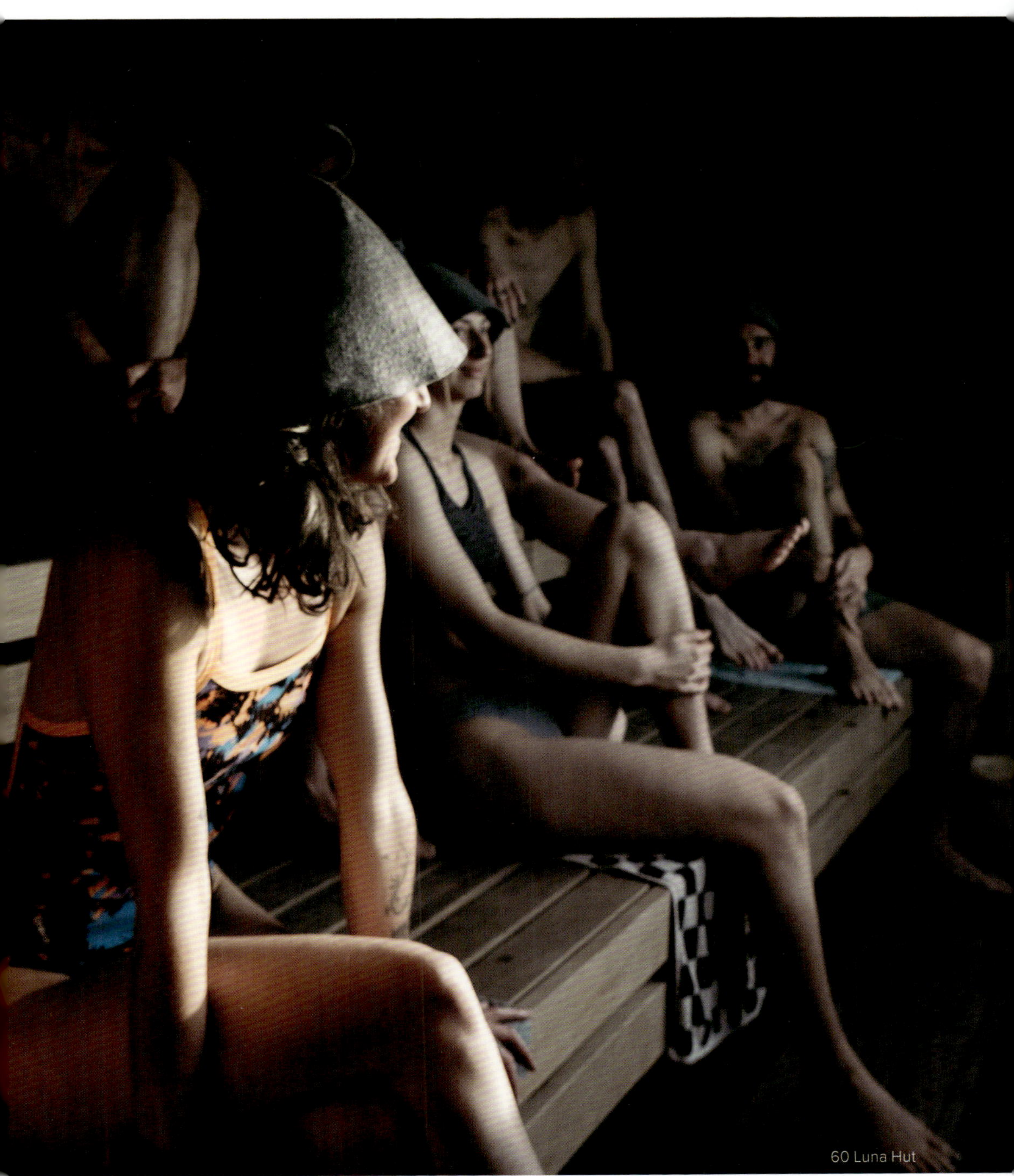

60 Luna Hut

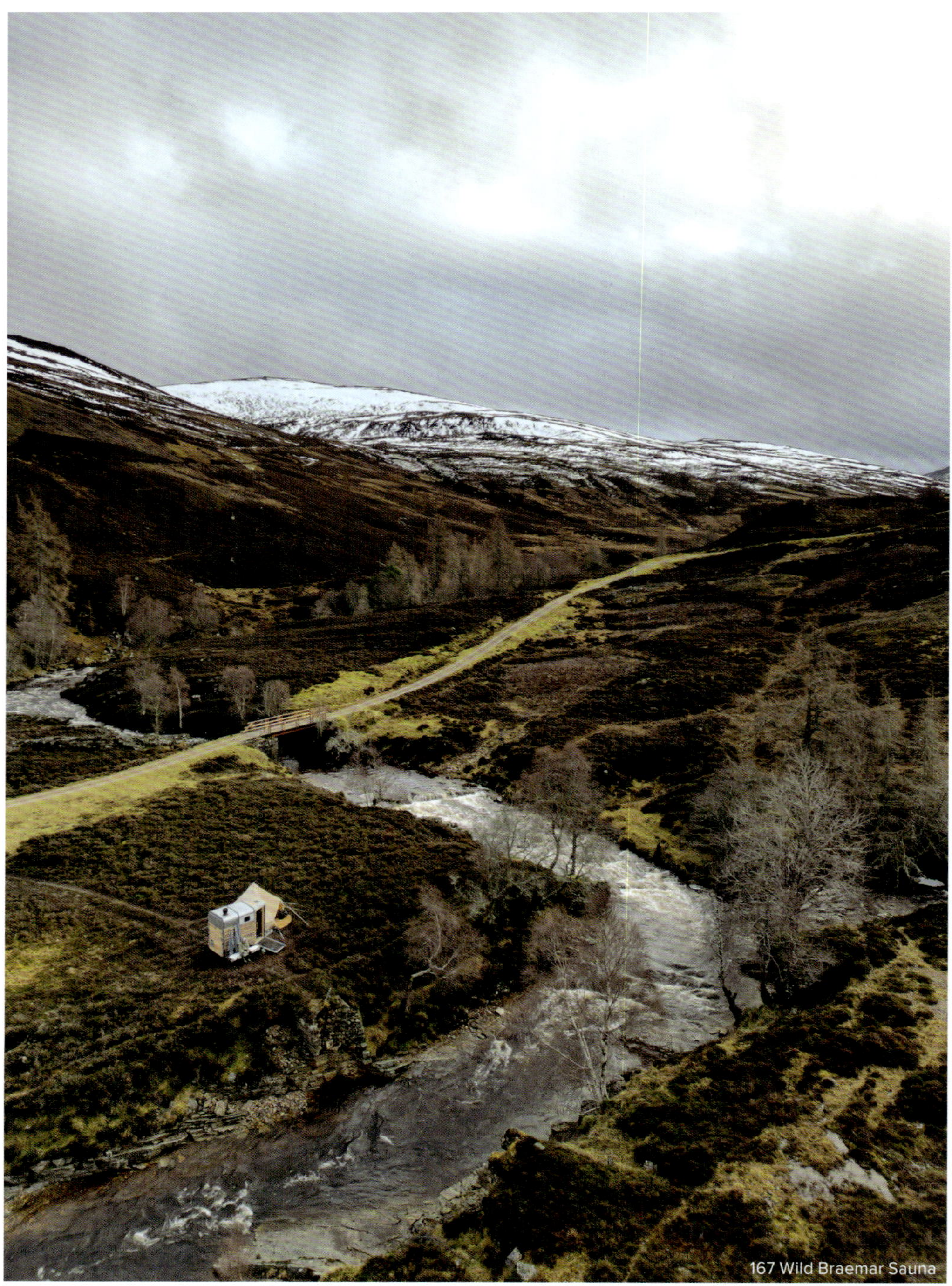
167 Wild Braemar Sauna

Introduction

What is a wild sauna? Let's start by saying what it's not. A wild sauna is not tucked away in a forgotten corner of a gym – dark, smelly, claustrophobic, with signs saying things like 'Don't pour water on the rocks'. It's not an add-on to a costly spa, where guests in fluffy robes and disposable slippers sip prosecco. It's not a space where bathers with gadgets 'optimise' their sweating and track their heart rates.

Many wild saunas perch – sometimes literally – on Britain's untamed fringes; they battle unpredictable elements to offer a healthy hit of outdoors and an exhilarating blast of hot and cold – with the latter coming from sea, lake, river, ice bath or outdoor shower. Often honed out of horseboxes or trailers, wild saunas are novel sanctuaries –where else can you while away an hour, semi-naked and sweaty, watching nature perform in glorious Technicolour?

The wild sauna 'movement' (we can call it that, now that there are more than 200, and counting, such saunas around the UK), takes most of its cues from Nordic bathing cultures, from Finland, Lithuania, Latvia and Estonia, where sauna is a way of life, and steam, or *löyly*, the nations' lifeblood. At the helm is a new generation of 'saunapreneurs', pioneering multitaskers who stoke wood-burning fires in all weathers in order to deliver a dose of health and happiness to others. These trailblazers cite studies that show how sauna reduces cardiovascular diseases, eases pain, boosts immunity and improves our mental health. They know that persuading bewildered authorities and undynamic councils to offer affordable 'wild wellness' for all is a form of quiet activism. It may also be the future for our nation's ailing health.

I visited tons of saunas for this book. On every trip, from Fife to Falmouth, no sooner had I boarded the train home, than another sauna opened behind me. The list just keeps on growing. I met a rich tapestry of bathers – women in wetsuits, teenagers, triathletes, recovering addicts, young, old, newbies and veterans. All of them told me how sauna helps them manage loneliness, pain, anxiety, depression; how they've made new friends, found new communities; how they've grown less awkward in their bodies, and learned to embrace the long, dark British winter. In every single sauna, bathers came out smiling, lifted, energised. And so did I.

I hope this book will tempt you to try a wild sauna or two. For when it does, the fire will draw you in, the warmth will feed your soul and the heat will wrap its arms round you like a long-lost friend.

EMMA O'KELLY

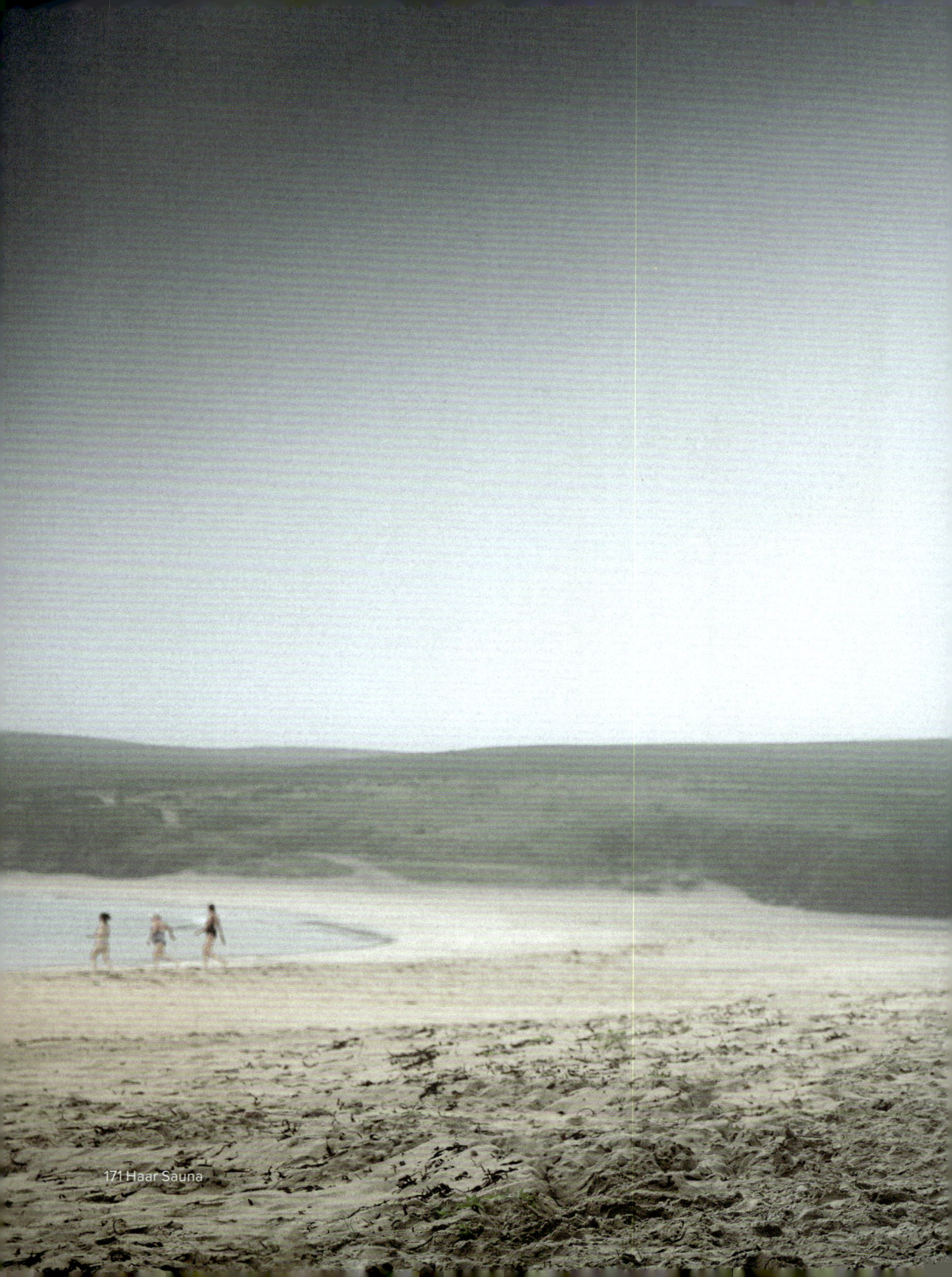

171 Haar Sauna

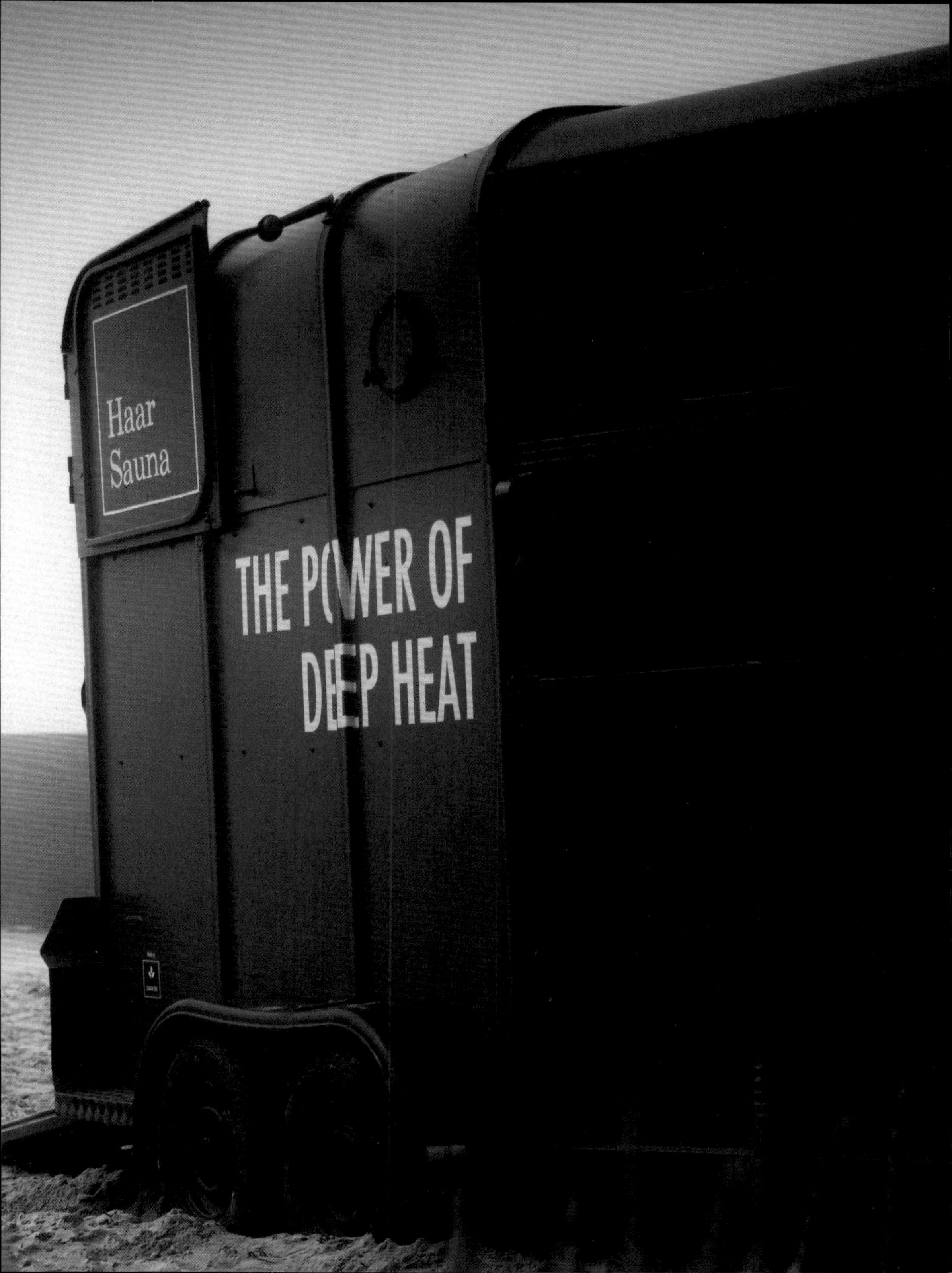

Haar
Sauna
THE POWER OF
DEEP HEAT

Hot and cold, body and soul

Those who are into sauna often pinpoint the moment when they 'got it'. And once you get it, there's no going back. Where else provides a comforting, cosy space that's neither work nor home (nor pub) that sends your blood pumping and fills you with endorphins, creating a buzz that can last for hours? Add to this the blast of wild beauty that beckons beyond the sauna door, and the whole experience is enticing, other-worldly and exhilarating.

WHAT HAPPENS TO YOUR BODY IN THE SAUNA?

The heart rate quickens and the temperature of the blood increases. Heat shock proteins are activated. These are essential components of all cells, and the heat helps these proteins to stabilise and repair. Warm, faster-flowing blood, carrying increased levels of oxygen and nutrients, travels to all the internal organs and muscles. Blood also flows through the capillaries to the surface of the skin to try and cool us down, which is why white skin turns red. We start to sweat to try and cool down. We produce around 0.5kg of sweat in a 30-minute sauna. Around 97 per cent of this is water, but some toxins and heavy metals are excreted too.

After sauna-bathing, the blood vessels relax and blood pressure drops. The effect can last for several hours. It often comes with a floaty feeling, caused by a lack of blood to the brain as the body prioritises sending it to the skin to cool us down.

Studies into sauna and heat therapy are scarce; most that have been conducted come from bathing nations, such as Finland, Japan and Germany. To date, no one has conducted a comparative study into hot and cold stress. But in 2019, a 20-year study by Finnish cardiologist Dr Jari Laukkanen revealed that regular sauna bathing dramatically reduces cardiovascular diseases. It has paved the way for further research. At the Montreal Heart Institute in Canada, Dr Earric Lee is incorporating sauna bathing into the cardiac rehab programme. Standard advice is for those with heart conditions to stay away from the sauna, but Lee hopes to discover that the cardiovascular workout it provides is good for everyone. Lee is also conducting a review on heat therapy, gathering together studies from the 1940s to the present day on the use of hot water immersion, sauna, steam rooms and more. He has uncovered some interesting acute findings in the realm of hot water immersion. 'There is good evidence that hot water immersion improves sleep duration and quality in female insomniacs. Similarly, hot water immersion acutely improves immune system response,' he says.

At the University of Portsmouth Dr Ant Shepherd, Associate Professor in Clinical Exercise Physiology, immerses volunteers with Type 2 diabetes into hot tubs, exposing them to heat stress. His findings show that heat shock proteins are activated, which in turn can help reduce inflammation. This can improve insulin sensitivity which can benefit those with Type 2 diabetes. He says, 'we don't know how long heat shock proteins go up for, but they stop the misfolding of proteins which cause many diseases. And for most people in the western world, burning energy is a good thing.'

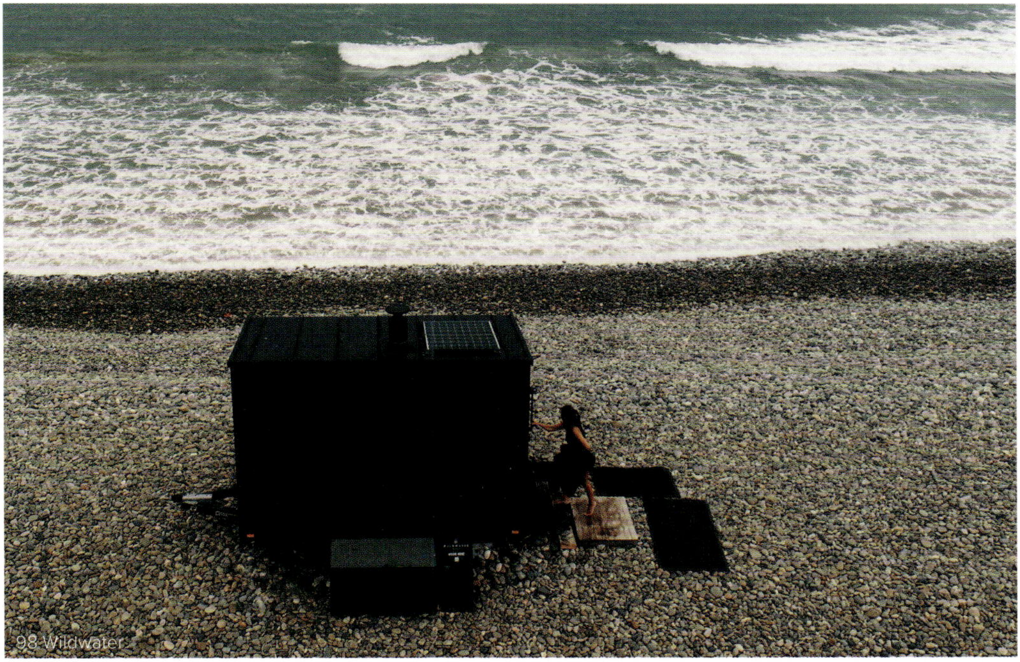

98 Wildwater

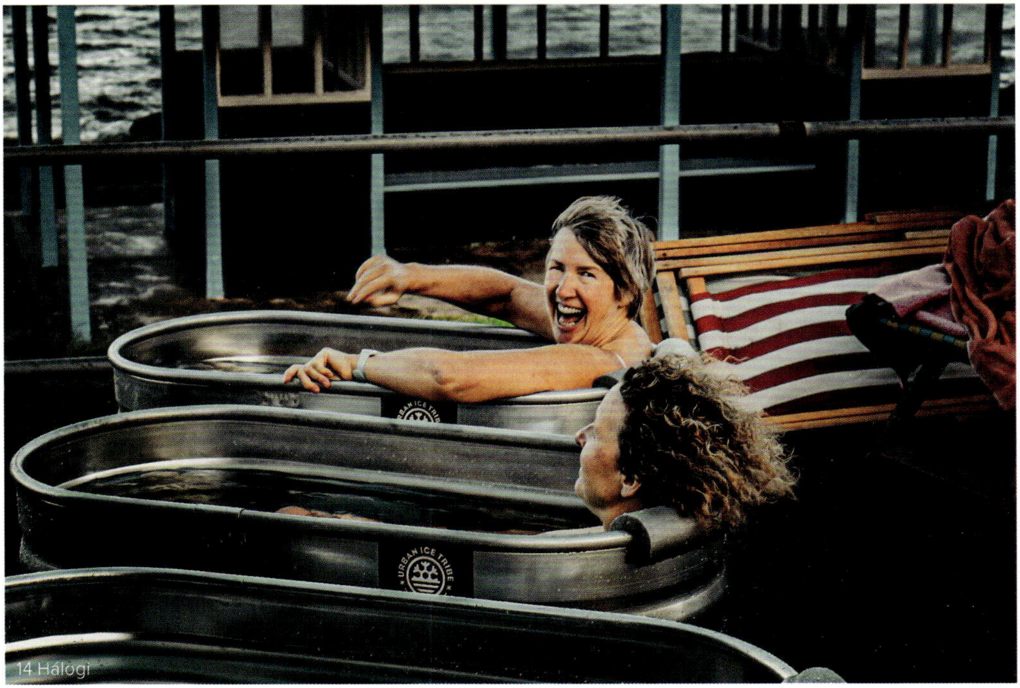

14 Hálogi

HOT AND COLD – CONTRAST THERAPY

But it's not just about the heat. Contrast therapy, or cycling between hot sauna and cold water, may be the buzzword among sauna bathers and cold-water swimmers today, but it's actually an ancient form of self-care. Roman baths would feature both cold frigidaria and the warm caldarium; and in the Nordic countries, a sauna has for centuries been complemented with a roll in the snow or a dip in an ice hole. Hot and cold go together like ... black and white, or heaven and hell.

And sometimes it really can feel like you're in heaven one minute, and hell the next. Studies show that it takes around seven sessions for our bodies to adapt to thermal stress, and extremes of temperature cause all sorts of reactions – both emotional and physical. The body has to be nimble to keep up; heartbeat and breathing yo-yo wildly, hormones and chemicals fly around. It's a thermoregulatory workout, a full system reset, and anyone who does it knows the euphoria it can bring. The Japanese call it *totonotta*. We don't have a word for it in English; maybe we need to invent one.

Dr Susanna Søberg is a cold-water swimmer and sauna-goer who has spent many years practising and studying contrast therapy. As founder of the Søberg Institute in Denmark, she runs courses in the Thermalist Cure™, a technique that outlines the science and best protocols on how to combine hot and cold. In recent research, Dr Søberg – like Dr Shepherd in Portsmouth – found that contrast therapy improves insulin sensitivity, which helps regulate glucose levels and protects us from Type 2 diabetes.

Dr Søberg adds that when we are exposed to cold stress, we activate brown fat or brown adipose tissue, which produces heat by breaking down glucose and fat to warm us up. She advocates brown fat activation as a calorie-burning strategy, which, combined with a healthy diet, can lead to weight loss.

In the book *The Power of Hot and Cold – From Sauna to Sea: The Finnish Way to a Happy, Healthy Life*, authors Katja Pantzar and Carita Harju write about how they enjoy contrast therapy. 'Neither the sauna nor winter swimming are about who wins,' says Katja. 'They're about taking time for self-care, and about the communities and friendships that develop around them.' Jamie Christopherson of Scenic Sauna in Oxfordshire adds: 'The cold is about enabling yourself to get through an external stimulus that doesn't go away; to tolerate pain and panic. Whereas the sauna, it's still an external stimulus, but it has a much deeper ability to enable a meditative state.' You can read more about how contrast therapy helped him heal from full-body paralysis in the Scenic Sauna entry 27.

THE NATURE CURE / CONNECTION

In the Nordics and Baltics in pre-Christian times, the sauna was a 'Church of Nature'. Ancient smoke saunas would be built near a sacred grove, or a holy well, whose waters would bless the stove. Local plants from the forest, 'the otherworld' would be used in healing, rituals and magic. Today, nature is still revered, and the sauna offers a connection with earth, fire, air and water in one small space. The smell of the wooden benches, birch whisks and essential oils, the crackle of the fire, the feeling of the steam as it rolls over the body bring all the senses to life. In the UK, the humble horsebox on a lonesome beach, or the modest barrel sauna shrouded by a wall of tall trees enhance these primeval beliefs and feelings and give us an opportunity to celebrate nature in its purest form.

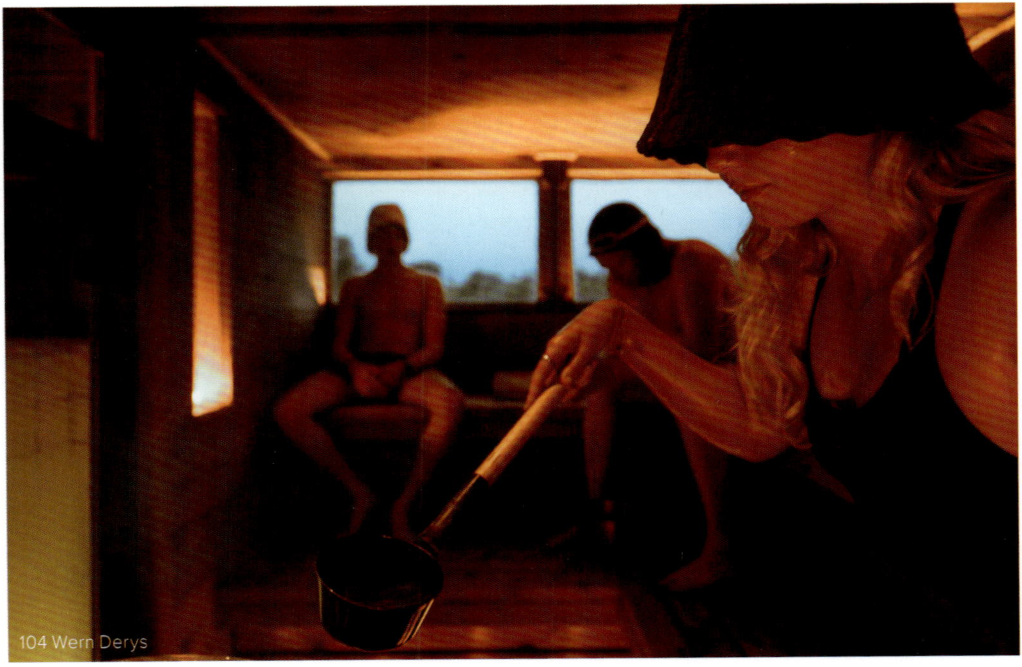
104 Wern Derys

ADDITIONAL HEALTH BENEFITS OF SAUNA HEAT

- In a proper, steamy sauna, the mucous membrane of the nose, throat, saliva glands and tear ducts increase secretion and capture pathogens such as cold coughs and viruses, which may help ward off colds.

- The skin is our largest and most complex organ, and because it eliminates toxins and waste products, it is sometimes known as the third kidney. Sweating gives it a good work-out, and scrubbing, sloughing and cleaning it in the sauna can help alleviate eczema, urticaria (hives), athlete's foot, acne and more.

- A study from the Karolinska Institute in Stockholm, Sweden, found that smelling human sweat or 'chemo-signals' from strangers may help alleviate social anxiety. Human sweat is made up of more than 300 compounds and is complex and variable in the way it carries information. Researchers hope to isolate these therapeutic molecules and put them to good use.

- Sauna warms up the whole body inside and out, and studies show that if we have warm hands and feet, we fall asleep more quickly and sleep more deeply.

- Heat causes blood flow to muscles and joints to increase. It carries raised levels of beta-endorphins – important pain relievers, which can ease pain and stiffness and make us feel good.

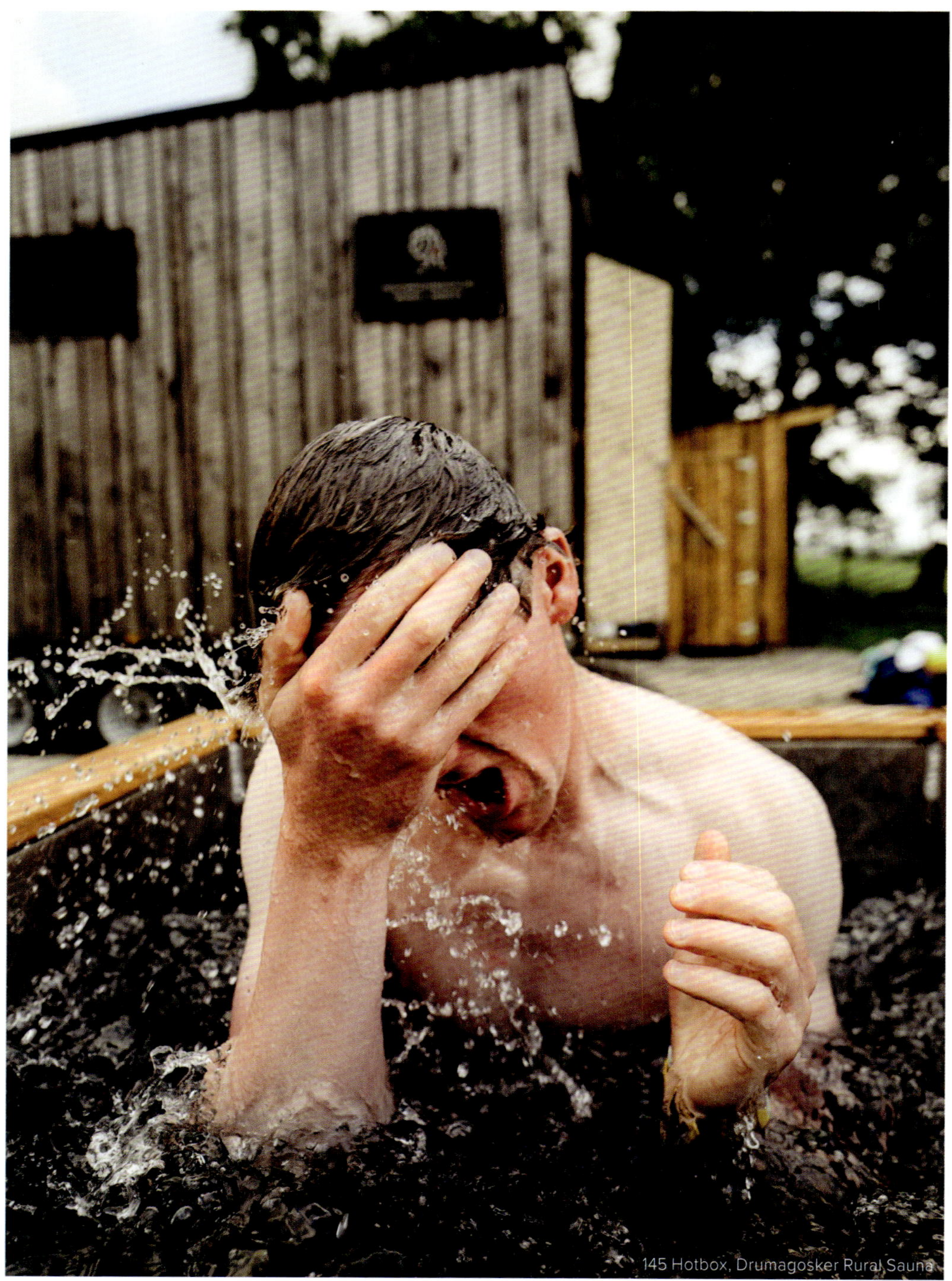

145 Hotbox, Drumagosker Rural Sauna

THE HEALTH BENEFITS OF COLD WATER PLUNGING

Improved Circulation:
Many studies over the decades have found that regular cold water immersion can improve blood flow and cardiovascular health by inducing vasoconstriction followed by vasodilation, helping to maintain a healthy circulatory system and improve blood flow to tissues.

Enhanced Mood and Reduced Stress
Research published in the *International Journal of Circumpolar Health* found that regular winter swimming (cold water exposure) led to an increase in well-being and reduction in stress, due to the release of endorphins and other feel-good neurotransmitters. Additionally, a case study published in the *BMJ* indicated that open water swimming helped reduce symptoms of major depressive disorder in some individuals.

Reduced Inflammation and Muscle Recovery:
Cold water immersion has been shown to help reduce muscle soreness after intense physical activity. According to a 2022 review, athletes who used cold water therapy experienced reduced muscle pain and faster recovery, as the cold temperature helps to reduce inflammation and decrease nerve transmission associated with soreness.

Strengthened Immune System:
A study published in the *European Journal of Applied Physiology* found that cold exposure may increase white blood cell counts, which can strengthen the immune system. This is thought to be due to the body's adaptation to the stress of cold exposure, which can increase resilience against infection.

Increased Metabolism and Fat Burning:
Research in the *Journal of Clinical Endocrinology & Metabolism* showed that cold-induced activation of brown adipose tissue (BAT) could increase energy expenditure and improve glucose metabolism, potentially contributing to fat loss. BAT burns calories to generate heat, which is activated through exposure to cold.

Better Sleep Quality:
Like sauna, cold exposure may aid in improving sleep by reducing cortisol levels and helping to reset circadian rhythms. Lowered core body temperature before bedtime is associated with improved sleep onset and quality, and this can be induced by cold water therapy, which promotes a calming effect and helps initiate restful sleep.

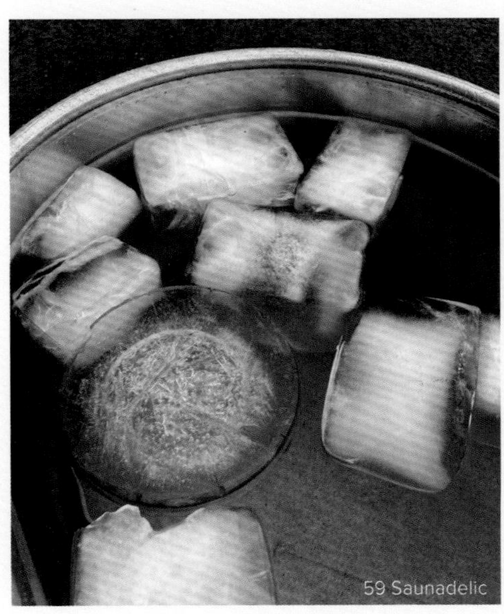

59 Saunadelic

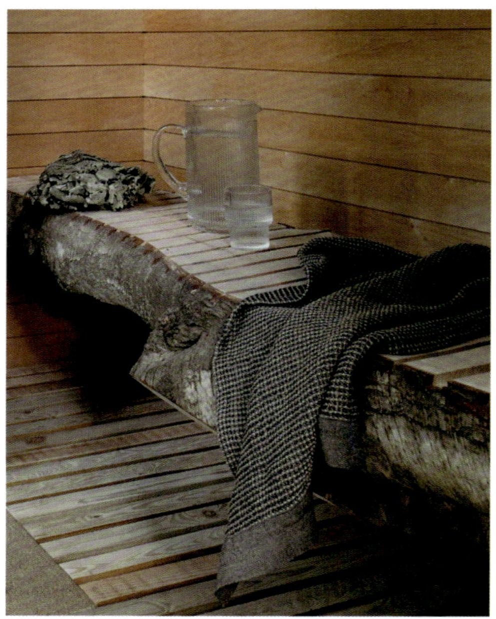

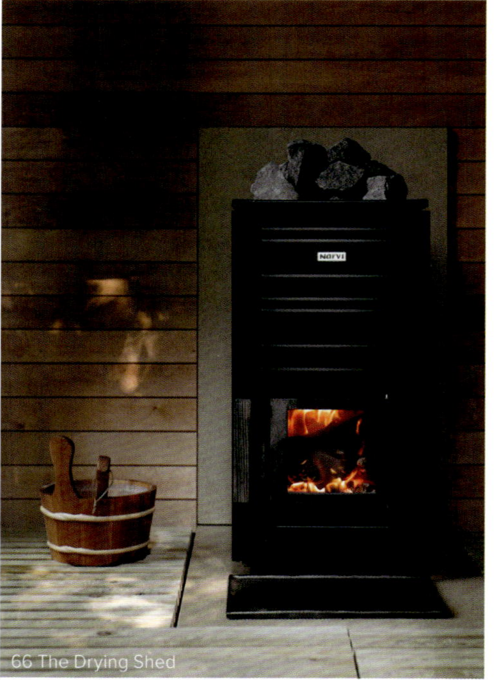

66 The Drying Shed

THINGS TO BEAR IN MIND

- Dehydration, which causes headaches and muscle cramps, occurs when we leave it too late to start drinking water. It takes two hours for water to hydrate the body, so drink 1-1.5 litres at least two hours before your sauna.

- If you are going to faint, then this usually happens on exiting the sauna, as a result of a blood pressure drop. If you have low blood pressure, start sauna-ing slowly to build up your tolerance, and always leave when you start feeling light-headed.

- After a sauna and cold plunge, white skin can look like a Battenberg cake, a pink and white patchwork of blotches; this is Livedo reticularis and is a harmless reaction to the cold.

- Sauna can inflame skin conditions such as eczema, psoriasis and other dermatological issues.

- Those with multiple sclerosis should not sauna, as it exacerbates the condition.

- Avoid the sauna if you have a pacemaker, and remove hearing aids before you enter.

- There are no fixed rules about having a sauna while pregnant, and women in the Nordic countries do it; if concerned, pregnancies are generally most robust in the second trimester and the early part of the third.

- Prosthetics, silicone implants, Botox or fillers are not damaged in the heat, though if you have the latter, it's advisable to stay out of the sauna for a few days after treatment.

- Regular sauna bathing temporarily reduces sperm count.

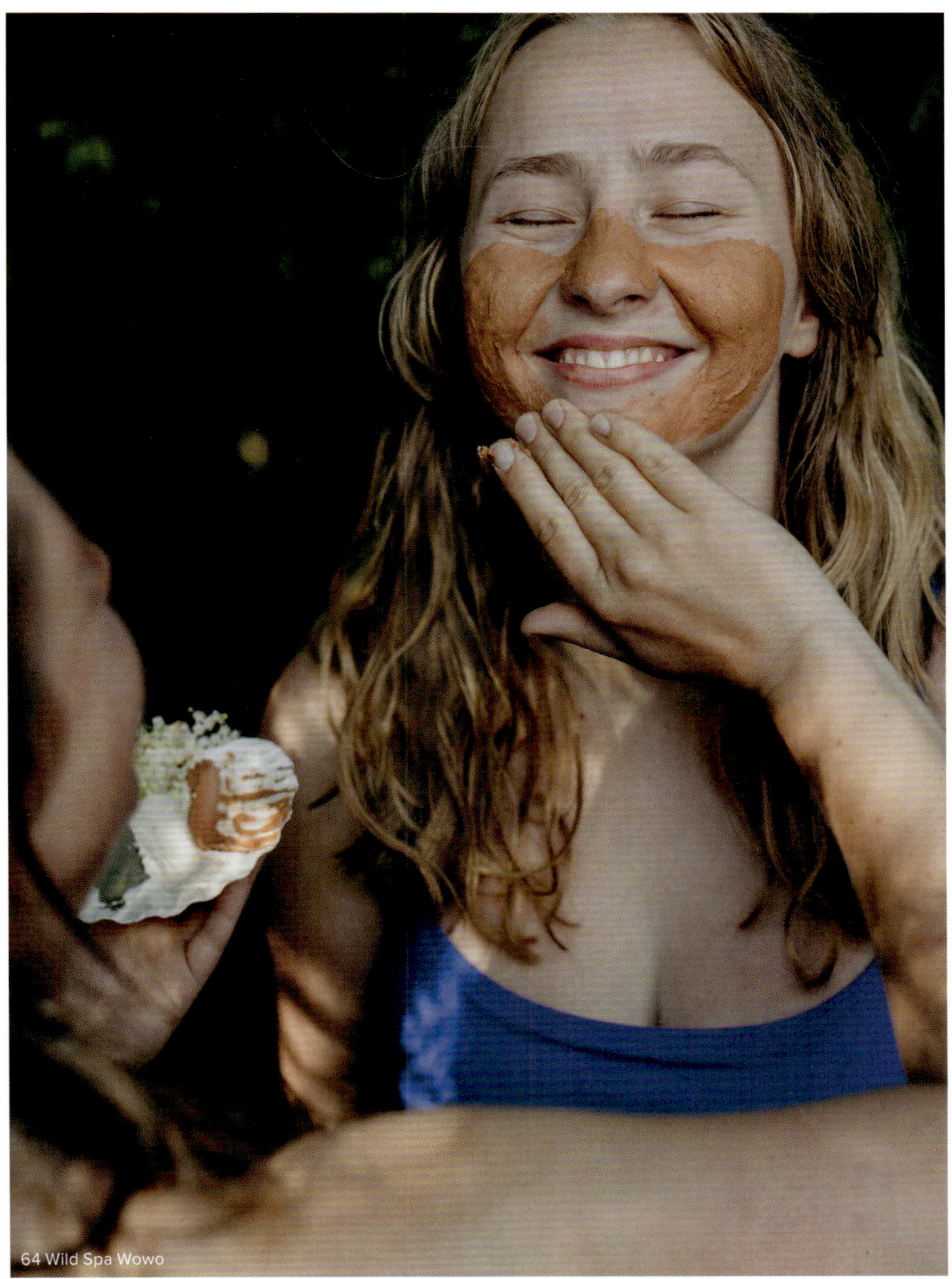

64 Wild Spa Wowo

History of sweat bathing

PREHISTORIC SAUNAS AND SWEAT LODGES

Sweat bathing knowledge is bit *Emperor's New Clothes*. Just when we think we have discovered something new about it, we discover that prehistoric man, our ancestral self, knew it already and had been practising it for millennia. Using the raw energy of heat and cold, combined with ritual, to cross boundaries and enter transformative, restorative realms has been enjoyed since time immemorial. In the UK, sweat bathing has ebbed and flowed over the centuries, and has appeared in many iterations since our Bronze Age ancestors on Orkney and elsewhere created the first sauna structures 5000 years ago.

In his cult 1970s book *Sweat*, author and photographer Mikkel Aaland embarked upon a sweat-bathing odyssey. He journeyed from Turkish hammam to Roman bath, from Finnish sauna to Russian banya, from Japanese mushi-buro to Native American sweat lodge, and in each culture, he noted the celebratory rituals and collective joy that arose in homage to the heat. Sweating, he concluded, 'is as essential to our health as eating and breathing.'

When it comes to sweat-bathing traditions, we tend to look to other cultures, such as the Native American sweat lodge (*inípi*), the Mexican *temazcal*, or the Korean *jjimjilbang*, for inspiration. But archaeological evidence from all over the UK and Ireland suggest our ancestors had their own sweat-bathing rituals. What exactly went on inside these dark, mysterious spaces is an increasingly hot topic on sauna benches.

SHETLAND'S BURNT MOUNDS

Some 1,900 so-called 'burnt mounds' – remnants of heat-shattered stones beside a rectangular water trough – dating from the Bronze Age have been recorded in the UK, with most being found in Shetland, Orkney and Ireland, where they are known as *fulachta fíadh* or 'ancient cooking places'.

The Fianna, a legendary band of warriors found in both Irish and Scottish mythology, used them; after a morning's hunting, they would find a spot, kindle fires and dig two pits in the clay. Some of the meat from the kill would be set to roast on the fire, and the rest set to boil in one of the pits which was heated by the rocks. The second pit would also be used for sweat bathing and reviving the warriors before the feasting began.

But beyond mythology, as more of these ruins are uncovered thanks to coastal erosion and geological shifts, academics are asking if burnt mounds had deeper, more spiritual roles to play.

'There are 30 burnt mounds on Fair Isle alone,' says Lauren Doughton, an academic from Shetland, whose PhD. is entitled 'A most curious class of small cairn – reinterpreting the burnt mounds of Shetland'. 'If they did indeed represent cooking sites, why was this performed on such a grand scale? And why, if they were used for feasting, are there few remnants of bone and waste matter at many of the sites?'

'What's more,' says Doughton, 'the Shetland sites are similar to Scandinavian burnt mounds, which are often found near rock art. This type of art often depicts how our ancestors understood the universe and is found in places of spiritual significance.' If, as experts believe, a sophisticated maritime culture stretched up to the Northern Isles and out to the Hebrides before the Roman conquest of southern Britain began, it's not hard to see that Scandinavia and Scotland would have shared ideas, beliefs and cultural practices.

Bronze Age man saw watery landscapes as liminal spaces, points of entry to the underworld; and burnt mounds are almost always located near running water. In 2015, on the Isle of Westray in Orkney, a 4000-year-old underground 'ritual building' was discovered next to the sea, thought to be a prehistoric sauna that was constructed for ceremonies, or as a place where women could give birth and bodies could be placed before burial. Other Neolithic and Bronze Age 'saunas' have been discovered from Yorkshire to Wiltshire.

'I don't know if we will ever really know what burnt mounds were used for,' says Doughton, 'but we need to think about them experientially, and the notion that they were used for sweat-bathing rituals is no less plausible than any other theory.'

TEACH ALLAIS – THE IRISH SWEAT HOUSE

To date, more than 600 *teach allais* – beehive-shaped stone structures – have been recorded across Ireland, notably in the northwestern counties of Leitrim, Roscommon, Cavan and Fermanagh.

Ireland's National Folklore Collection (NFC) collects, preserves and disseminates the country's oral traditions. In it, many uses of the *teach* which means 'house', and *allais* which means 'sweat' in Irish, are recorded. For centuries, those who were sick, in pain or needed a good scrub went to the sweat house to be cured and cleaned. It was used to treat everything from 'pains in the bones' to pleurisy, lumbago, sciatica, fever, pneumonia

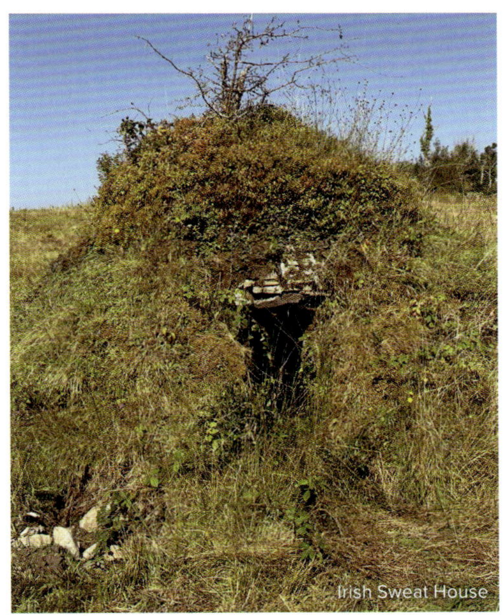
Irish Sweat House

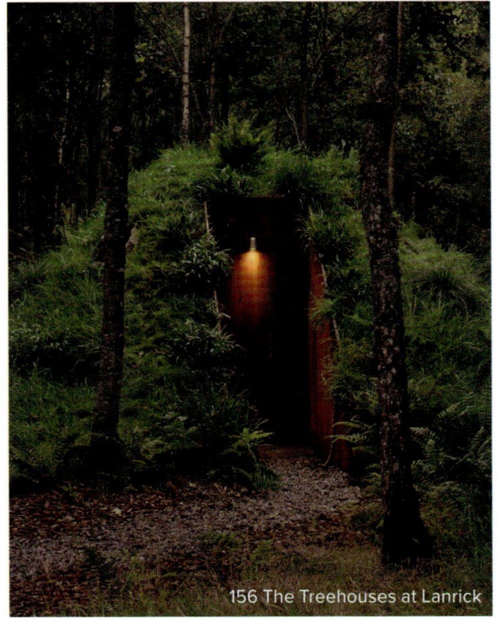
156 The Treehouses at Lanrick

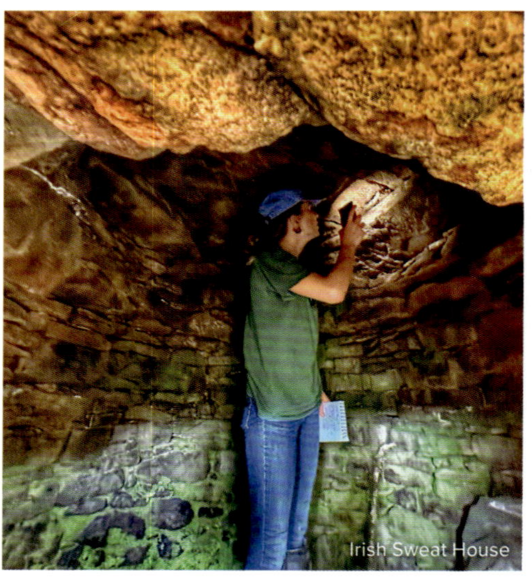
Irish Sweat House

and influenza. Patients would also be 'bled' at the sweat house if sweating was not able to bring relief; (perhaps this alludes to miscarriage and abortion too?) and women went to the sweat house to improve their complexions.

Bathers would crawl, often naked with a pitcher of water for hydration, through a tiny entrance. Inside, the space was pre-heated by a peat fire and the ash removed before they entered. The igloo-shaped structure was typically big enough for up to three, and bathers would sit on rush matting in the dark, often for many hours, before rinsing off in cold water – sweat houses were always located next to a water source. Sometimes, a professional 'sweat man' would assist with treatment, and in certain places people would pay to visit the sweat house. Often the space was managed by women, who would procure the turf and tend to the fire. One oral account tells of Old Martha Douglas, a healer who had a sweat house on her land and guided patients through sweat treatments with special herbs. Martha kept her medicine a secret, and it died with her.

The Creevaghbaun Sweat House in Galway is one of the best-preserved examples of its kind in Ireland. It was built in the early 1700s with limestone stolen from a nearby monastery, has space for eight people and is located next to a holy well, believed to have curative powers. The last reported use of a sweathouse was in 1934 in County Longford, but many of them are listed on tourist maps and are free to visit, although none have been fired up. Yet.

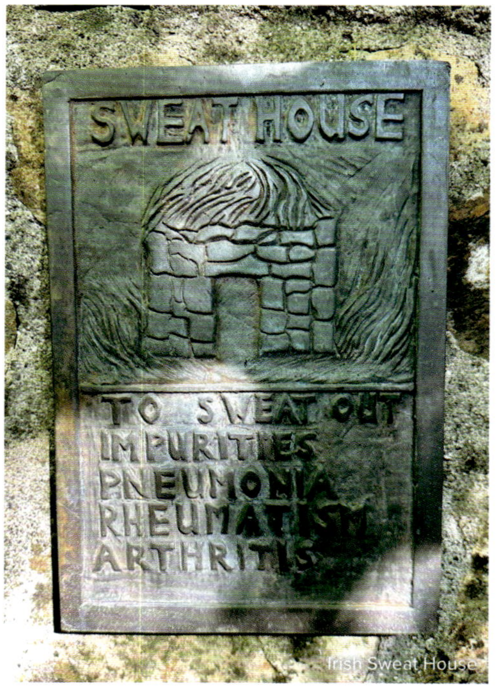

Irish Sweat House

In her book Sweat House, Irish author Rosanna Cooney threads together the history of sweat bathing in Ireland from 3000 years ago when the people of Kilkenny were building sweat lodges in the shadow of ancient burial grounds to the enigmatic sweat houses of today. She seeks to find the 'missing pieces of the sweat house story'. She says, 'The knowledge of sweat houses, where they came from, what they were used for, was ruptured so quickly. They went from being a central part of community life in rural Ireland to relics within half a century. We were severed from our culture by The Great Famine, in which half the population died, and the destruction of the Irish Language, which would likely have held rich oral histories of sweat houses.' It is known by some as The Great Forgetting.

While there's no evidence to date that Irish sweat houses were also places of ceremony and spiritual transition, in every other sweat-bathing culture this is the case, so why would Ireland, with its landscape rich in myth, superstition and magic, be any different? Could it be that the people were too afraid to speak of otherworldly activities? Sweat houses were often built away from the view of the village, in magical, liminal places; was their semi-visibility necessary to protect them from being interfered with, to keep them safe from land agents and authorities if altered states were being induced? Or was it to protect the people using them? Perhaps solitude was important, to create a sense of separation from the world and deepen the connection to nature? So many questions, so few answers, many of them tragically lost for good thanks to the lack of written history.

FROM THE ROMANS TO THE VICTORIANS

The Celtic connection also extends into England, as far south as Bath. The twists and turns of history have never stopped the flow of this sacred city's thermal waters. It was here, almost 3,000 years ago, that the Celts built a shrine to Sulis, the goddess of healing, wells and waterways. In the first century, the Romans merged Sulis with their equivalent goddess Minerva, and built the temple Sulis Minerva. They also built Aquae Sulis (which translates as Waters of Sulis), which was Britannia's most luxurious bathing complex.

The Romans believed that good health came from bathing, eating, massage and exercise and the large *thermae* and smaller *balnea* offered them all. Citizens would go regularly for a long, many-phased ritual. First, a vigorous workout to stimulate the circulation and loosen the body, then a meander through three rooms, moving from warm to hot and hotter still. The *tepidarium* (warm room) was the largest and most luxurious; this was followed by the caldarium (hot room), which had small stalls for private bathing and the option of hot or cold water. The final room, the *laconicum*, was the hottest (at 50°C) and the place for massage and exfoliation. This journey was followed by a dip in the cool pool of the *frigidarium*, after which bathers would head to the outer areas to read, hang out, eat and drink. Some baths featured a sudatorium, a dry sweating room like a modern-day sauna and the entrance fee was minimal so that everyone could visit. This affordable, vast, multi-layered bathing model has never gone away; it's something Therme Spa currently offers in Romania and Germany and is bringing to Manchester in the near future.

Historians argue that the act of joining Sulis and Minerva to create a communal place of worship in Bath was key in helping Celts adapt to the culture of the Romans. This cements the idea that communal bathing can bring different cultures together in a mutual space; yet when the Romans retreated, so did their bathing culture. Britannia's bath houses fell into decline, and the statue of Sulis Minerva was pulled down. It wasn't until the 1700s that the Georgians rediscovered the wonders of Bath, and 'taking the waters' became a healthy pastime. At this time, hot and cold bathing was said to alleviate nightmares, plague, rickets, inflammation of the eyes, 'female complaints', hysteria, gout, constipation, blows to the head, numbness, bronchitis, cancer and flatulence. Sea-bathing hospitals sprang up around the coast from Scarborough to Margate, as the ocean was believed to cure a myriad of illnesses and ailments. And in 2018, when Haeckels opened Margate's Sea Bathing Machine, a free community sauna that takes its cues from Victorian bathing contraptions, its aim was to reacquaint the community with the health-giving properties of their local waters.

However, when the first Turkish bath opened in Manchester in 1857, no hot-air baths had been built in England since Roman times. It quickly caught on, and 600 opened over the next century. Although they were called Turkish baths, they were more akin to Roman thermae than Islamic hammam. Like the Roman visitors of Aquae Sulis, bathers progressed through a series of hot rooms, with temperatures ranging from 45°C to 110°C, before receiving a 'shampooing' and relaxing in a cold room. Many doctors, in the absence of medication, advocated a trip to the baths to relieve gout and rheumatism.

While Victorian bathers enjoyed the so-called Turkish steam, Russian Jewish immigrants were bringing their own sweat-bathing culture to London's East End. By 1888, there were five exclusive Russian bathhouses in London, the most famous of which was Schevzik's Russian Vapour Baths opposite the synagogue in Brick Lane. Today, Banya No. 1 and The Bath House are authentic, contemporary versions.

At the same time, the use of hot and cold water became a way to treat mental health. In psychiatric hospitals, patients would be doused under cold showers and wrapped in wet sheets, topped by a rubber sheet and then left to sweat for hours, or even days, in a warm bath. Physicians believed this eased congestion in the brain or eliminated the toxins that caused insanity. Hydrotherapy eventually fell out of favour, but it was one of the first treatments that focused on changing the body to treat the mind, suggesting a biological origin of mental illness – an idea taken almost for granted today. Anyone who's into contrast therapy knows it works.

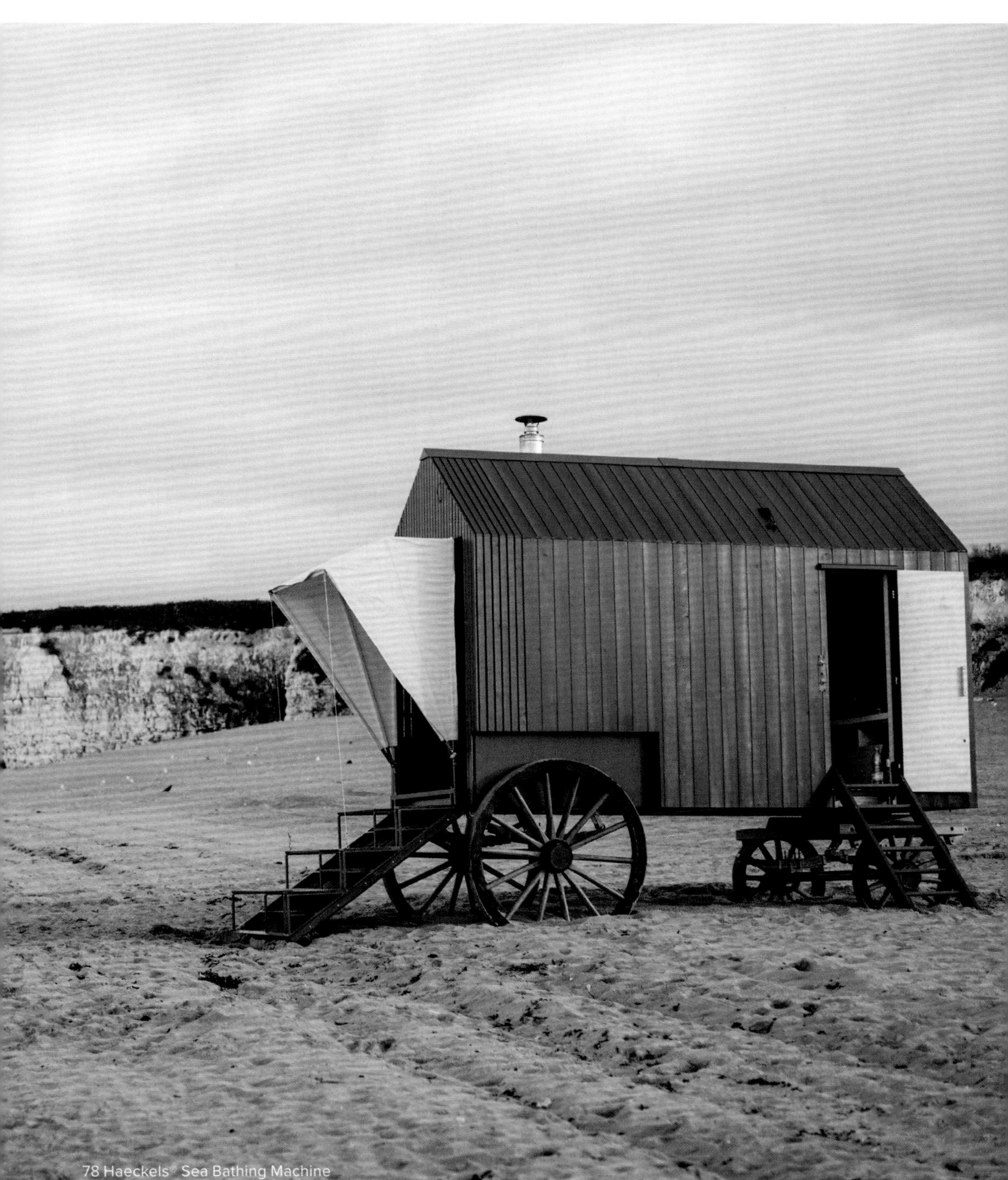

78 Haeckels® Sea Bathing Machine

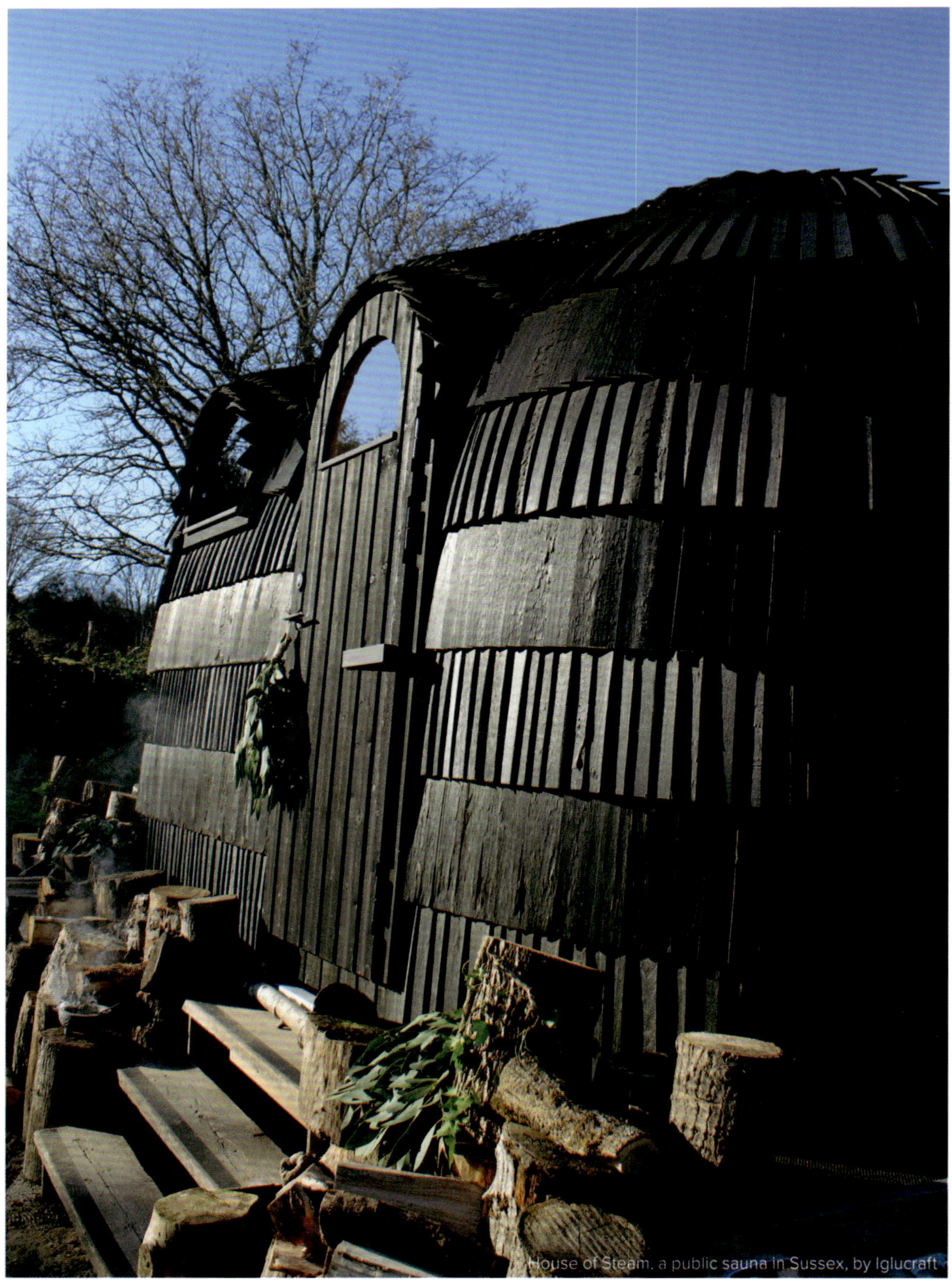

House of Steam, a public sauna in Sussex, by Iglucraft

20TH-CENTURY SAUNA

As the understanding of disease and public health advanced in the early 20th century, public bathing became a key priority for many local authorities, and with it came communal baths and washhouses, lidos and tidal pools. Over time, the rise of domestic bathrooms and the focus on private, cleansing rituals eclipsed public baths. In 1948, the birth of the NHS and free medication for all, meant the focus shifted to treatment rather than prevention of illness. By the 1970s, many communal bathing facilities had closed down or been demolished.

FROM ESTONIA TO SCOTLAND

In a mirrored sauna on the shores of Loch Lomond, a group of Estonian and Scottish sauna lovers discuss the cultural connections between their countries. From a bespoke Estonian tartan and love of Burn's Night to trade routes dating back to the Middle Ages, Scotland and Estonia have a long, fond history. Who knew?

According to archives, food from Estonia kept Scots alive following the Battle of Bannockburn in 1314 and, perhaps because they are small states next to dominant foes, they have shared a mutual understanding ever since.

Estonia has consuls all over the UK, including in Edinburgh, Glasgow and Aberdeen, and dignitaries from all three were in attendance at the soirée (or 'sweaty', as one guest called it) at Loch Lomond to showcase Estonian sauna makers ÖÖD House, Iglucraft and Haljas Houses. As the Scottish sauna scene booms, these high-design saunas are popping up at distilleries, on retreats and on private estates from Fife to Fair Isle.

1948 – THE FINNISH OLYMPIC SAUNA

England's oldest purpose-built sauna – which may also be the oldest Olympic sauna in the world – dates back to 1948 and is in Kent. This is not as random as it sounds. Finnish Olympic officials commissioned it for their athletes competing in the 1948 British Olympics as a recovery and relaxation facility complete with a sauna, hot room, cold showers, massage tables and a kitchen.

After the games, it was gifted to the UK and acquired by a Kent-based paper company with links to Finnish timber, who used it as a staff social club. Until 2020, it was lovingly maintained and enjoyed by a group of former employees, known as Cobdown Sauna Club. These passionate bathers followed authentic Finnish principles; naturist, men and women on different days, affordable – guests could sweat it out for £3 a session or pay an annual membership of £150.

Though badly in need of refurbishment, the sauna retains its original features, right down to the mid-century floral tiling, red leather massage beds and timber-lined walls decked with photos from the 1940s.

In 2024, its members fought to get the complex Grade II listed by English Heritage in recognition of its stand-out prefabricated design by Finnish firm Puutalo Oy. This was a smart move, because the Olympic sauna finds itself in the middle of a battle between developers who want to build houses around it and locals who are objecting. Former Cobdown club member Richard Young is running a campaign to raise the £40,000 needed to restore this slice of Finnish history and bring it back to life. Meanwhile, the sauna sits, protected and unused, while the battle rages on.

If you'd like to know more, you can visit Cobdown Sauna Club's Facebook page, or to arrange an actual visit, email Richard at richwyoung@aol.com

FINNISH DIPLOMACY

Rather like British cuisine, the wild sauna scene takes a magpie approach to sweat bathing, scooping up the bits that are easiest to digest and adapting them for British audiences. And while many barrel saunas are imported from Latvia and Lithuania, most cultural cues come from Finland. In sauna circles, Finland is still the mothership, the go-to destination offering authentic, unforgettable sweat-bathing experiences. After all, which other country has more than 3.3 million saunas (for a population of 5.4 million), and where else has 80 saunas in its embassies and residences?

A fundamental Finnish belief is that everyone is equal in the sauna. Negotiating while semi-naked in the heat breaks down barriers, builds trust and creates solid bonds; and what happens in the sauna stays in the sauna.

Since it opened in 2022, the sauna in the Finnish embassy in London has hosted around 150 guests, among them Mika Meskanen, the Finnish co-founder of the British Sauna Society. Mika is happy to report that the UK wild sauna scene is adopting many Finnish attitudes, such as 'a connection to nature through treatments and being outdoors, and the idea of sauna as a communal and social space', as well as a physical and spiritual appreciation for *löyly* – the vapour drawn by pouring water on hot stones. According to Mika, sauna 'boils down to a powerful trinity: *löyly*, hot and cold, nature.'

SAUNAS TODAY

'When people say to me that sauna is new to us, I remind them that we have had a bathing culture for millennia,' says Gabrielle Reason, general secretary of the British Sauna Society. The current bathing renaissance, which sees hordes of open-water swim groups flock to beaches, rivers and lidos, and saunas popping up to service them, is bringing many of these old facilities back to life. The Eastway Baths in Hackney, closed for 40 years, is now the headquarters of Community Sauna Baths which has sites all over London; in Fife, a band of locals raised funds to renovate the Cellardyke tidal pool and brought in Scottish Seaside Saunas; when locals spearheaded a fundraiser for the repair of La Vallette bathing pools in Guernsey, along came Hot Haus sauna. Across the country, venues such as FIX in Manchester, Kernow Springs in Wadebridge, Saunassa in Newquay, PAUS in Cambridge and ARC in London offer saunas, hot tubs, cold plunges and ice baths dedicated to hot and cold therapy.

Real-life connection, the need to be outdoors and an age-old desire to sweat are the pillars of the wild sauna movement. As Mikkel Aaland puts it, 'In our rapidly changing world, the growing need for physical, social and spiritual wellness is inspiring people to look for alternative lifestyles, and the sauna/sweat bath fits this yearning.'

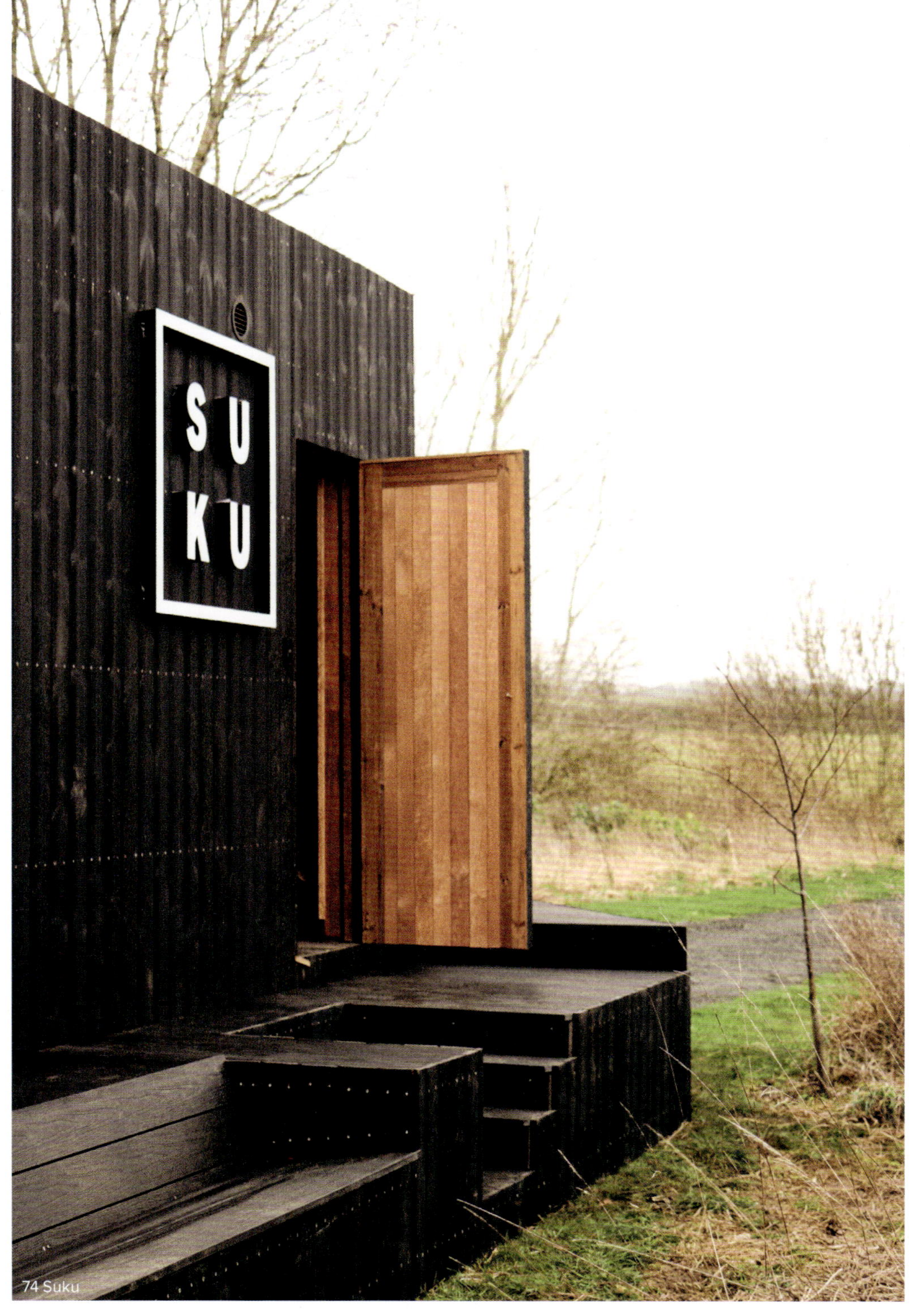

74 Suku

Sauna rituals & therapies

'It's not about a furious effort to slow down. It's about getting out of the way and discovering the pace that was there all along.'

On Connection, Kae Tempest

The sweat lodge of history was a spiritual and emotional therapy, just as much about ritual as the physical intensity of the heat and cold.

'Hot, cold, rest, repeat', has become a sauna catch phrase, but it's not always easy to switch off and be in the moment, despite our best efforts, and many saunas offer guided rituals to help us unplug from the outside world and connect with ourselves. Add to this the collective effervescence that arises on the benches, and sauna is a ready-made arena, an event space where engagement is a given. From sauna yoga to gong baths to full moon sauna parties and aromatherapy journeys, a ritual can create a safe atmosphere that can lead to transformation, a release and a profound sense of joy.

SONGS, STORIES AND MYTHS

Traditional sauna healing in the Nordic countries was based on folklore, and spells, poems, chants, laments and lullabies were used to change fortunes, bring luck and summon spirits into the sauna to ease suffering and pain. (Our ancestors were on to something, because humming is known to stimulate the vagus nerve, which moves us out of fight or flight mode into rest and relaxation.)

British and Celtic sauna stories, if they existed, have been long lost, but in the Irish myth 'The Romance of Mis and Dubh Ruis', Mis' madness is cured by bathing over and over in hot water and animal fat. British-born Tim Jago has spent 30 years running Celtic sweat lodges; he's an artful storyteller, bringing to life legends and myths from Ireland and Wales in deep, transformative rituals. The Celts belived in reincarnation and many gods; they found divinity in rivers, hills, sky and sea. Birth, death and rebirth form the foundation of Tim's lodges.

At Community Sauna Baths in Hackney (69), Myth Mondays puts a new spin on tales of old, and bathers are asked to visualise stone giants from Chile, Norwegian trolls, Scottish fairies, and the goblins, sprites and elves of Celtic folklore. It's a creative exercise that's easy to bypass in the age of Netflix. In the sauna all our senses can come alive, and even cross over, to the point where we can 'taste' colours, 'feel' sounds and chart curious mental maps. This (harmless) process is called synaesthesia, and 'saunasthesia' at CSB is a multi-sensory session in which temperature, sound and scent synchronise in a HiFi-equipped blackout sauna.

GRIEF SAUNA

In Nordic cultures where the sauna, not the church, was the heart of the community, the dead were honoured in the steam. Often they would be taken to the sauna to breathe their last after which they would be prepared for burial on a 'corpse board' that was placed on the bottom bench. Mourners would come together to chant, sing and sweat out their pain, calling on their ancestors for comfort.

Film director Anna Hints documents the lives of bathers in the smoke saunas of southern Estonia, where she grew up. 'When my grandfather died, granny and my aunties went to the smoke sauna, where granny released all these emotions – pain, frustration, anger and hurt – and we were there witnessing it. We stayed in the sauna for several hours, and when we came out, I felt granny had made peace with grandfather.'

Heat forces thoughts and feelings, sometimes long locked away, to the surface; and in expert hands, sauna can be a space in which to heal. 'It's a safe space where all our emotions and experiences can be heard and shared without judgement,' says Anna, who spent seven years filming the award-winning *Smoke Sauna Sisterhood*, where real women laugh, cry and sweat together. 'In the sauna, I never fear being uncomfortable.'

When Irish sauna practitioner Saorla Wright started hosting rituals in England, they noticed grief would often surface. The loss of a friend in London left Saorla, who grew up in Dublin, reeling. 'In Ireland, death is dealt with when it comes up. Before Christianity, in pagan times, funeral traditions were raucous. At the Irish wake, people were getting off with each other, playing sexy parlour games; it was almost like a Bacchanalia. There was an open coffin; there still is. Everyone comes over, and traditionally, you stay awake with the body.'

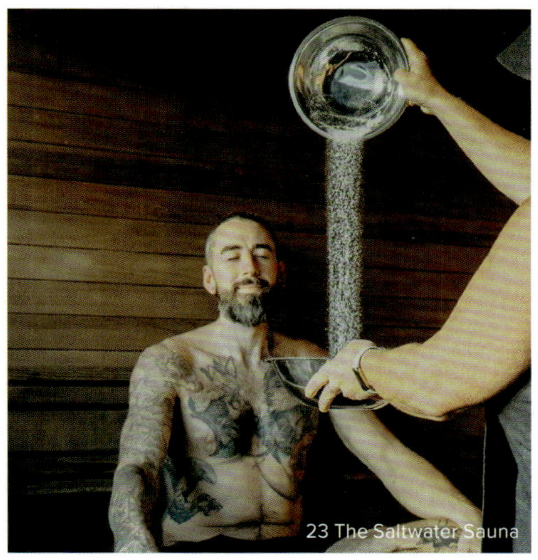

23 The Saltwater Sauna

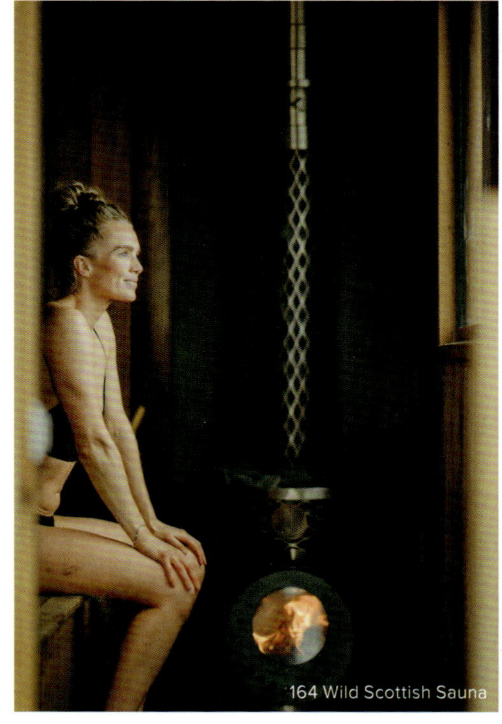

164 Wild Scottish Sauna

Britain's medicalised, bureaucratic approach to dying, which can be seen as starting in 1836 with the Registration Act (creation of a national register for births, marriages and deaths) 'makes the process sterilised and distant, and means it's easy to stay in denial for a really long time. If you don't see the body, you don't feel it's gone. It can all seem unreal,' Saorla explains.

To this end, they started running grief sauna sessions, using myths and stories as emotional hooks, at the Community Sauna Baths in Hackney, and they now lead them in other saunas around the country. 'When a group of people who don't know each other come together under the name of grief, something really magical happens. You're in a darkened room, you're listening to a story, and you're allowed to cry without saying why.' In the past, Saorla had frequented Death Cafés, where strangers gather to eat cake and drink tea, but they would often leave feeling overburdened with other people's losses. Saorla devised the grief sauna as an alternative, less intense space. 'You don't have to open your mouth if you don't want to. You don't have to say why you're there.'

In the grief sessions, people are free to let it all out – to stomp their feet, clap, cry, shake. 'If you did that on the street, or even at home, people would be really worried. Sometimes, it's just about giving people permission. But there's no pressure. You can come to a grief sauna and sit slumped in the corner with your eyes closed and have a nice skin scrub, if you want to.' Anna takes comfort from her grandmother's wisdom: 'Granny used to say "We consist of water, and when we experience trauma, this water freezes inside us and doesn't have the potential to flow." The physical heat of the sauna, and the emotional heat too, can warm up those frozen waters.'

The heat may work its magic and soothe our inner depths, but grief doesn't disappear after just one session. According to Saorla, 'Once people know the sauna portal has been opened, they just want to keep coming back. Some of the most beautiful things I've seen were inside the grief sauna. It's just so moving and deeply affecting.'

LEAF WHISKING

In Lithuania and Latvia, the sauna, or pirts, is not a static space; it's buzzing with whooshes of steam and the swooshing of whisks. And everyone has a whisk. Birch is a popular choice as it contains saponin, a soap-like liquid that exfoliates and cleans the skin, but other trees and plants – oak, eucalyptus, juniper, elderflower and mint – can be used, and each has its own healing properties. In Irish sweat houses, heather was dipped in water from a bucket and shaken on the stones to create steam.

In a dedicated ritual, a bath master will work with two whisks, spiralling the branches to create heat peaks like an expert conductor and 'slapping' bathers with the leaves. Far from being painful, this feels like a gentle massage. The smell of fresh leaves and the hypnotic swoosh of the whisks in action is mesmerising and addictive, and whips the senses into life.

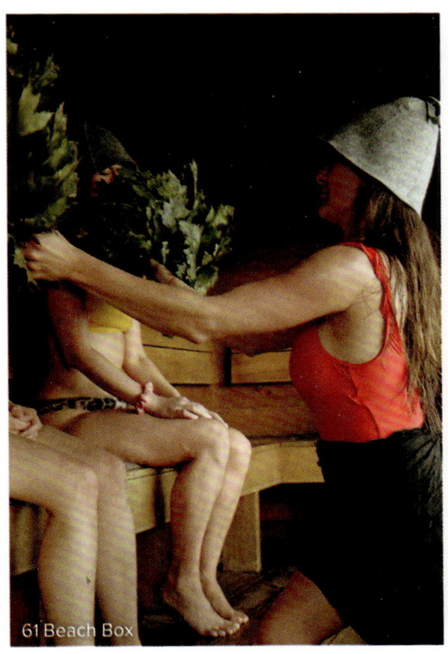
61 Beach Box

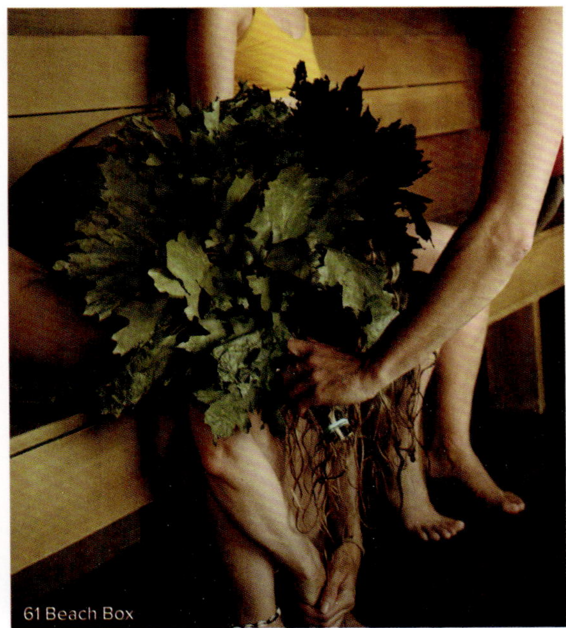
61 Beach Box

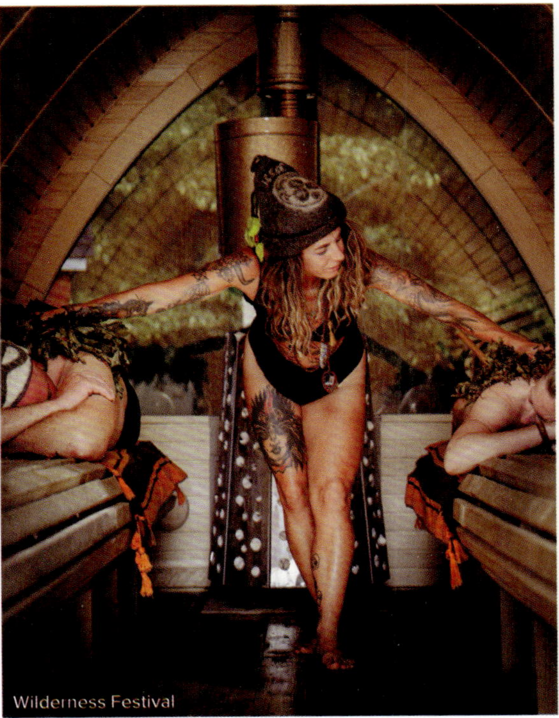
Wilderness Festival

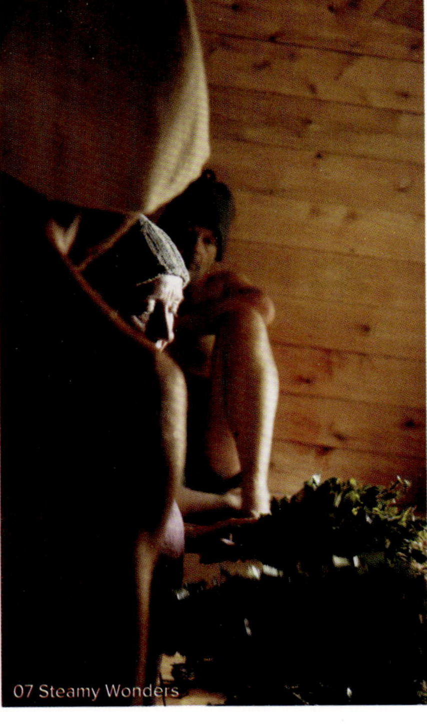
07 Steamy Wonders

SEAWEED BATHING

'In the same way that there are superfoods for the body, seaweed is a superfood for the skin,' says Helen Atherton, founder of Edinburgh-based beauty brand Dook. Together with Kirsty Carver of Edinburgh's Soul Water Sauna, Dook has created clay face masks made with Scottish dulse, Irish moss and spirulina. They are a signature treatment at Soul Water and Granton Wild Spa.

Given that there are over 650 seaweed species dotted around the UK's rugged coastlines, it's no surprise that seaweed and its rich bounty has found its way into the sauna. The question is, what took us so long?

Packed with vitamins, antioxidants and lipids, the common red, brown and green seaweeds improve skin elasticity, tone and texture. Brown seaweeds are particularly high in the polysaccharide fucoidan, which has anti-coagulant, antiviral and anti-inflammatory properties.

In the heat, we sweat out harmful metals – mercury, lead and cobalt – and our skin soaks up the nutrients that all seaweeds contain, from collagen-boosting vitamin C to sleep-enhancing magnesium.

Sauna practitioners Molly and Sam run Heal Saunas and specialise in nature-based rituals using plants that they have foraged. They make whisks with seasonal plants – oak, eucalyptus, elderflower – and a body wrap from seaweed. Sourced from clean beaches, the seaweed is heated up in a bowl of water on the sauna stove until it forms a gloopy, clear liquid that is neither sticky nor smelly and has a texture like aloe vera. It's packed with goodness, and bathers are encouraged to smother it all over their bodies, heads and hair. Open pores drink it up, and the skin is left feeling baby-soft.

On the northwest coast of Ireland, seaweed baths have long been used to provide relief from rheumatism and arthritis. Meanwhile, at Anglesey sea-salt makers Halen Môn, soaking in a bath full of bladderwrack is a smart use of warm water left over from the manufacturing process. Wooden barrels are filled with 40°C water and bladderwrack is supplied by local seaweed farm Câr-y-Môr. The baths are particularly popular with swimming and cycling groups who want to ease sore muscles, and those with skin conditions can soak under the stars while Snowdonia reaches skywards in the distance.

AUFGUSS – INFUSION THERAPY

If you've visited a typical European spa with a large sauna, you may well have come across *aufguss*. It's a German word meaning 'infusion' and is also a ritual held by an '*aufguss master*' – someone who pours water or puts essential-oil infused ice balls onto the hot rocks, and then distributes aromatic steam over sweat bathers with a towel, often in a graceful rhythmical dance set to music. If you've ever seen it, you'll know exactly what this is, and if you haven't you probably won't believe it until you do...

At its best, *aufguss* is entertaining, engaging, beautiful even – and the deep sweating it delivers makes you feel cleansed. Anyone who has sat through a well-choreographed aufguss ritual will want to go back for more. And, what's more, it's very easy to forget you're in a sauna, which is good news for people who might otherwise struggle with the heat. A 2017 study from University College London's Psychological and Language Sciences Department found that when watching a live theatre performance we can synchronize our heartbeat with others in the audience, regardless of whether we know them or not; if the performance is strong enough, the different social groups overcome their differences and engage as a whole. Likewise, in the heat of the sauna, good storytelling can amplify collective empathy.

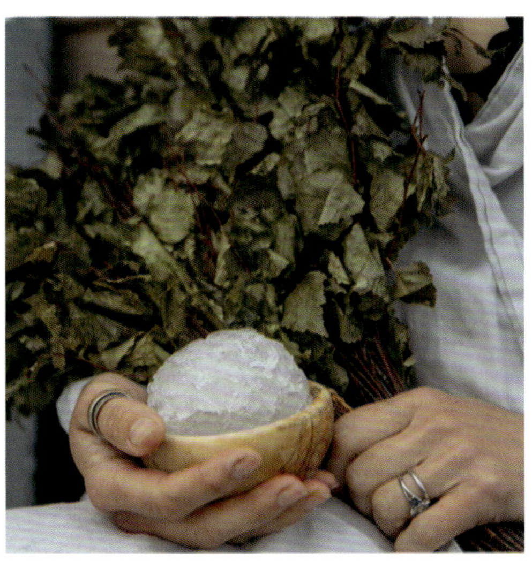

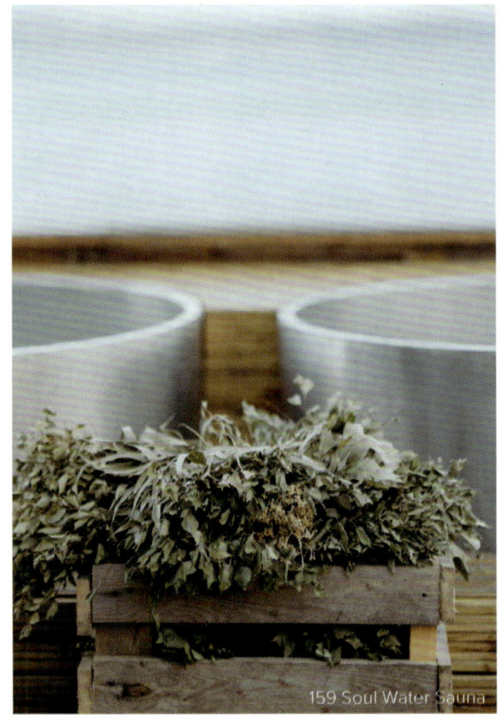

159 Soul Water Sauna

And then there's 'Show Aufguss' – the Eurovision of sauna. This loud, gold-sequinned, bells-on version of *aufguss* attracts serious fans who love its humour, jazzy costumes and Las Vegas kitsch. It's performance-art-meets-musical-theatre in the steam. At the annual Aufguss World Championships, more than 100 participants gather in a European mega-spa to flex their skills in a large 'event sauna', complete with sound system and digital screens. Naked audiences are captivated by shows on topics from *Dracula* and shipwrecks to life in a Tokyo bakery and warring siblings. Costumes, lighting, storylines, aromas and, of course, towel-waving skills are scored by an international panel of judges.

And if this sounds totally mad and Not Very British, be surprised, because in the past three years the UK has got in on the act. Thanks largely to Deborah Carr of Anada (anada.co.uk) and Rudding Park (ruddingpark.co.uk) hotel in Harrogate, we are developing our own Show Aufguss, underpinned by our own particular brand of British humour. Shows to date have ranged from the rebirth of Boris Johnson to British fry-ups to Celtic witchcraft and spells. And although Show Aufguss has its roots in the big, hi-tech spas, its impact is reaching the wild sauna scene as more and more enthusiasts hitch their horseboxes to the *aufguss* wagon. The 2025 UK *aufguss* championships took place in ARC, London's new 70-seater sauna and bathers gathered to watch entrants perform over two days.

SAUNA MASTERS

The heat melts away barriers and allows bigger, deeper things to surface. Emotions can run high and sauna masters need to be emotionally tuned in to be able to hold the space and keep bathers safe. It's a delicate role, and in Russia and the Baltics, being a 'bath master' is a respected profession. Organisations such as the International Bath Academy (bath.academy) and the Latvian Pirts Spirit (pirtsspirit.com) offer deep-level training where becoming an esteemed bath master is akin to becoming a Buddhist monk; it takes years of spiritual, as well as practical training.

In the UK, Wild Spa Wowo (64) and Anada offer sauna master training courses to those eager to lead journeys into steam. Participants learn about leaf whisking, *aufguss* and the psychological and physiological effects of thermotherapy. To date, there are around 100 trained sauna masters in the UK. Like the Nordic sauna healers of old, many, among them Nick Tettersell, move from sauna to sauna. Nick says, 'I see so much anxiety, low self-esteem, self-doubt. Talking therapies only go so far; in the sauna, body-based, somatic work brings releases to the surface in passive ways.' The late psychoanalyst Carl Jung called these releases 'unforgotten wisdoms' that lie at the core of the psyche. Our fast-paced, digital lives have no time for them, and offer no space to process them, so when they surface in the steam, it can be profound.

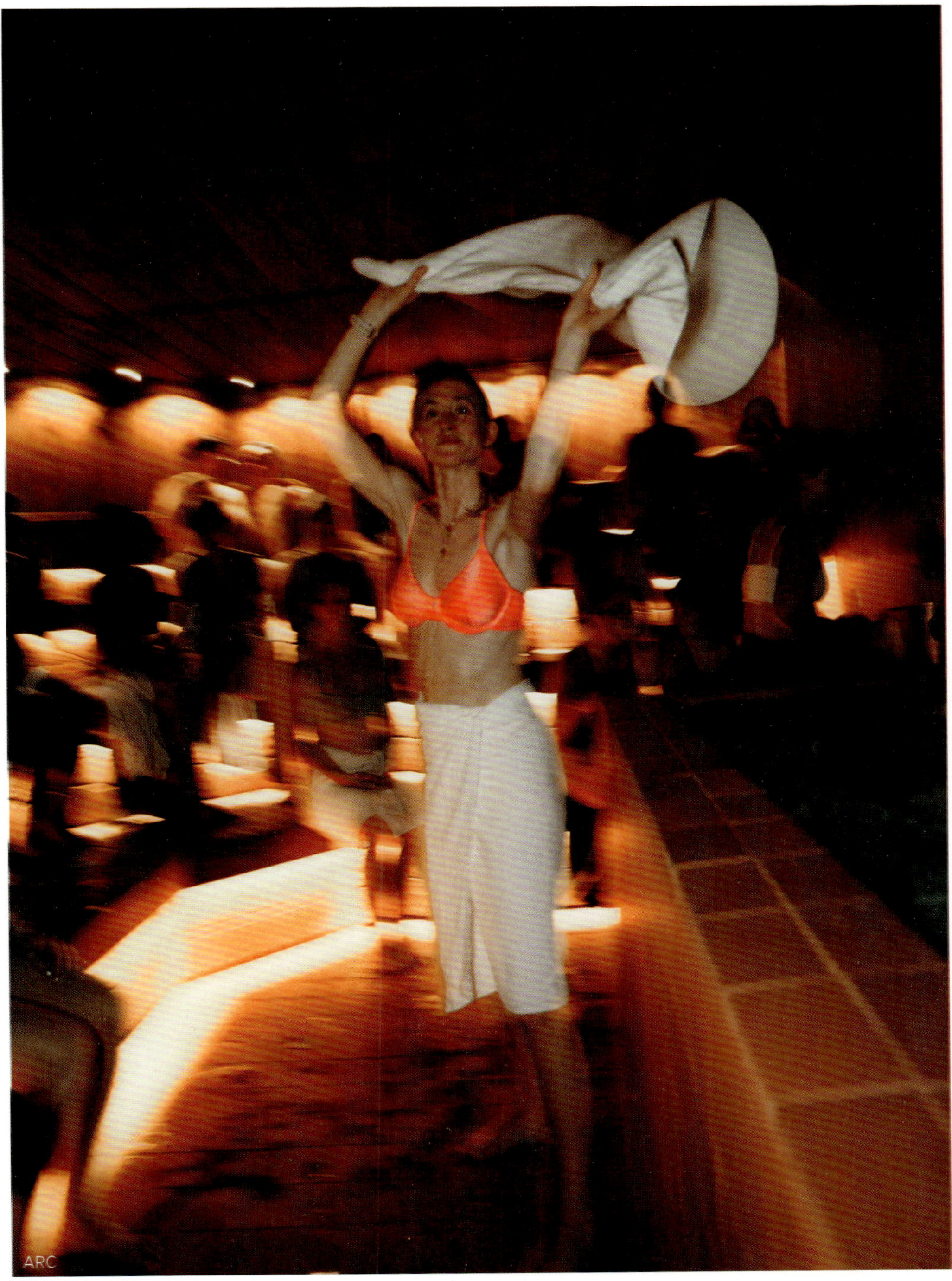
ARC

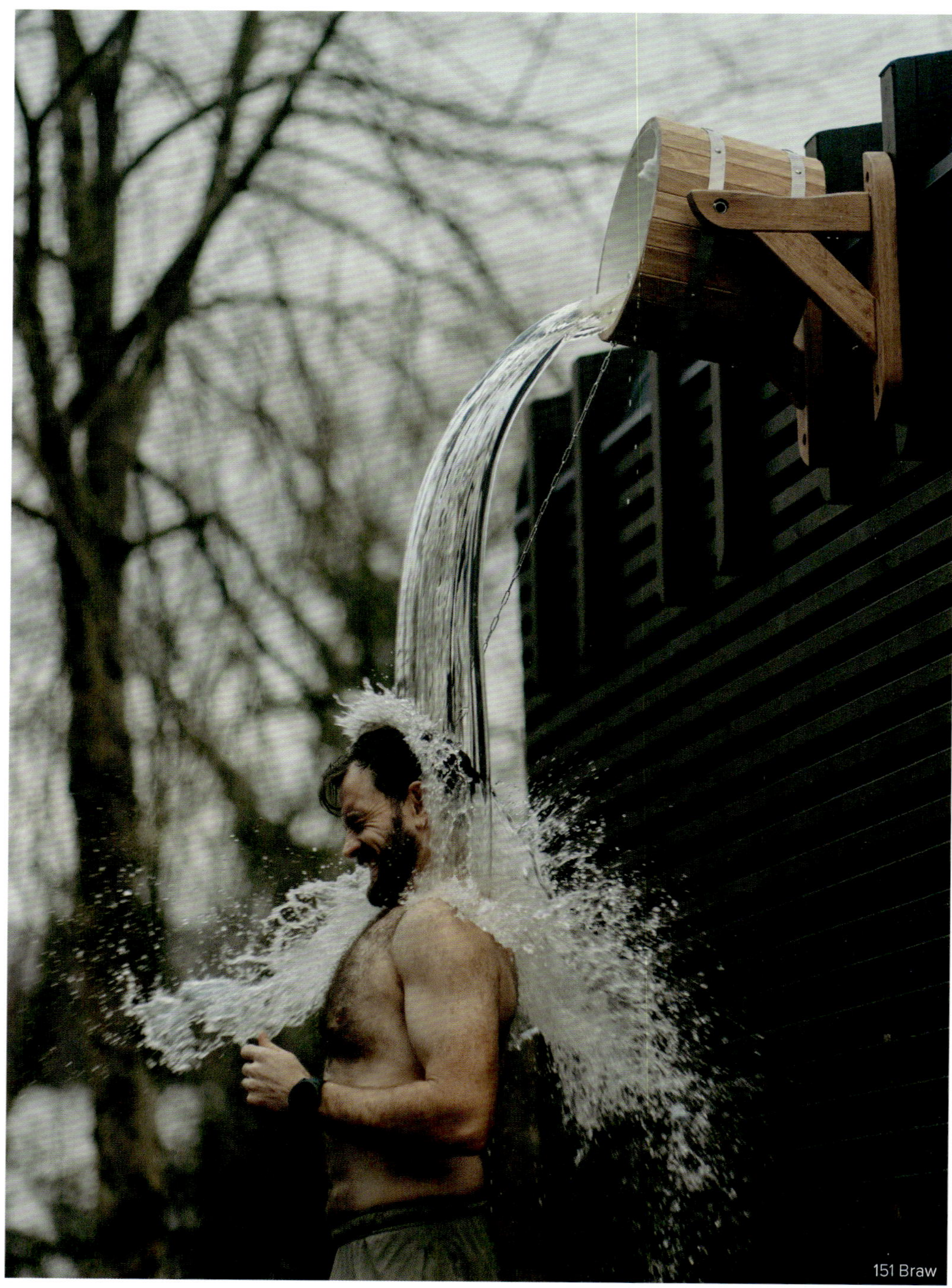

151 Braw

Etiquette and how to sauna

Yes, sauna etiquette is a thing. Here, we'll briefly cover the dos and don'ts of sweat-bathing.

WHICH COMES FIRST, HOT OR COLD?

Whichever you prefer – there's no right or wrong. Listen to your body and go with your mood. But what you shouldn't do is go straight from cold to hot and hot to cold without pause, because that means you're constantly repeating the hermetic stress.

If your window of tolerance is slim, if your nervous system is hyper-aroused, or if you haven't done contrast therapy before, extreme stress may not be the answer. Treat yourself more gently. A cold shower is a good middle ground, so you can adapt slowly. Or just splash cold water on your face, or put your hands into cold water, then wrap yourself up. You don't want your body to hijack itself before you get to the good bit.

Yoyo-ing back and forth between hot and cold takes effort, and it's easy to get caught up in the mechanics without shifting gear mentally. Take time to find headspace and make room for interoception – the eighth sense that notices the inner workings of the body and how this makes us feel. Turn your mind's eye inwards.

If you have had a long swim in cold water, don't go straight to the top bench of the sauna. Acclimatise outside first, so you can keep vasodilation (widening of blood vessels) under control. The blood needs to warm up before it starts pumping quickly around the body. Sit with a hot drink on the bottom bench and reheat slowly.

'Afterdrop' – when you carry on cooling down after you have got out of cold water – and 'after sweat,' – when you carry on sweating after a hot sauna – are unpleasant and can be unnerving. Whether you end on hot or cold, be sure that your core and your extremities feel in balance. Søberg advises ending on cold to increase your metabolism. And once you're used to the cold, it's good to have the body work a little harder to warm you up.

THE PRE-WASH

Rinse, rinse, rinse. In other sauna cultures, it's compulsory to shower before you begin, and it's nice to start with wet, clean skin. The first sweat is the toxin-heavy, dirtiest one, so wash this (and subsequent sweats) off under a shower or in the sea, not in a communal pool. After all, who wants to jump in a cold plunge filled with someone else's sweat?

HOW LONG SHOULD I STAY IN?

Ignore the pundits on social media who like to impose time limits on hot and cold immersions. Even if you only last a few minutes, that's okay. The top bench can be up to 10 degrees hotter than the bottom bench, so if you're new to sauna start low and work your way up, and never force yourself to stay in until the timer has run out (most last 15 minutes). Some sauna owners have taken timers out of their spaces, as bathers have been known to lie on the floor until time's up rather than stepping out. A sauna session is not a test, it's a safe space in which you can relax and reset. If you listen to your body, you will know when it's time to stop. Leave when you're 'comfortably uncomfortable'.

Typically, a sauna session involves around three rounds of hot and cold. It's tempting to dart between the two to maximise the time slot, but doing so without a break can put stress on the body, and keep it in fight or flight mode. Between cold water and sauna, take a pause. Enjoy the space between. Drink some water, sit back and tune into yourself.

Ultimately, there are no rules, no optimal timings or temperatures. Sauna and contrast therapy at its most pure is about being out in the elements, relaxing and de-stressing. Treat it as an easy form of self-care, not a competition.

WHAT TO (NOT) WEAR?

To strip or not to strip? This is a big question in the UK, where most would rather poke our eyes out with a stick than be seen naked in a public space. Unlike other sauna cultures where nudity is compulsory, among British bathers, anything goes – from wetsuits to running gear to hen and stag-do fancy dress – and anything, it seems, is better than nothing. 'Textile-free' sessions are unusual, but increasingly, sauna operators are hosting naked, single sex sessions. The more you sauna, however, the more you realise that it's so much more hygienic to sweat naked on a towel than swaddled in neoprene.

One traditional item of Baltic clothing you might consider is a felt sauna hat – which sometimes has a loop on the top so you can hang it up. A sauna hat can generate hoots of laughter from the uninitiated. Who wants to look like a garden gnome in swimwear? But once you get used to this comedy headgear, you won't look back. In the Irish sweat houses of old, bathers wore a cabbage leaf, and current versions are made from felt or breathable linen and shaped like a tea cosy. Counterintuitively, the sauna hat keeps the head cool and protects the face and hair from any over-zealous swooshes of *löyly*. And, if you don't feel like talking, you can pull it down over your nose with a Do-Not-Disturb shrug.

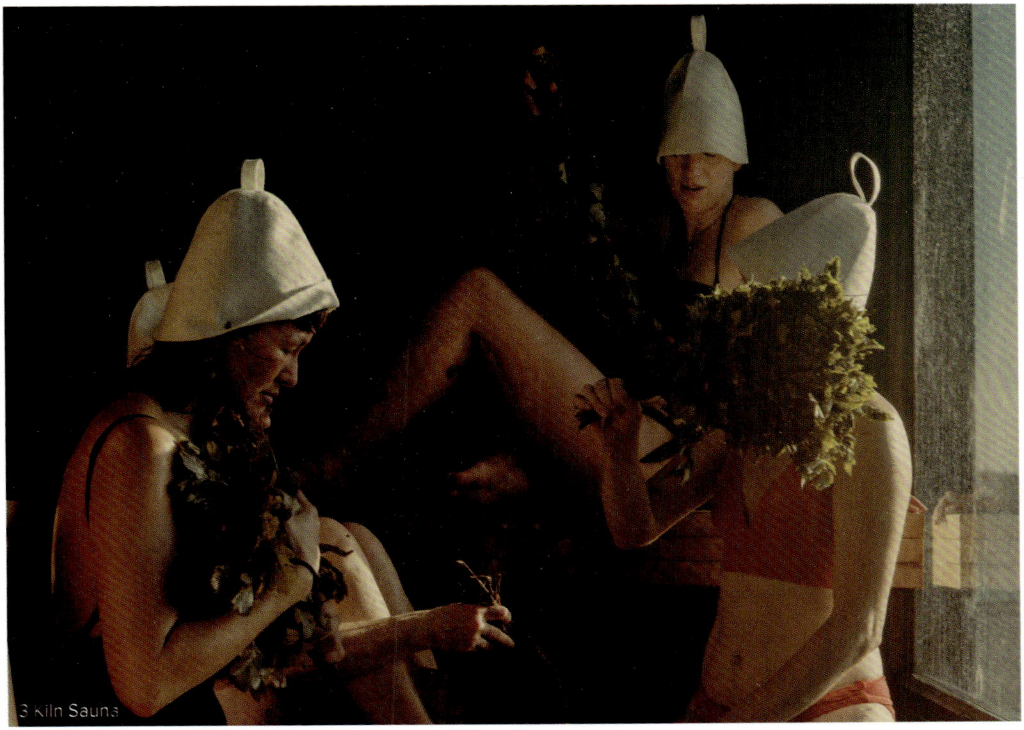

3 Kiln Sauna

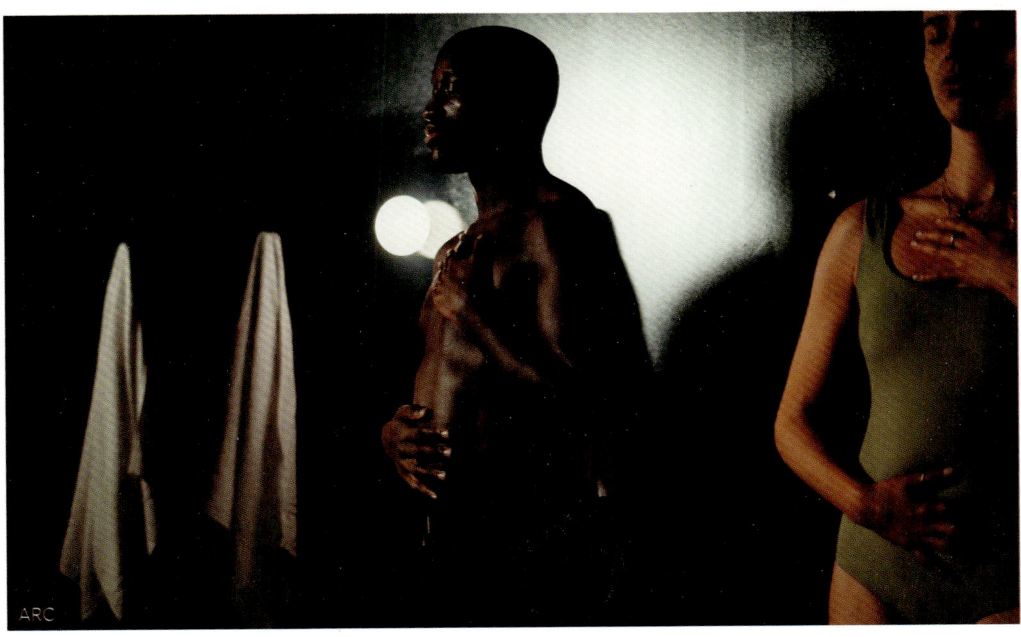

ARC

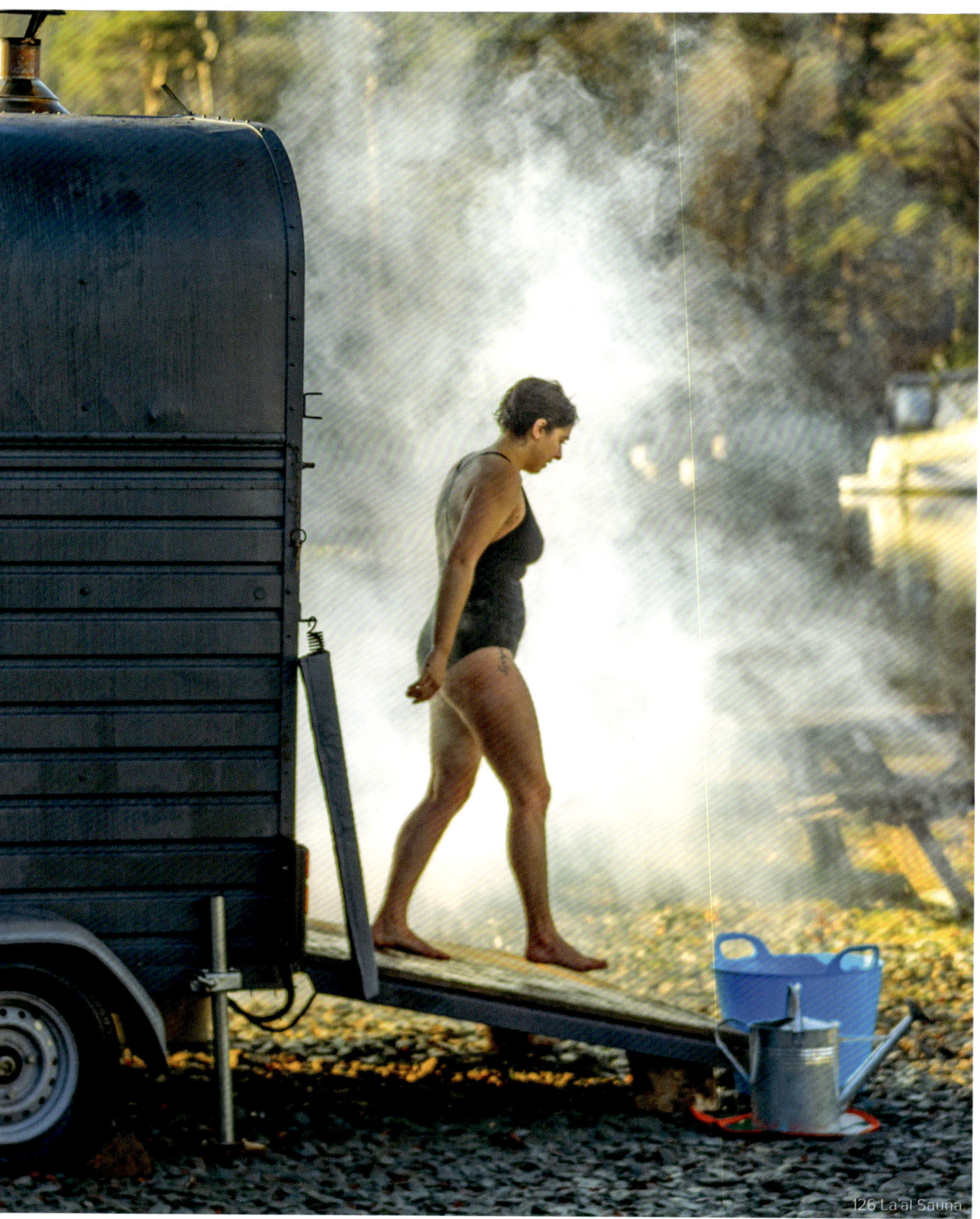

126 La'al Sauna

RESPECT OTHERS

Remember to close the door when you step in and out. Don't bag a spot by leaving your towel in place when you're not sitting on it; the sauna is a shared, fluid space and everyone should expect to move around.

Brits tend to be a rowdy bunch, and the community atmosphere of the sauna is often compared to the pub. But, unlike the pub, it's a small space where everyone can hear each other, so speaking quietly and being mindful of what is discussed is basic courtesy. In Finland and Estonia, thorny issues such as politics and religion are kept firmly outside its walls, and in Finland, silence is often preferred.

The same obviously goes for phones. Sauna is one of the few spaces that allows a quick and easy digital detox. Respect it as a tech-free zone and leave your phone outside.

Sauna brain is that disconnected, floaty feeling that comes after a good sweat; with it comes forgetfulness. Sauna operators have so much lost property they do regular charity runs to get rid of it. Don't leave your belongings behind.

STEAM

Steam (*löyly* in Finnish) is the sauna's beating heart. A sauna is not a proper sauna unless you can pour water on the rocks to create steam. Pour a small ladle full of water slowly and evenly around the top rocks. Apply little and often, and ask other bathers before you pour. In Nordic nations, it's rude to throw water on the rocks without asking permission or to create mass evacuation by steaming everyone out. Adding essential oils to the bucket and ladle is tempting, but be warned: many contain ingredients that wreck the sauna rocks and cause allergic reactions in other bathers. And they can be flammable too.

REHYDRATION

If you need to eat before you sauna, keep it light. Trying to digest a heavy meal while sweating puts extra strain on your system. And don't sauna if you're under the influence of drugs or alcohol; on average, we lose about a pint of water in a 10–15-minute session, and dehydration and headaches are not uncommon. Opt for electrolytes rather than alcohol, or go Nordic with pickles, salmon and kvass (a cereal-based sweet and sour drink).

What makes a good sauna?

BRITISH SAUNA SOCIETY SAUNA QUALITY GUIDELINES

The British Sauna Society (BSS) is a non-profit organisation of volunteers, who are committed to developing authentic sauna culture in the UK and bringing its wellbeing benefits to everyone.

ELEMENTS OF GOOD SAUNA EXPERIENCE:

- Immersive heat and good steam – sauna stove with hot stones, so that bathers or practitioners can create enjoyable steam (*löyly*)
- Health and safety – quality construction that minimises the risk of slips, falls, fires and burns
- Well ventilated space, drained floor and insulated shell for comfort, safety and energy efficiency
- Furnished with good facilities, adequate space for changing, storage, showers, toilets etc.
- Clean and hygienic – regularly cleaned, odour-free space maintained with care
- Access to open water, ice baths, cold plunges or cold showers
- Access to outdoor space, nature and fresh clean air for cooldowns, rest, reset and relaxation
- Easy and free access to drinking water for hydration
- Accessible: designed for all abilities
- Safe space free of judgement and argument, where everyone is welcome
- Sustainably and responsibly built and operated
- Educated and hospitable staff who understand sauna practice and can guide bathers on how to use sauna
- Community engagement – encourage communal use, which promotes social interaction and wellbeing within the community. Sauna connects everyone.

TO HELP KEEP THESE SPACES CLEAN AND HEALTHY:

- shower, or rinse in the sea before you start your session
- bring two towels, one to sit on and one to dry off with
- wear flip flops or rock shoes in the sea or on sand
- bring your own toiletries
- cold-water swimmers should take off neoprene boots and gloves before entering the sauna
- use the (hopefully provided) footbath at the entrance to rinse feet when going in and out
- Rinse off between rounds – but never in the plunge pool or the ice bath

CLEANLINESS AND HYGIENE IN THE WILD

Many wild saunas in the UK operate in locations where there's no running water. Instead, the sea or watering cans are on hand to cool bathers down between rounds, and people are encouraged to bring their own drinking water to stay hydrated. Often there's no changing room either, which means a hasty scramble in and out of swimwear under a changing robe.

This no-frills approach is part of the experience, but it's a challenge to keep floors, doors, windows and benches free from mould, sweat and salt stains. And a dirty sauna is a no-go. In Nordic cultures, before the invention of domestic bathrooms, the sauna was the wash house. It was a clean space and government officials would close down community saunas that fell short of expected hygiene levels.

SAUNA HEAT

A 40-60°C sauna is too cool to bring on a strong sweat, but it's a good temperature for children and newcomers, and for exercises such as sauna yoga and stretching. The average sauna is 70–90°C, and upwards of 90°C, the heat can feel intense. When it hits the 100°C mark, it can feel as though your forehead is melting, and it is actually possible to sear an outer layer of skin if you sit too close to the stove; a well-designed space will have a handrail or barrier round the stove to protect bathers. A spot on the lower bench, farthest away from the rocks, is always the coolest option.

SAUNA SAFETY

All sauna operators are first-aid trained, and on the beaches, many of them are lifeguard trained too. Safety is a top priority, especially as many Brits talk about how the sauna makes them feel claustrophobic. This is usually because we have only experienced a poorly ventilated space (which is often dark and pokey), where the heat sits heavily on the skin, burning it instead of swirling around and caressing it. In a well-ventilated space, you don't feel like you're trapped and basting like a turkey. But, whatever the circumstances, if you do start to feel overheated and panicky, it's time to leave.

A PROPER SAUNA MUST BE:

- hot
- well-ventilated – oxygen rich
- clean
- furnished with well-stacked, good quality rocks so it's easy to create good steam
- accessible
- odour-free
- made of simple materials
- run by welcoming staff who understand sauna and provide proper, responsible instructions on how to use it
- furnished with good facilities (changing room, drinking water, storage)
- supplemented with a cold plunge – ideally in a natural body of water and places to cool off, rest and reset
- a safe space, free of judgement and argument, where everyone is welcome
- see Britishsaunasociety.org.uk for more information

Types of sauna

There is no shortage of sauna builders in the UK creating spaces in all shapes and sizes. But what's the difference between the options, and what can you expect in terms of sauna experience?

SWEAT LODGE

Deep, dark, hot and often lasting for several hours, the sweat lodge ceremony is the mother of all sweat-bathing rituals and its history goes back millennia. It's also the simplest sauna to build, if you know what to do: Basic Guidelines: create a dome structure from bendy green saplings or tent poles stuck into the ground, cover with lots of blankets and rugs and place hot stones in a central pit and sprinkle with water. But to do it properly, in the traditional way, takes years of practice, and requires the guidance of a 'shaman' or 'sauna sage'. Typically, young green branches of alder, willow, rowan or hazel are cut and tied with string to make an igloo-shaped, bendy frame. Igneous, shatter-proof rocks that can withstand being heated on a fire until they glow red are required. In the UK, granite is a good option – but watch out for river rocks that can explode as trapped moisture rapidly expands. A large fire outside heats these rocks, which are brought into the lodge at different intervals – the only time light enters the pitch-black space.

Then the ceremony itself can begin; bathers crawl in through a tiny west-facing entrance on hands and knees (a symbolic act of returning to the womb) and sweat for hours while the host guides them through life, death and everything in between, dousing the glowing rocks with water, plants and herbs to create a deep, perfumed steam in which transformations can occur. When the ceremony is over, bathers crawl out of an east-facing exit, having been 'reborn'. It's often hard to put into words what happens in a lodge; it can take time to process; but those who want to try gather round the fire afterwards to share their experiences.

Sweat lodges can be life-changing; they can challenge the status quo and rewire our psychological pathways. They require physical and mental preparation, stamina and recovery time. Take note: joining one if you're not heat-adapted is like diving into the deep end before you have learned to swim.

MEXICAN TEMAZCAL

The *temazcal* is to Mexicans what sauna is to Finns. Many households have a hotbox in the yard where families and friends enjoy sweat-bathing rituals: kids go after school, women join until late pregnancy, and *abuelas* don't stop until the day they die. This most ancient of sweat-bathing rituals originated with the Mayans (the name *temazcal* comes from the Nahuatl words *teme* to bathe, and *calli*, house) so when a Mexican *temazcalero* came to Somerset to host a ceremony at eco-retreat 42 Acres, it was too good an opportunity to miss. How would this far-flung ritual compare to our own, ancestral sweat lodges (which are being reignited in certain sweat-bathing circles)?

In appearance, this *temazcal* looked similar to sweat lodges. It has a tiny entrance, an earth 'altar' and a domed igloo-like structure. Ahau, the *temazcalero*, makes his lodge with tent poles (much simpler than willow branches) covered in thick felt blankets. Inside, it's pitch black and cramped; 30-odd people sit cross-legged in a circle, cheek by jowl. And the rounds begin, each one honouring an element: earth, water, wind, fire. Between each, the door is opened and glowing red rocks, heated on a fire outside are passed in on antlers. Gradually, the heat builds and the energy shifts. Ahau uses drums, shakers and his powerful voice to sing and chant incantations in Spanish. He sprinkles herbs and pours buckets of water onto the rocks to create powerful, scented vapour that Mexicans traditionally use to heal ailments. 'In Mexico, the *temazcal* supports wellbeing in so many ways,' says Ahau. 'Medicinal, physical, mental and emotional. It's also a form of traditional bathing, spiritual growth and strengthening.'

The ceremony lasts a few hours. Ahau brings about a communal, trance-like state, amplified by the darkness and the relentless heat, which leaves people singing, sobbing and writhing around the floor. Like the Celtic sweat lodge, the *temazcal* digs deep into our psychological, emotional and physical reaches in a way that daily life prohibits. It reminds us, as it has since time began, that whoever we are and wherever we are from, our similarities are greater than those things that divide us.
Rootofthegods.com

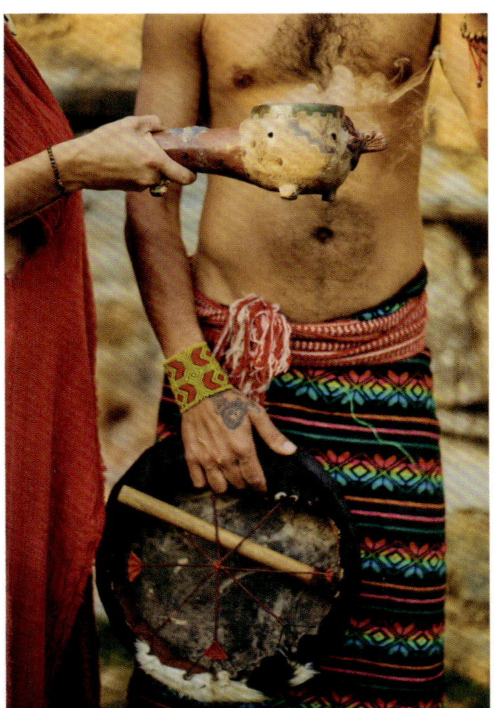

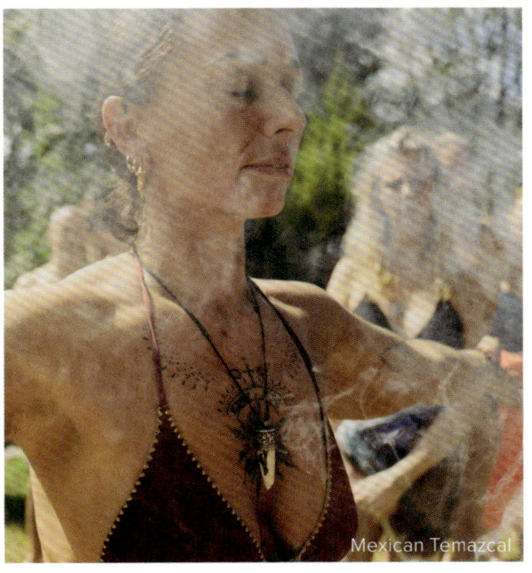

Mexican Temazcal

TENT

Popular with Baltic armies and Chinese ice-fishermen alike, the tent sauna is a genius invention. A metal frame, a few layers of non-permeable fabric, some wooden benches and a wood-fired heater make up the tent sauna, which can reach upwards of 70°C in around 30 minutes. Popular brands include Mobiba, Arctinar, Morzh, Portasauna and Savotta, and can hold from two to 30 people. Although they are mobile, tent saunas are not backpack-portable – stove rocks alone can fill a supermarket trolley – and they take about an hour to set up. But they're an affordable pop-up option and produce an unexpectedly good steam.

YURT

Because the yurt sauna is circular and dome-shaped, it comes with a stove in the middle so that the steam rises and falls in a spiral, creating a gentle undulating heat that typically sits at an easy 70°C. Some have a transparent crown that lets light in, while others are dark inside. Its canvas façade means weather conditions affect the temperature, but if there's no wind or rain and plenty of steam, it can reach 100°C. Red Kite Yurts in Scotland make yurts and yurt saunas based on Turkic styles from Uzbekistan, Kazakhstan and Tajikistan. They come with bentwood frames in larch, pine, American white oak and Scottish ash, and the largest seats eight.

HORSEBOX

The horsebox sauna is a quintessentially British concept, and one that has come to symbolize the wild sauna movement. Quirky, creative and resourceful, the idea of turning horseboxes into saunas really took off during lockdown, when a generation of 'saunapreneurs' was born. Innovative design ideas abound, from built-in speakers to cool paintwork and logos, and a delightful mix of woods. Benches, windows, doors and stoves vary hugely and are a testament to what can be done with a small space. And, of course, they are easy to tow, have a ready-made ramp and are low to the ground, making them a very accessible mobile option.

BARREL

Shaped like a barrel, this is affordable, simple and easy to assemble. Many are imported from Latvia and Lithuania and are made with wood that has been thermally treated to remove moisture, resin and bacteria and topped with an asphalt-tiled roof. Benches come with back support and typically hold four to eight bathers, and there's a window at one end. A wood-fired stove is fed from either inside or out, and better versions have a small ante-room that acts as a thermal gate and offers a space to shelter or change.

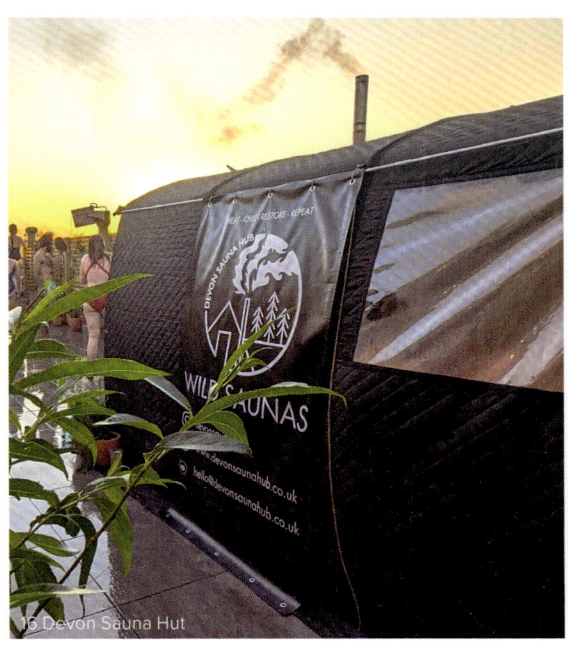

16 Devon Sauna Hut

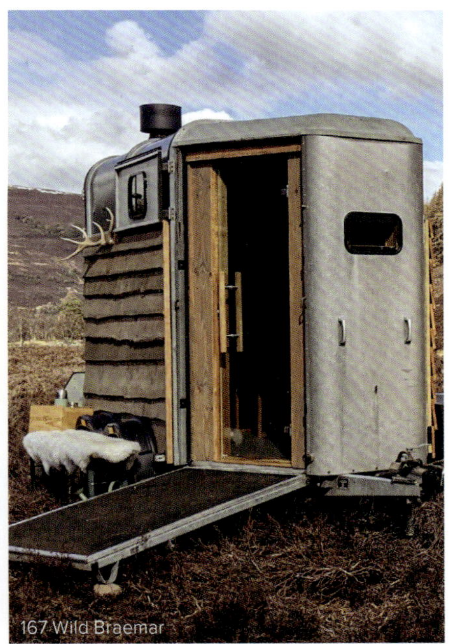
167 Wild Braemar

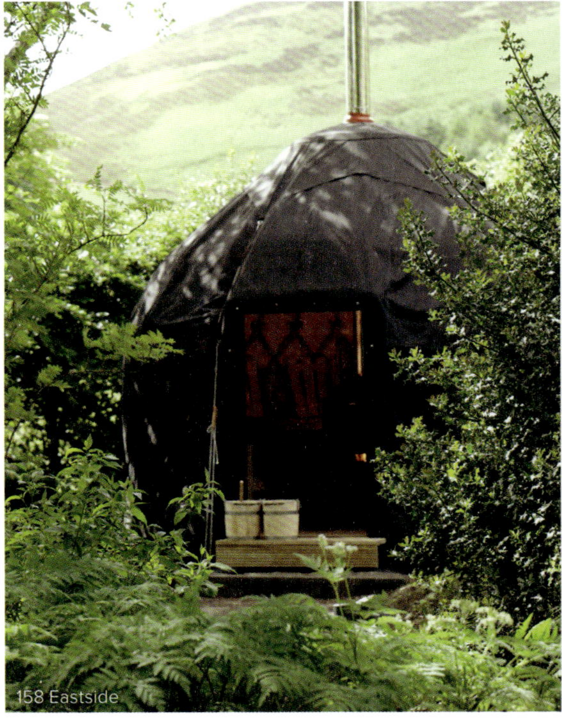
158 Eastside

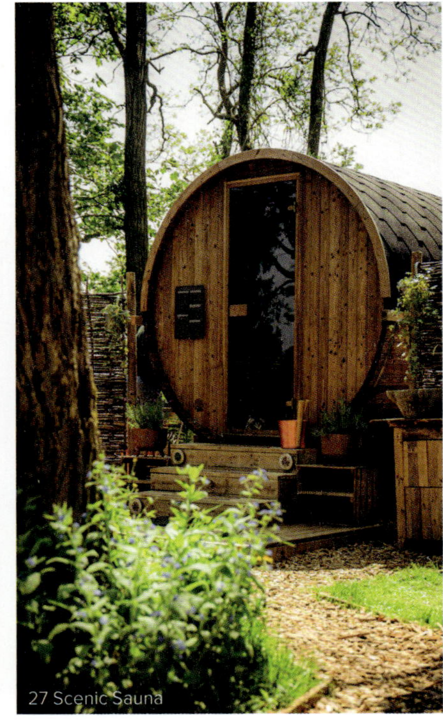
27 Scenic Sauna

FLOATING SAUNA

Erifting down a lake or a fjord with the sauna stove gently chuffing is the ultimate bathing adventure in Norway or Finland, and the UK has joined in. Revive Wild sauna in Portland Marina, Slomo at Tapnell Farm on the Isle of Wight, and Wyld, a 24-person floating sauna in Liverpool's Princes Dock have set sail, and more will surely follow.

SMOKE SAUNA

Pitch black and sooty, with a tiny window and no chimney, the smoke sauna sits somewhere between a sweat lodge and a regular sauna. It takes many hours to heat up and provides the gentlest of steam, which in the Baltics and Finland is loaded with spiritual and cultural significance. Before bathers enter, the smoke is let out, and a session typically lasts several hours, with food and drink enjoyed between rounds. In 2014, to honour an age-old, sacred tradition, UNESCO added Estonian smoke sauna culture to its List of Intangible Cultural Heritage. Most smoke saunas are found in the Võro region of the country, and it was here that the award-winning documentary *Smoke Sauna Sisterhood* was filmed. To date, there are only a couple of smoke saunas in the UK. Both are privately owned and invite-only, but such is the enthusiasm among sauna aficionados to try this deep, transformative experience that it won't be long before there are more.

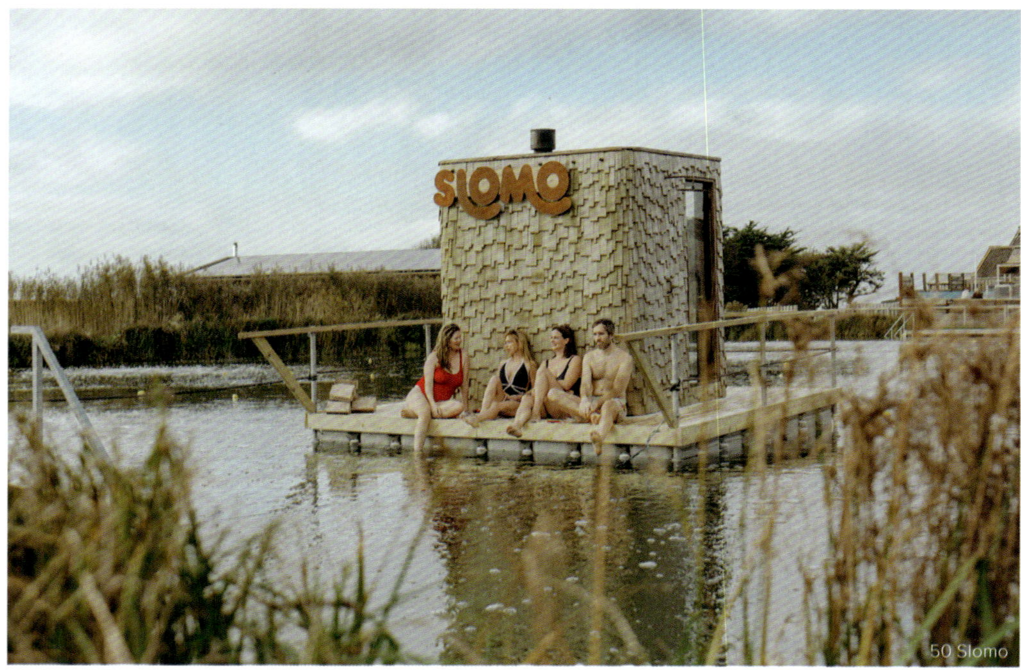

50 Slomo

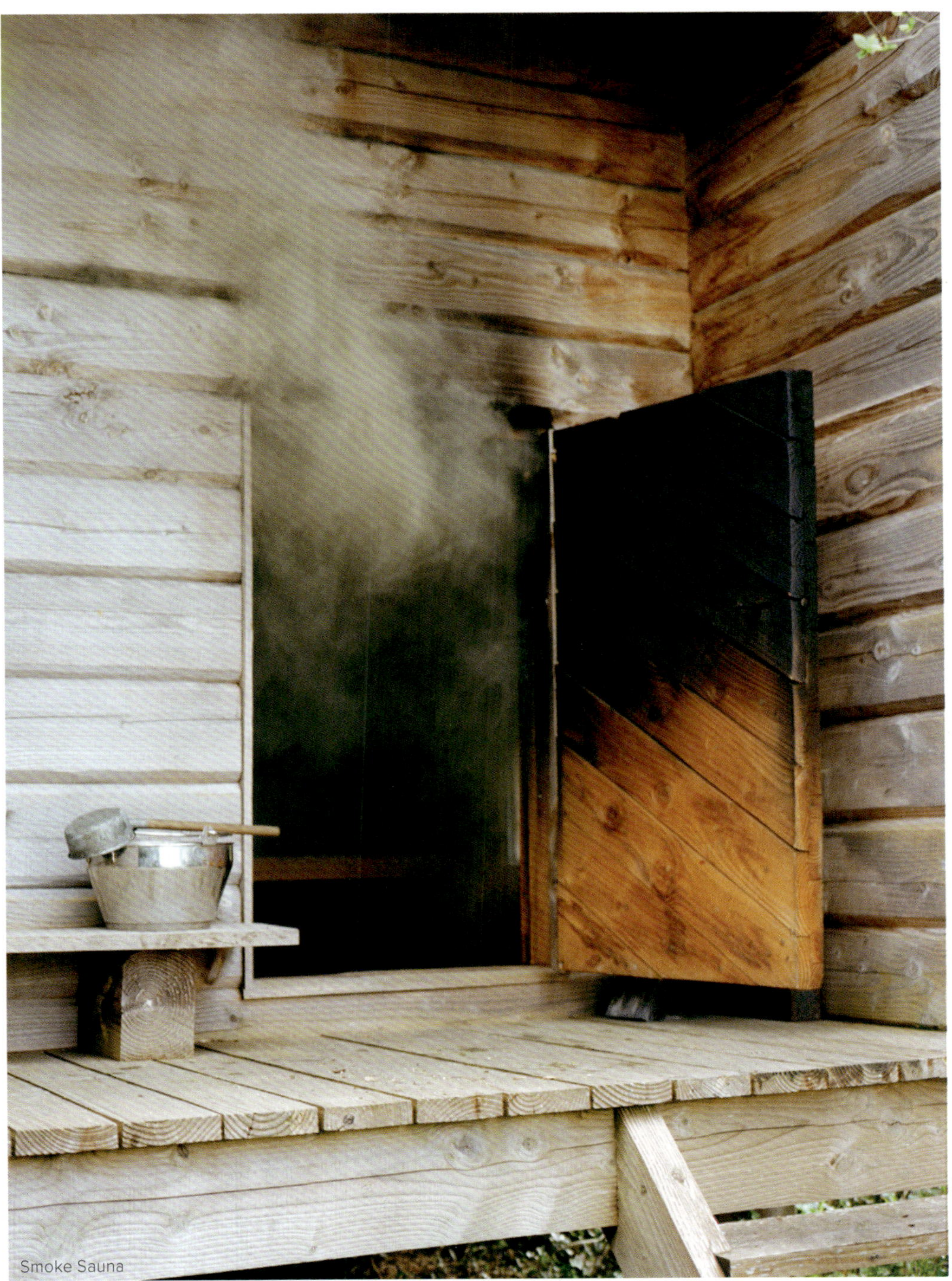
Smoke Sauna

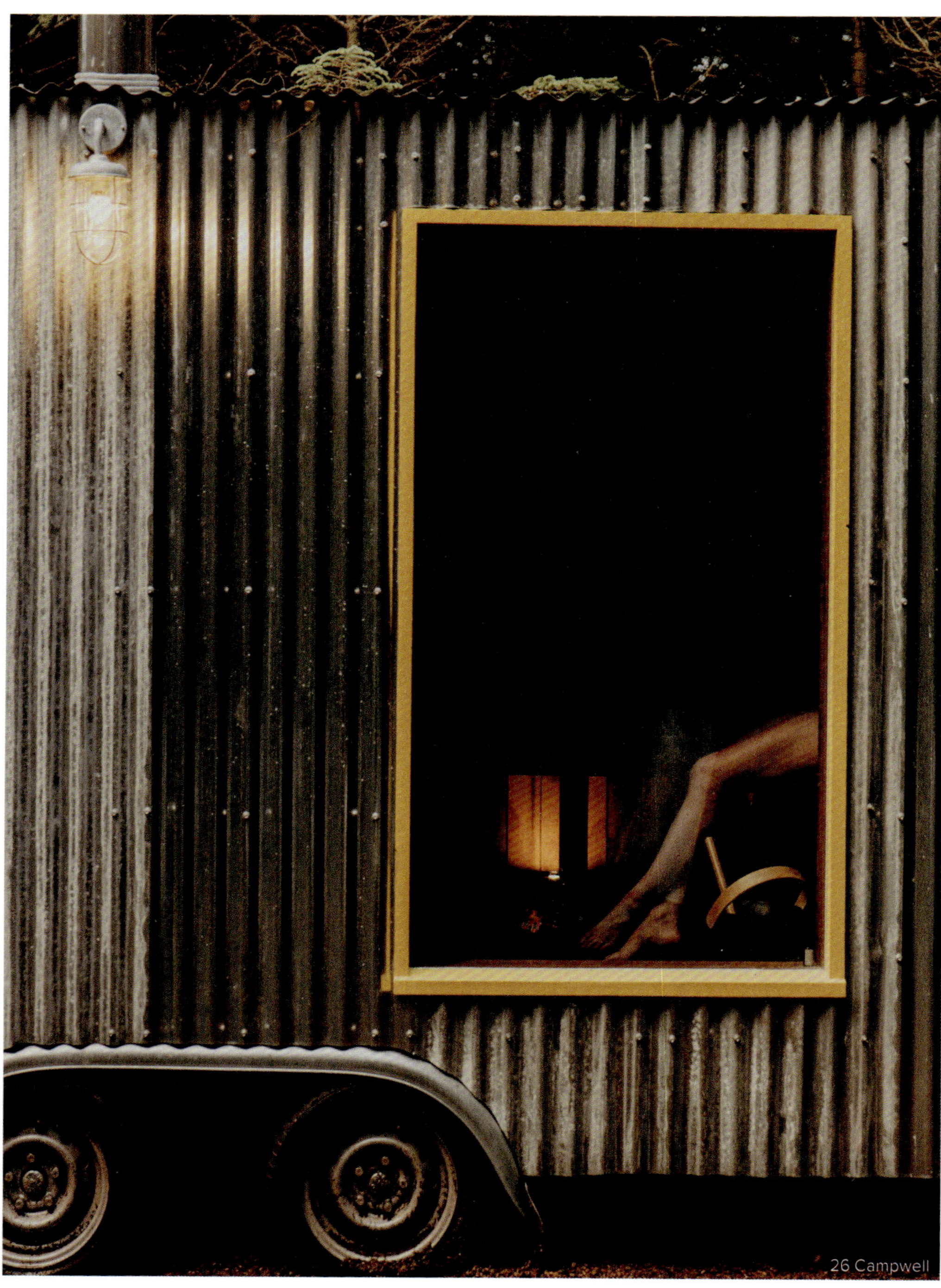

26 Campwell

EVENT SAUNA

Event saunas that seat up to 200 people are popular in the large spas of Europe, such as Thermen Bussloo in the Netherlands, Satama in Berlin and Therme in Bucharest. In the UK, Galgorm in Northern Ireland and Rudding Park in Yorkshire are among a handful of spas thinking big, but event saunas are on their way. First up is The Wildwood Spa in Cornwall which has a 30-seater sauna-in-the-round in the forest; open to the public and guests staying at the resort, it was built by local sauna makers Kernow Springs, who use it to host special events and rituals. ARC in London has an event sauna for 50+ people along with ice baths, and offers collective contrast therapy and *aufguss*.

TRAILER

Bigger than the barrel and the horsebox, the trailer sauna can hold up to around 20 people, making it a popular choice for operators with bigger audiences and builders who prefer to start from scratch. Many trailers have a minimal, clean-lined aesthetic that blends into the natural surroundings, and in certain sites, they are robust, semi-permanent structures that have been built onto a trailer largely to circumvent planning restrictions rather than because they are going anywhere.

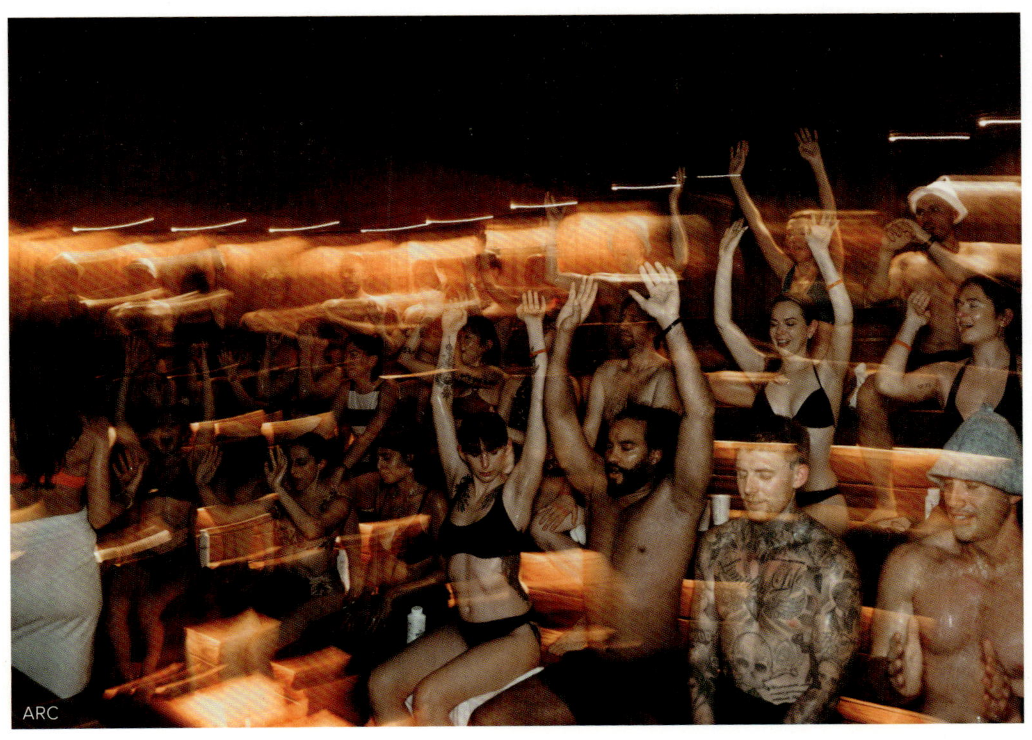

ARC

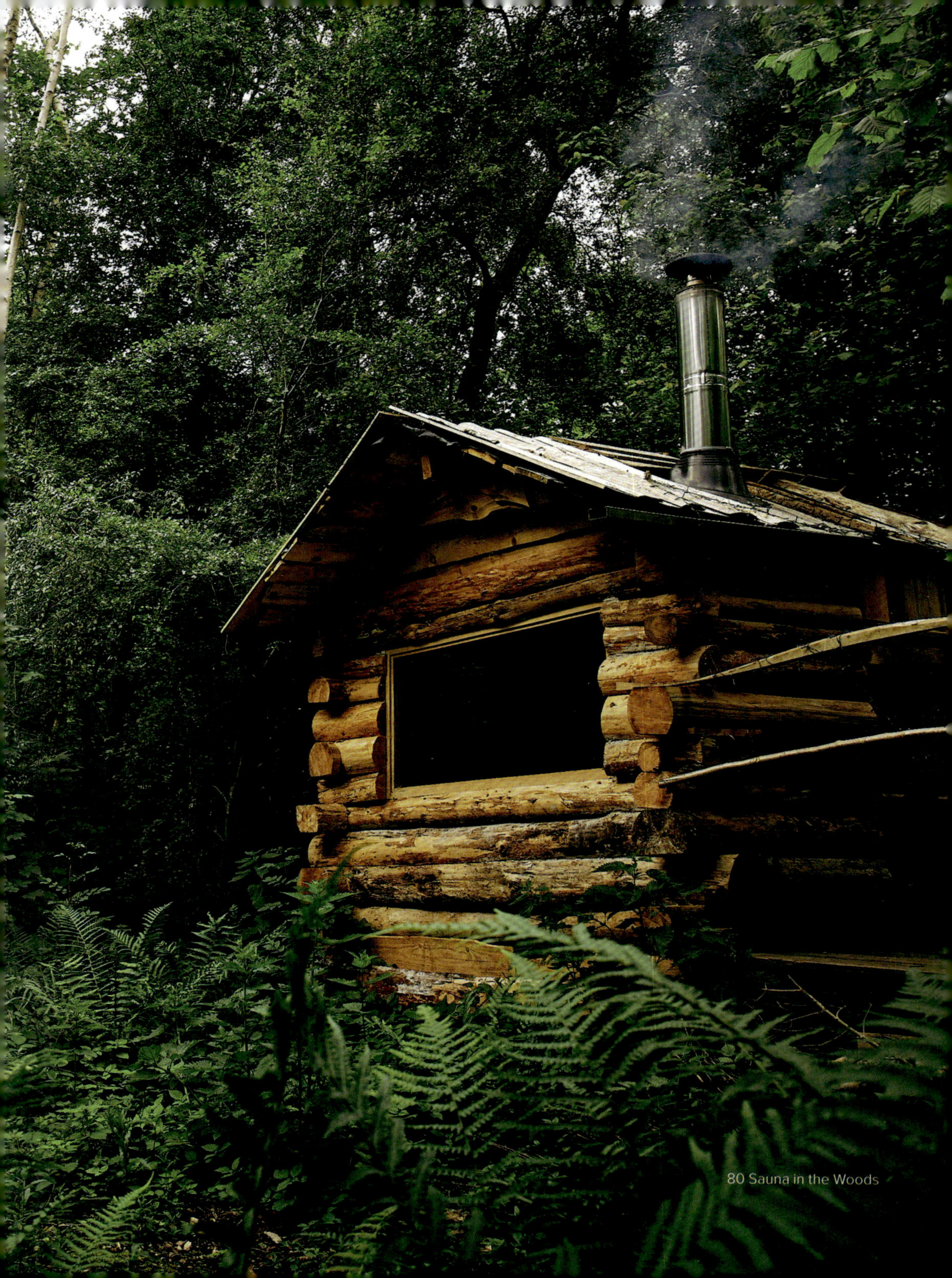

80 Sauna in the Woods

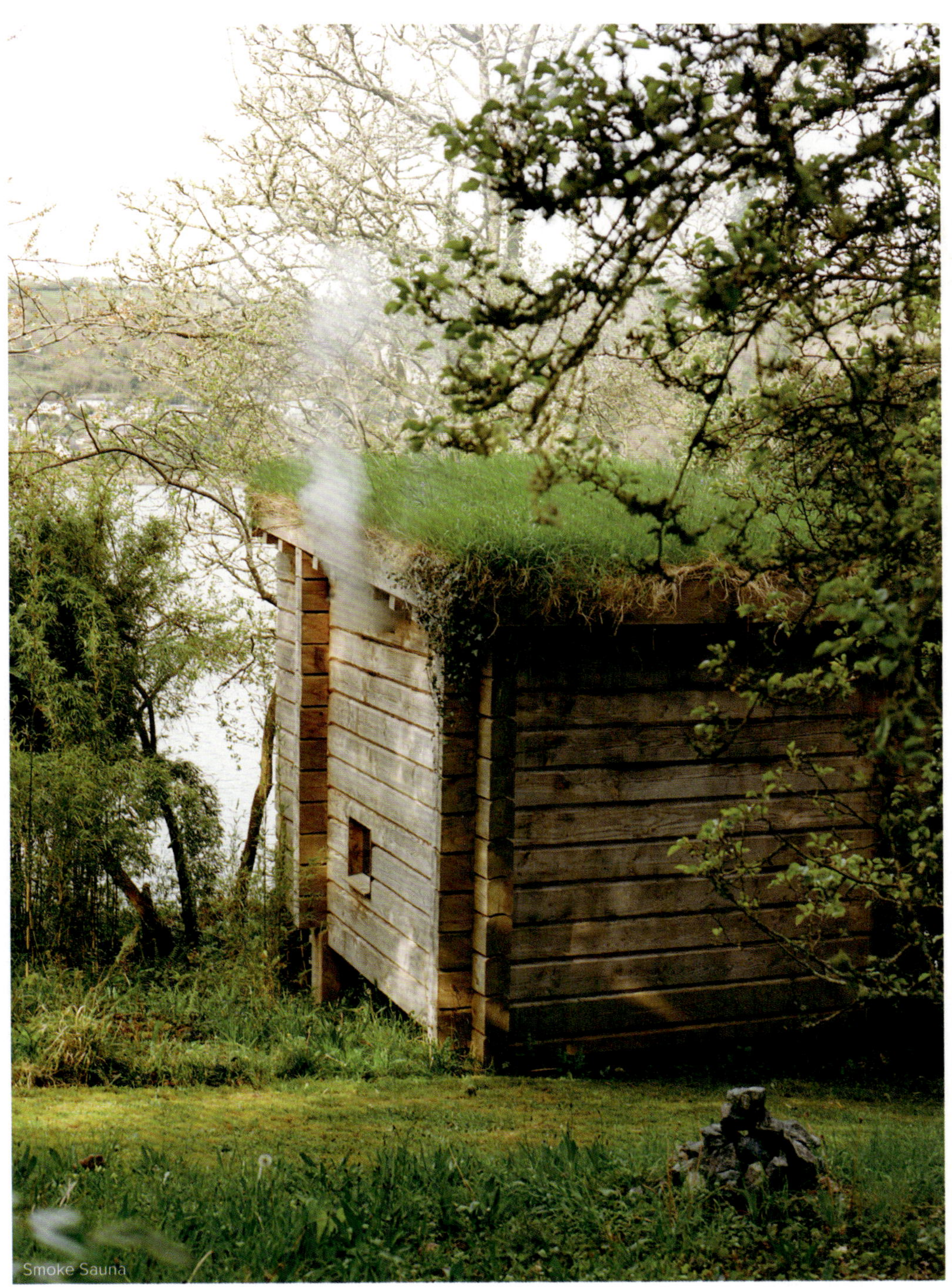
Smoke Sauna

Sauna shack

DESIGN AND BUILD YOUR OWN SAUNA

I've been fortunate enough to experience many incredible saunas, some built by ingenious enthusiasts, but I have increasingly wondered how do you build your own? And what makes a good sauna? I'm rubbish at DIY, and our small London garden offers no space to play. I had no idea how or where to start building a sauna, so it was serendipitous that an opportunity fell into our laps. My husband's old schoolfriend Murray was struggling with bouts of depression, and we knew from our own experience that contrast therapy could help him. He had also built a garden shack at the bottom of his Somerset garden, which was hardly used and housed little more than a broken pinball machine. And so, with only a little persuasion, the Sauna Shack project was born in early 2024. The goal? To convert Murray's 2-metre by 4-metre shed into a sauna before the next long winter when the inevitable mood swings would set in. Despite the shack's tricky trapezium shape, sloping sedum roof, and central door, measuring up and drawing the optimal way to divide the space into a three or four-person sauna with a separate changing room was actually simple and quickly agreed upon. Still, we called on our friends at Finnmark (finnmarksauna.com) to advise on the design and build details and to supply everything that was going to be needed.

So, what are the sauna essentials? Converted horseboxes, bespoke trailers, caravans and barrel saunas are all popular in the UK and have proven that almost anything can be turned into some sort of sweat box. But what they are made from does affect the quality of both the experience and their longevity. Softwoods are often used on the exterior because they withstand the British wet weather; for instance, in Scotland, larch is plentiful, durable and a popular choice. Then, on to insulation and the vapour barrier. In lieu of natural sheep's wool, Finnmark supplied specialist aluminium-backed insulation boards. These were easily cut to size and packed between the structural stud timbers. We then sealed the joints, corners, edges and door frame with aluminium foil tape and cut a couple of 12.5cm ventilation holes through the entire structure. These were ducted and sealed again with aluminium tape before attractive wooden covers were attached. The internal alder cladding was simple to install over all of this, and voilà – or siella, as they say in Finland – we had a sauna room.

For benches and wall panelling, hardwoods such as alder and aspen are ideal as they are porous and sap-free (nobody wants their hair glued to the back wall or roof). Cedar, with its spicy aroma, works well, while anything that warps or drips resin is a no-go. The boys chose specialist alder for its beautiful honey-coloured finish and reasonable cost. The sauna experience is also determined by where you sit, and benches should be at the optimal, or 'correct,' height. In general, this means that ideally, those on the top bench should have their feet level with or above the top of the stove. Other things to think through include a safety rail around the heater, adequate drainage for water and steam, lighting (we used a simple off-the-shelf LED kit), and the right stove or heater. The UK imports most of its stoves from Finland and Estonia, with Huum, Harvia, IKI, and Narvi being popular choices offering both wood-burning and electric solutions. We chose a Kota Kuru wood burner, which seemed perfect for the compact space. The debate about which is better – wood or electric – rages on, and while a crackling wood fire with a smoky smell is always pleasant, the Finnish saying 'the rocks don't know what's heating them' comes quickly to mind. Either way, the sauna stones do need to be the same size and should be stacked carefully so that steam can pass through them smoothly and the electrical elements are not on view. Given the wonky-walled original shack, the complex benches were made to order off-site at the Finnmark workshop. Nevertheless, the team did the whole thing for around £5,000. There were some minor bungles along the way; Murray managed to install the alder cladding inside out on the ceiling before being informed. 'Who knew that?' he protested. And without the help of Gwynn, the carpenter next door, the boys would have struggled to get the door in. Luckily, Max Newport, Finnmark's co-founder, was on hand for panicky video calls throughout the job and gave up a weekend onsite to cut a hole in the roof and install the heater (be warned – this is by far the most difficult moment of alignment). Without his help, there would have been many more mishaps, maybe a lost finger or two, and the boys would definitely have run out of patience with each other. Forty years of friendship severely tested and in serious need of some sauna diplomacy! The project took about 100 hours in total. They finally installed the benches in October and immediately wanted to share Sauna Shack with friends, many of whom had thought the whole thing was daft and vowed they would never set foot in a sauna. But every sauna operator in the UK has heard that before and then seen 'hell yes!' moments unfold before them.

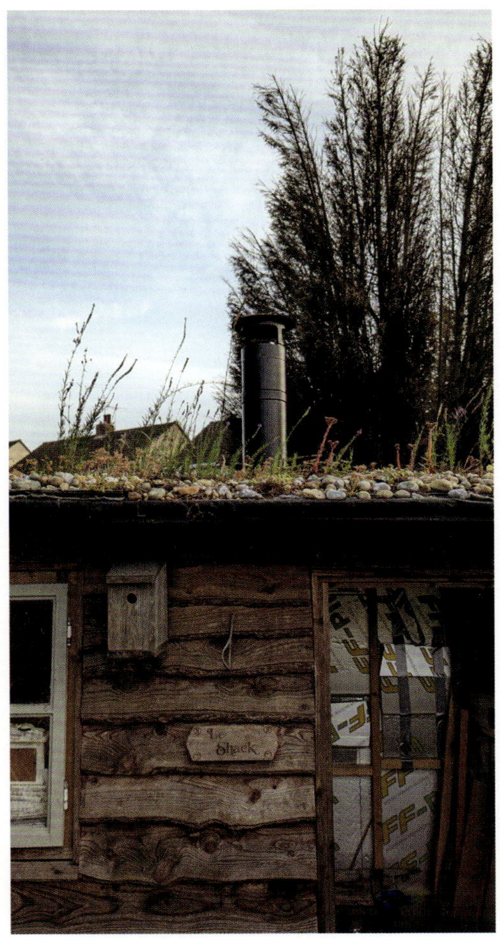

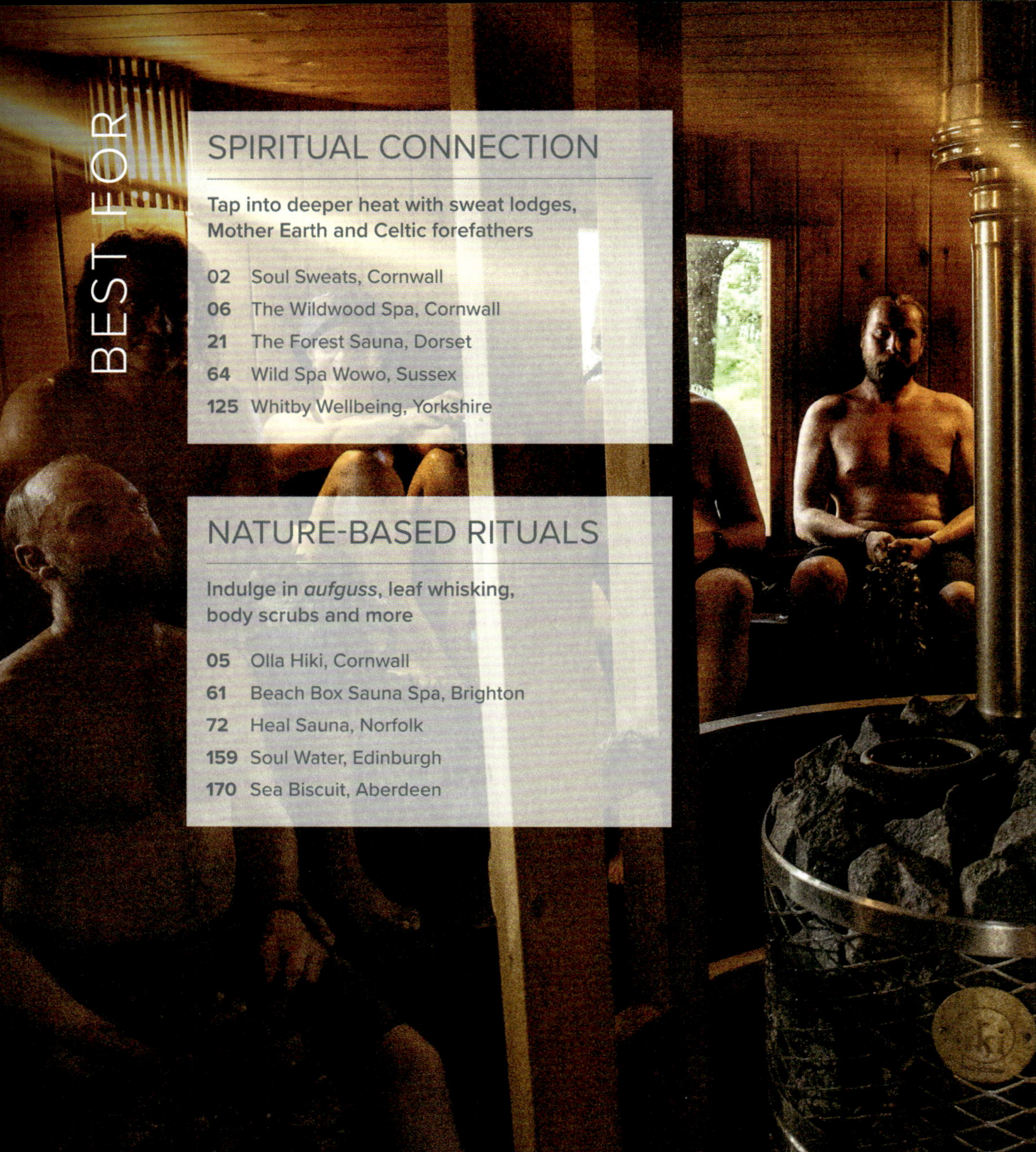

BEST FOR

SPIRITUAL CONNECTION

Tap into deeper heat with sweat lodges, Mother Earth and Celtic forefathers

02 Soul Sweats, Cornwall
06 The Wildwood Spa, Cornwall
21 The Forest Sauna, Dorset
64 Wild Spa Wowo, Sussex
125 Whitby Wellbeing, Yorkshire

NATURE-BASED RITUALS

Indulge in *aufguss*, leaf whisking, body scrubs and more

05 Olla Hiki, Cornwall
61 Beach Box Sauna Spa, Brighton
72 Heal Sauna, Norfolk
159 Soul Water, Edinburgh
170 Sea Biscuit, Aberdeen

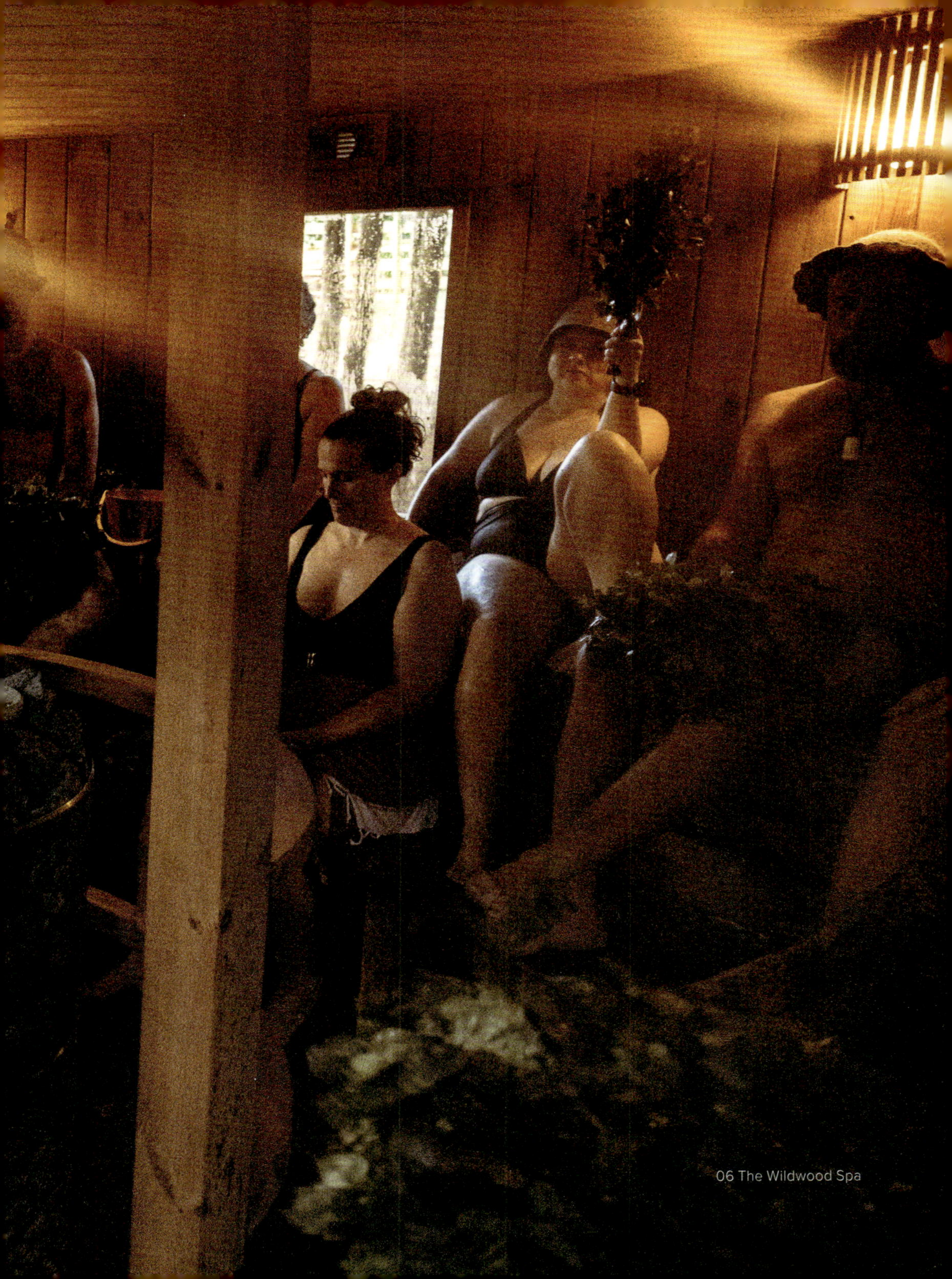

06 The Wildwood Spa

BEST FOR

OCEAN DIPS

Bob in the waves and gaze at horizons

09 Saunas by the Sea, Baby Bay Cornwall
29 Sauna Society, Jersey
77 Sea Scrub, Kent
129 Hotbox Benone, Londonderry
131 Kishtey Çheh, Isle of Man

REMOTE AND WILD

Switch off and sweat in the splendid isolation of nature's church

98 Wildwater, Pembrokeshire
103 Sawna Bach, Anglesey
150 Saltbox, Outer Hebrides
168 Watershed, Moray
171 Haar Sauna, Shetland

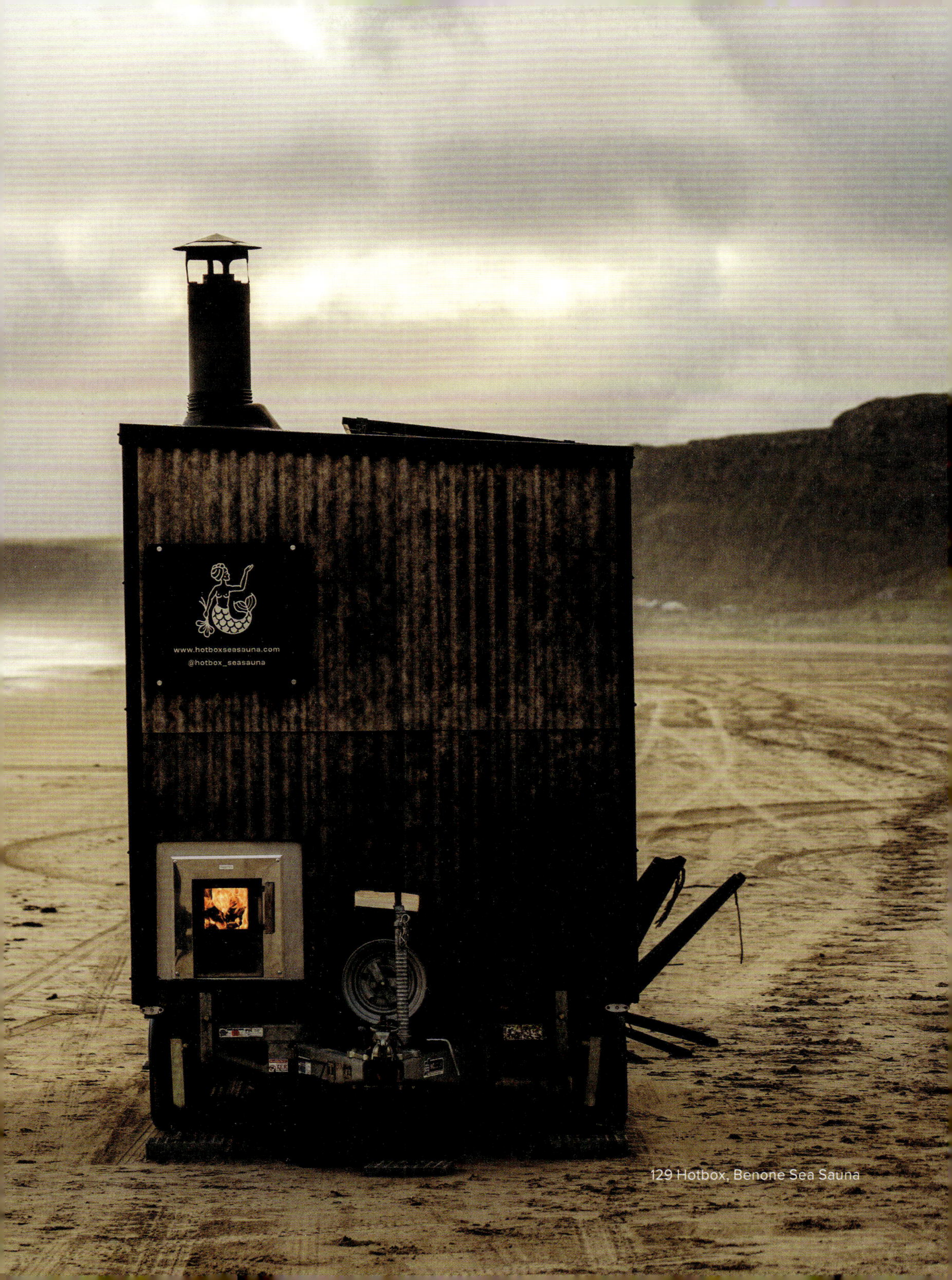

129 Hotbox, Benone Sea Sauna

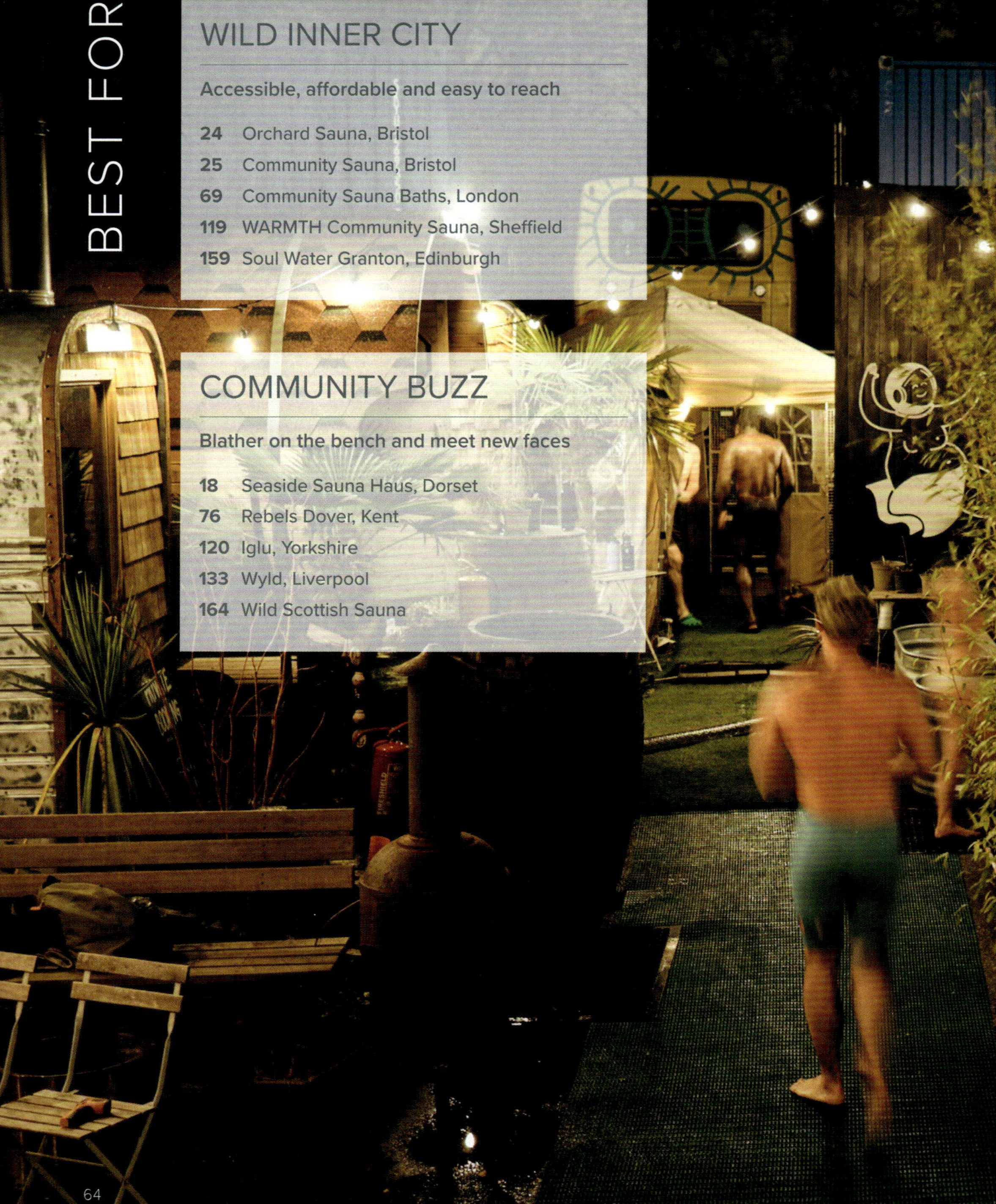

WILD INNER CITY

Accessible, affordable and easy to reach

24 Orchard Sauna, Bristol
25 Community Sauna, Bristol
69 Community Sauna Baths, London
119 WARMTH Community Sauna, Sheffield
159 Soul Water Granton, Edinburgh

COMMUNITY BUZZ

Blather on the bench and meet new faces

18 Seaside Sauna Haus, Dorset
76 Rebels Dover, Kent
120 Iglu, Yorkshire
133 Wyld, Liverpool
164 Wild Scottish Sauna

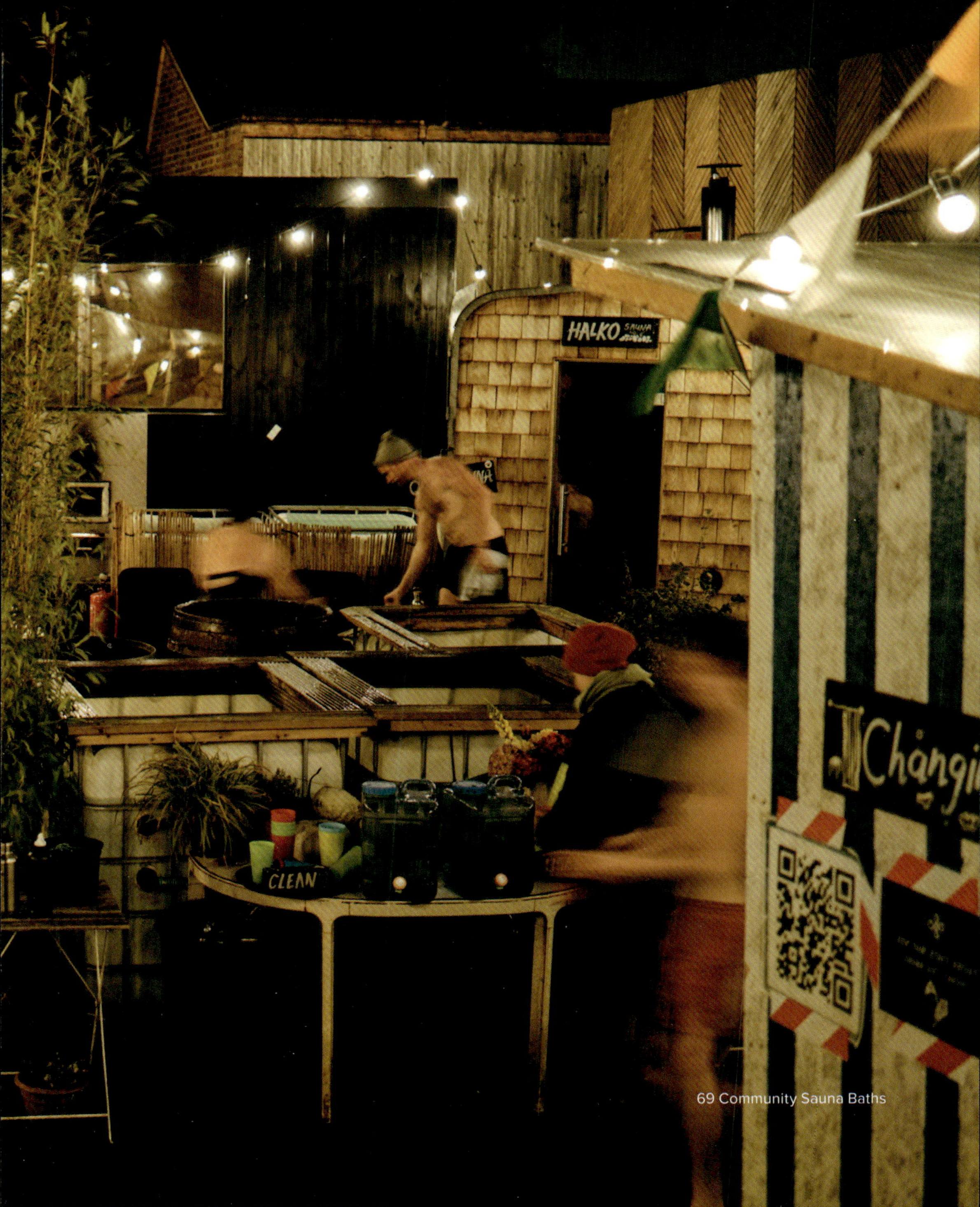
HALKO
CLEAN

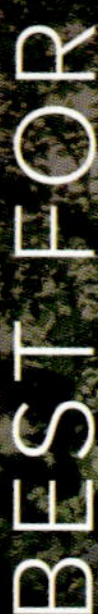

SAUNA RETREATS

Make a sauna weekend of it like the Scandinavians do

07 Steamy Wonders, Cornwall
55 The Wild Sauna, Oxfordshire
66 The Drying Shed, Sussex
79 Secret Sauna, Suffolk
104 Wern Derys, Hereford

FRESHWATER DIPS

Cool off in a river, stream, lake or pond

51 Tuhka Talo, Hampshire
122 Pool Bridge Farm, Yorkshire
126 La'al, Cumbria
127 Finn Lough, County Fermanagh
155 Hot Tottie Sauna, Argyll and Bute

DESIGN

Building a sauna offers a multitude of ways to get creative

15 The Somewhere Sauna, Devon
23 Saltwater Avon, Dorset
50 Slomo, Isle of Wight
57 The Nomadic Sauna, Sussex
127 Finn Lough, County Fermanagh

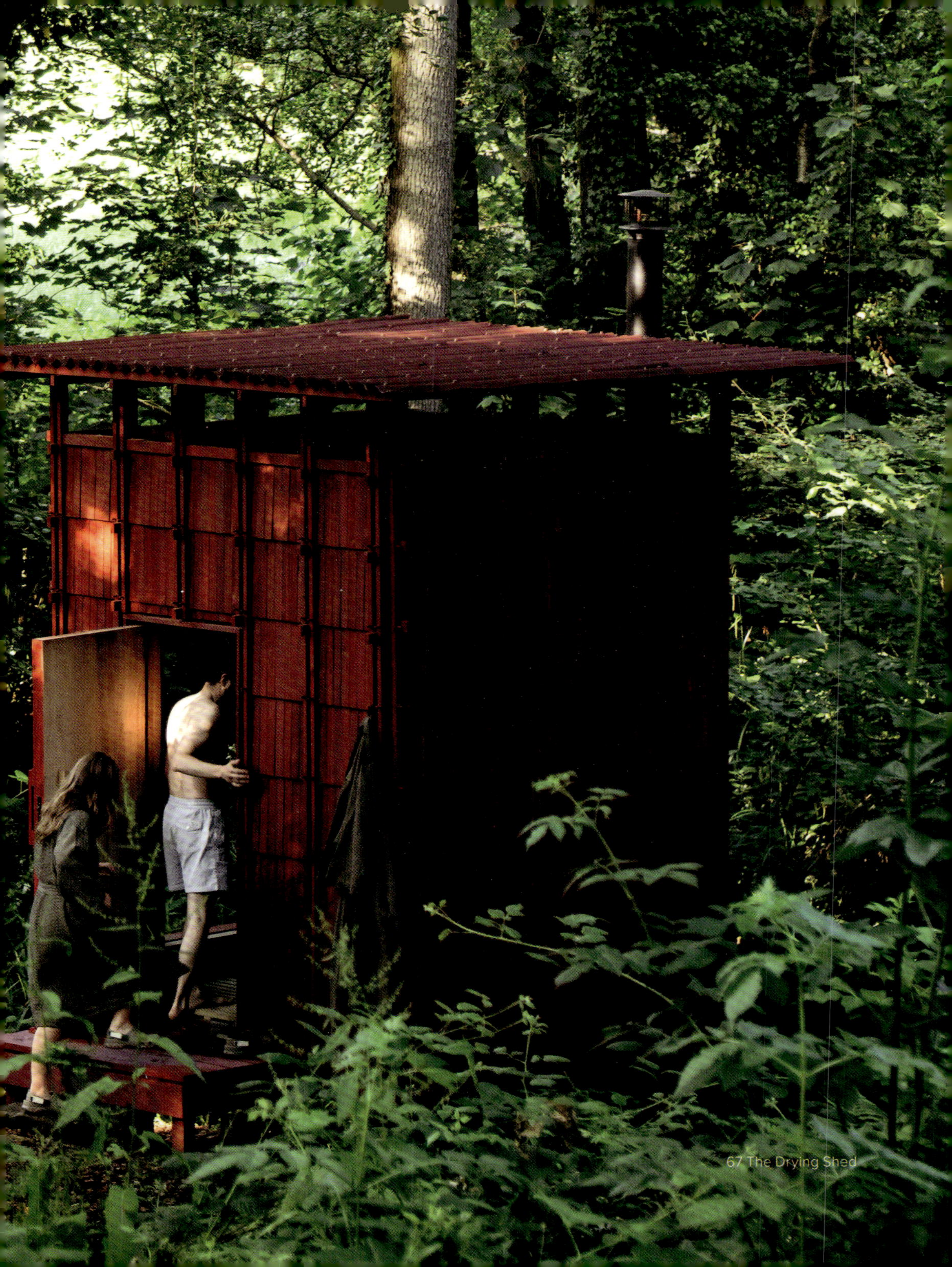

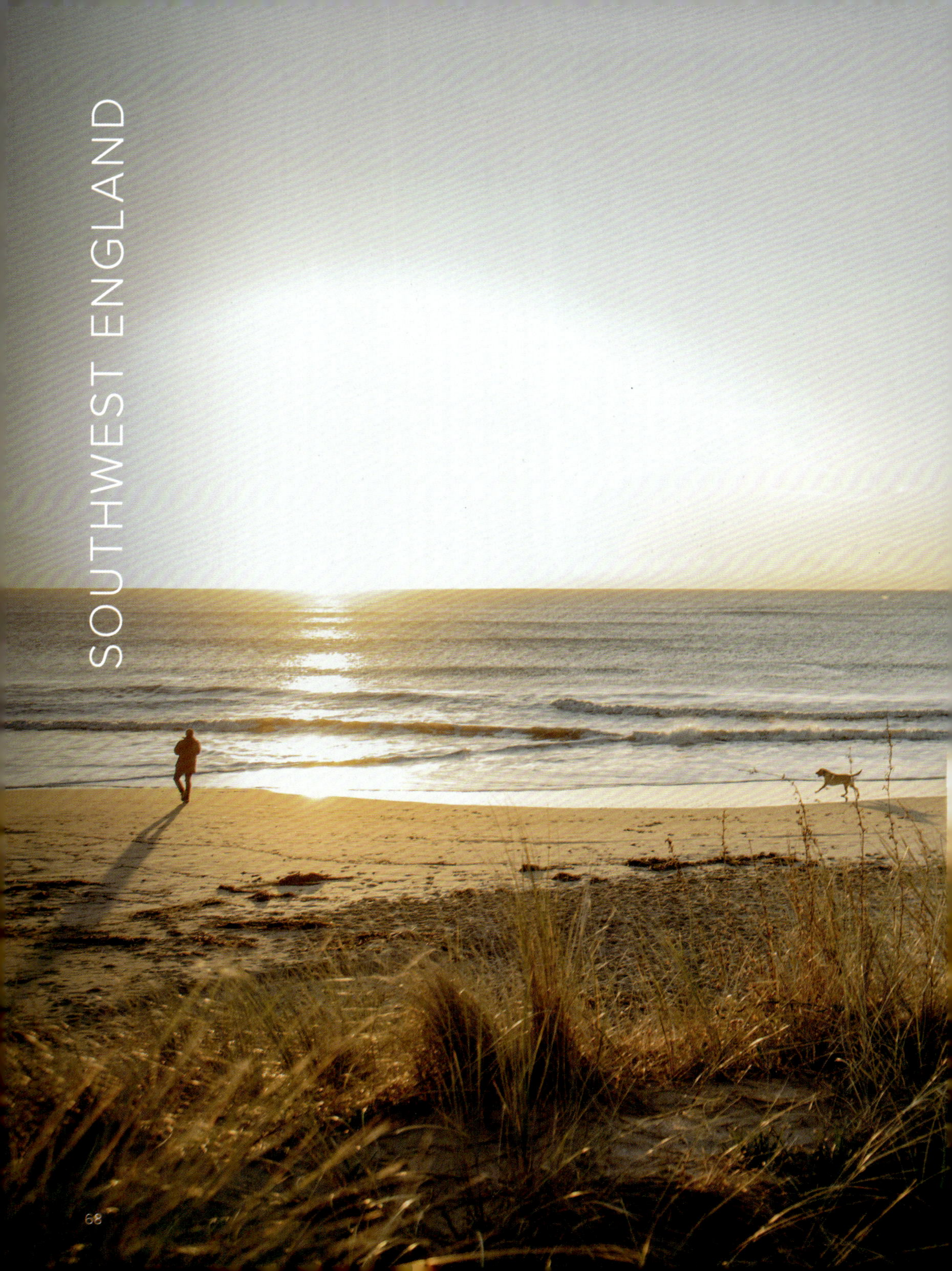

SOUTHWEST ENGLAND

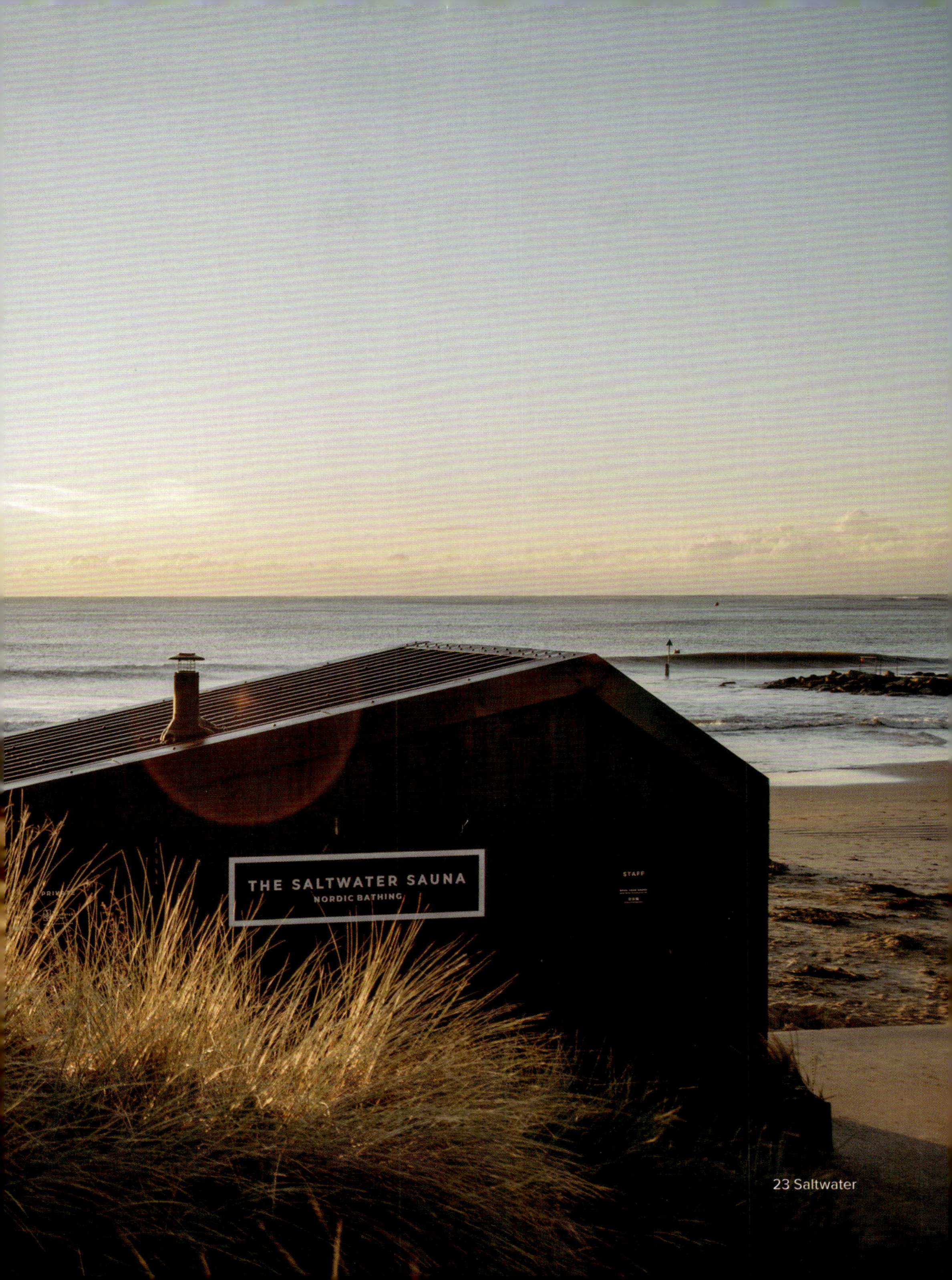
THE SALTWATER SAUNA
NORDIC BATHING
STAFF

01

Mor Holan Wild Spa

PORTHLEVEN ❦ CORNWALL

Mor Holan sauna, nestled into a Grade II listed, disused lime kiln above Porthleven, is a shining example of what can be done with a patch of scrappy land. Perched on a scaffold, under a limestone cliff teeming with birds, this six-seat sauna feels tucked away and private, while offering stunning views over the bustling harbour below. Cold dip tanks, a plunge bucket and warm showers are on offer for those who don't want to jump off the harbour wall at high tide – although this is highly recommended as the sea is deep, calm and clean.

Porthleven's harbour is privately owned, and Mor Holan is just the sort of young, quirky business that its owner encourages; all around the harbour's edge is an energetic buzz of people, bars and restaurants. Mor Holan's founder Simon Thomas welcomes locals and tourists, and works with local GPs to socially prescribe his sauna to their patients. Mor Holan means 'sea salt' in Cornish, and Morlanow ('high tide') is a mobile sister sauna that pops up at events all around west Cornwall

➔ Morholan.co.uk
❄ Sea/ice bath 📍 50.0838, -5.3173

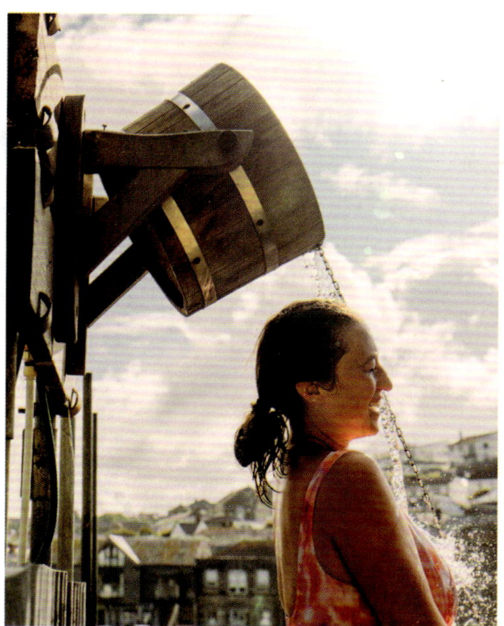

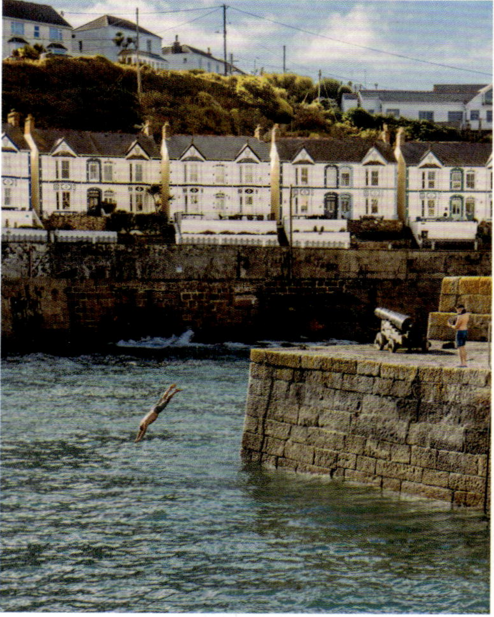

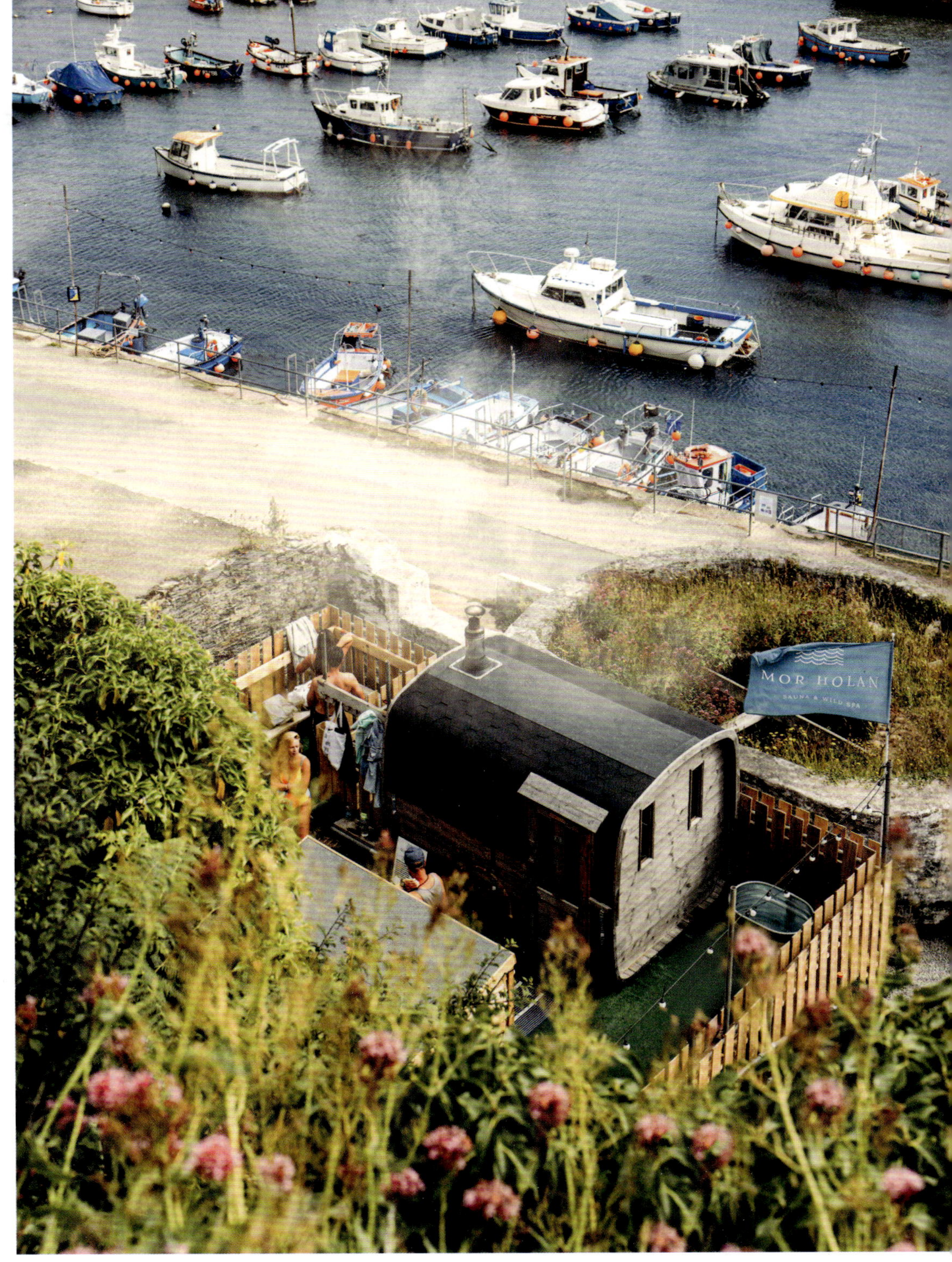
MOR HOLAN
SAUNA & WILD SPA

02

Soul Sweats

PORTHTOWAN ❦ CORNWALL

Some years ago, Sam Boot lived and surfed on the west coast of Canada, and this was where he started using tarpaulins to construct makeshift sweat boxes on the beach. Since 2018, Sam, an advanced Wim Hof instructor, and Jana a yoga teacher, have been connecting people to themselves in retreat venues across Cornwall. In 2024, their Wild Sauna and Holistic Health Hub opened at Mount Pleasant Eco Park near Porthtowan Beach. Two saunas, cold plunge baths and a geodome make up the space, and, inspired, by her German roots, Jana hosts weekly *Aufguss* and *Yin* yoga, while Sam's hot and cold therapy, breathwork and sound healing sessions draw people from all walks of life. Also on offer are weekly communal sauna and cold plunge sessions, workshops and retreats.

soulsweats.co.uk
Ice bath 50.2765, -5.2347

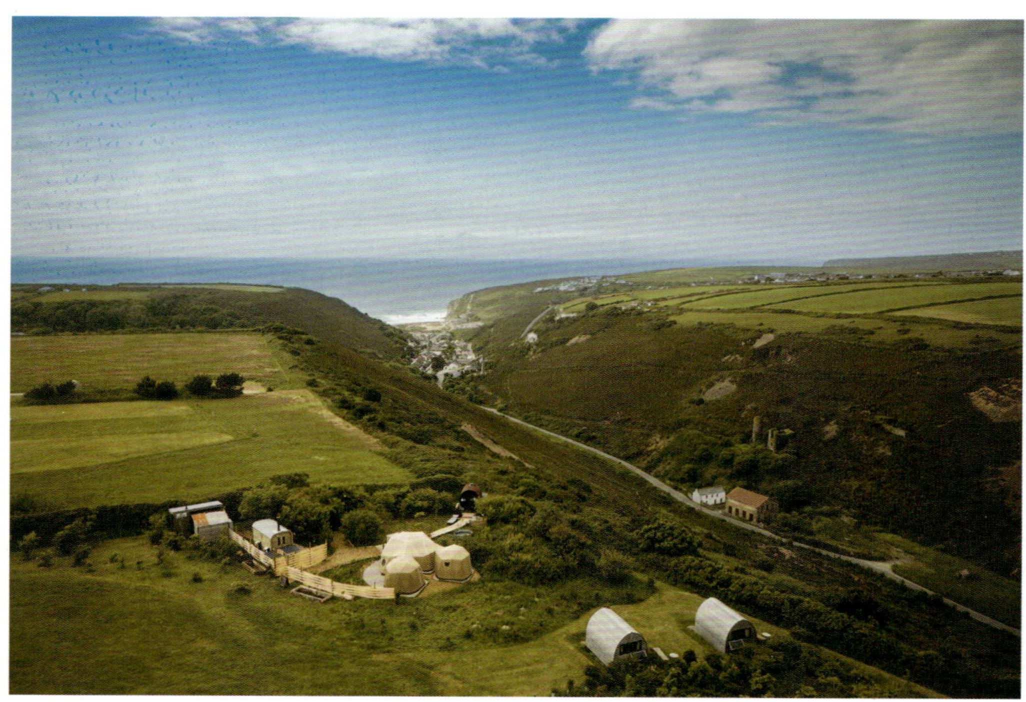

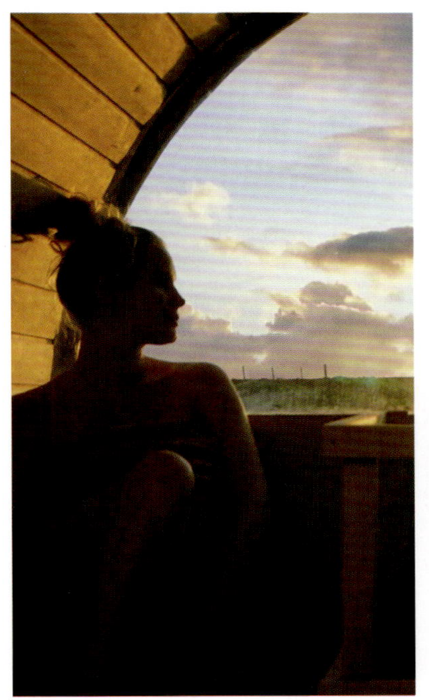

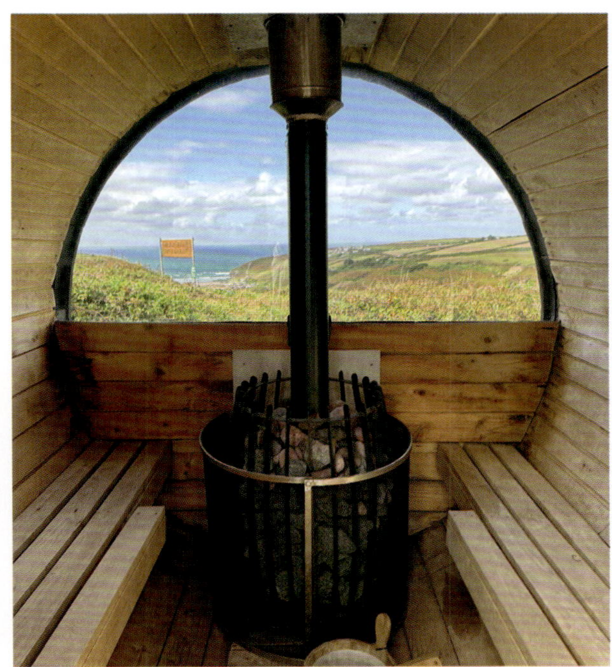

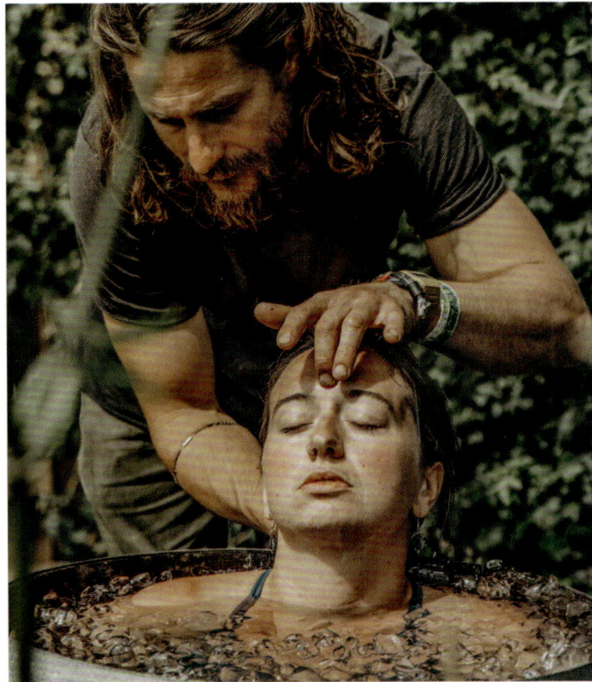

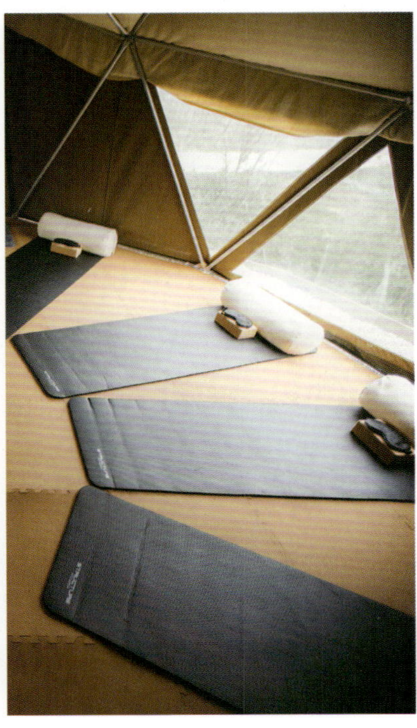

03

Kiln Sauna

FALMOUTH, MYLOR, HELFORD ❦ CORNWALL

Kiln sauna occupies a picturesque corner of Gyllyngvase beach (Gylly to locals), one of Falmouth's white sand, crystal-blue water jewels. It's a tranquil swimming spot at sunrise, and a gathering place by night – as such, Kiln caters to a mixed crowd of all ages. This is also one of the few saunas in the UK that allows children to enter. This, in part, is due to owner Kathryn Tyler's sauna experience as a child. 'I was in Sweden and got stung all over by horseflies. The adults coated me in honey and took me to the sauna.' It worked as a cure. In Scandinavia, honey and children are both commonplace in the steam. Attracting young bathers is something Kathryn wants to encourage at Kiln, so parents (like herself) and their families can enjoy a sauna session together.

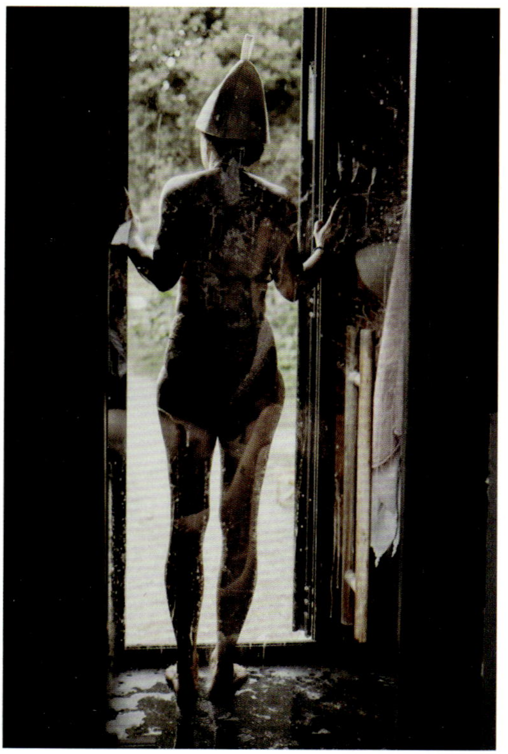

Kathryn is a known figure on Gylly, having designed the award-winning Beach Café in 2005. Even so, it still took six years to get permission for their elegant black sauna to get its spot. The second Kiln Sauna will appear in early 2025, touring the Ferryboat Inn on the Helford Passage, Kiln Quay at Flushing Beach, and spending summers on the Carrick Roads at Coastland campsite in Mylor Churchtown.

The name 'Kiln' is a nod to Cornwall's limeburning heritage of the 18th and 19th centuries, and ancient kilns dot the coast and tidal rivers. (It felt poetic that Kiln was first launched at Kiln Quay, Flushing.) But there's a cultural backstory to kilns and sweat bathing too. In Japan, *kama-buro* is a steam sauna in an earthen kiln used to cure various ailments, and in South Korea, *hanjeungmak* are charcoal kilns used after hours as sweat houses by local villagers as they cool down.

➔ kilnsauna.com ❄ Sea
50.1763, -5.0480 Coastland, Mylor,
50.1435, -5.0691 Gylly Beach, Falmouth
50.1624, -5.0598 Kiln Quay, Flushing
50.1004 ,-5.1287 Helford Passage

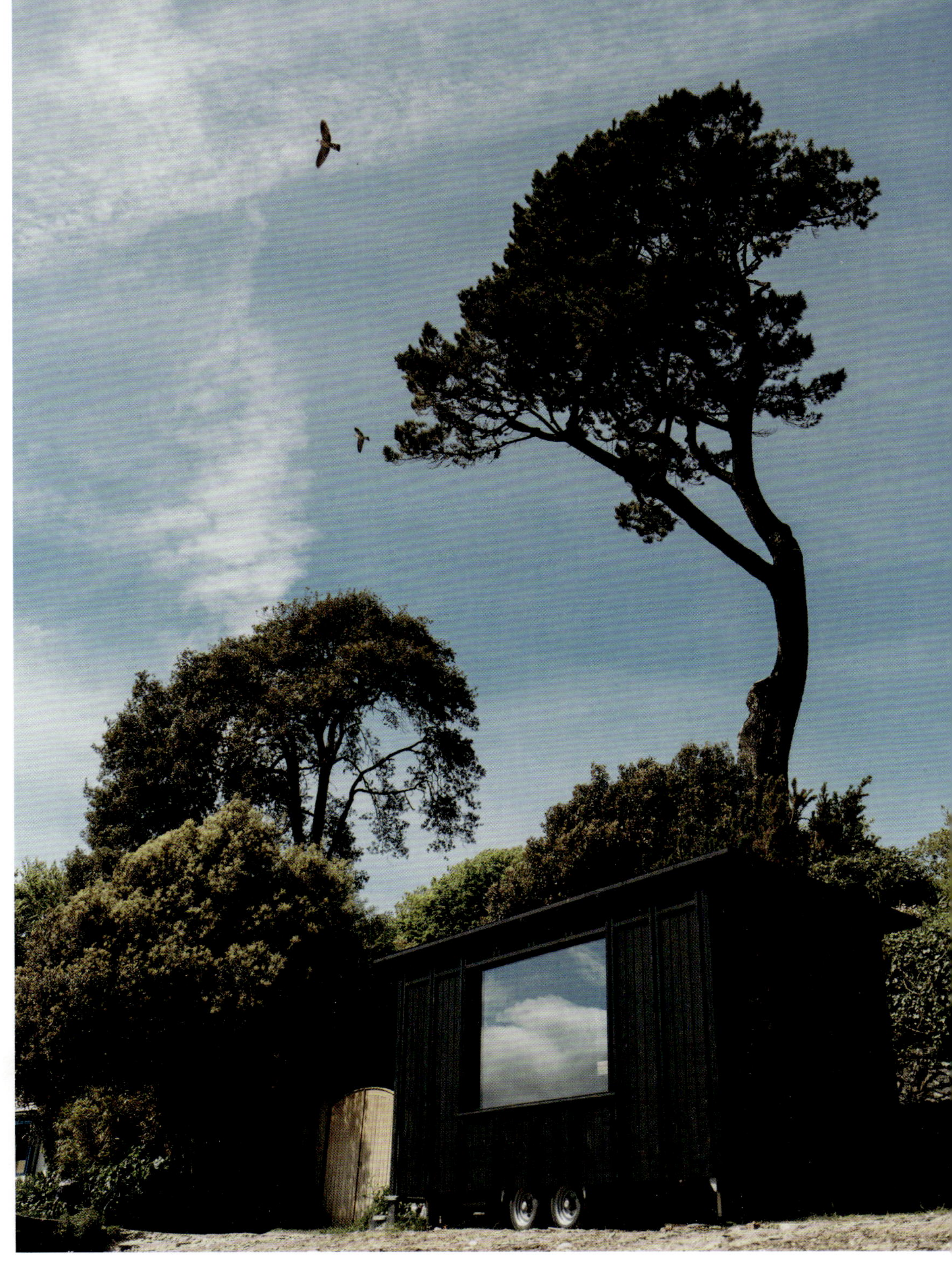

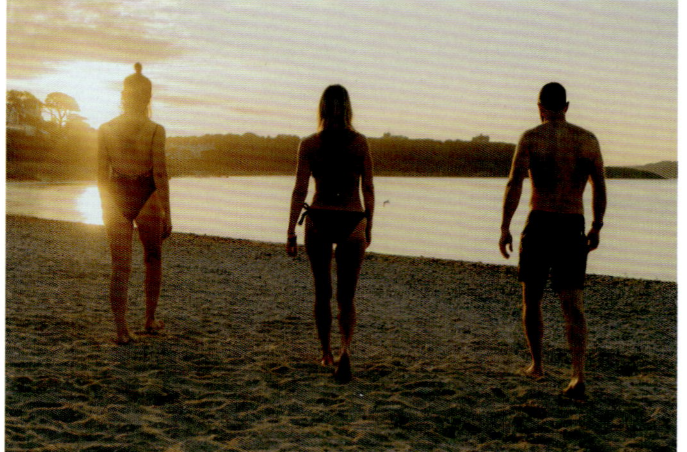

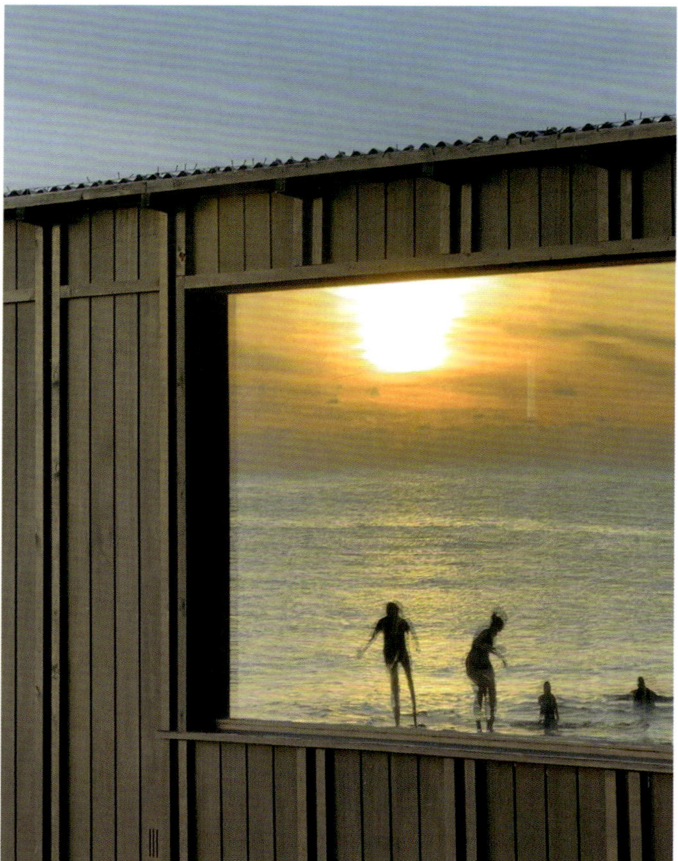

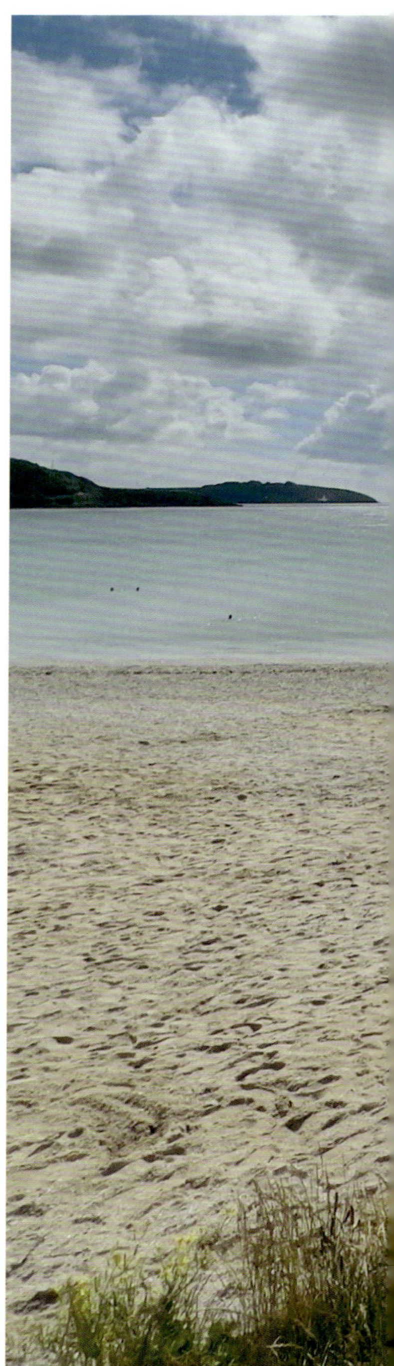

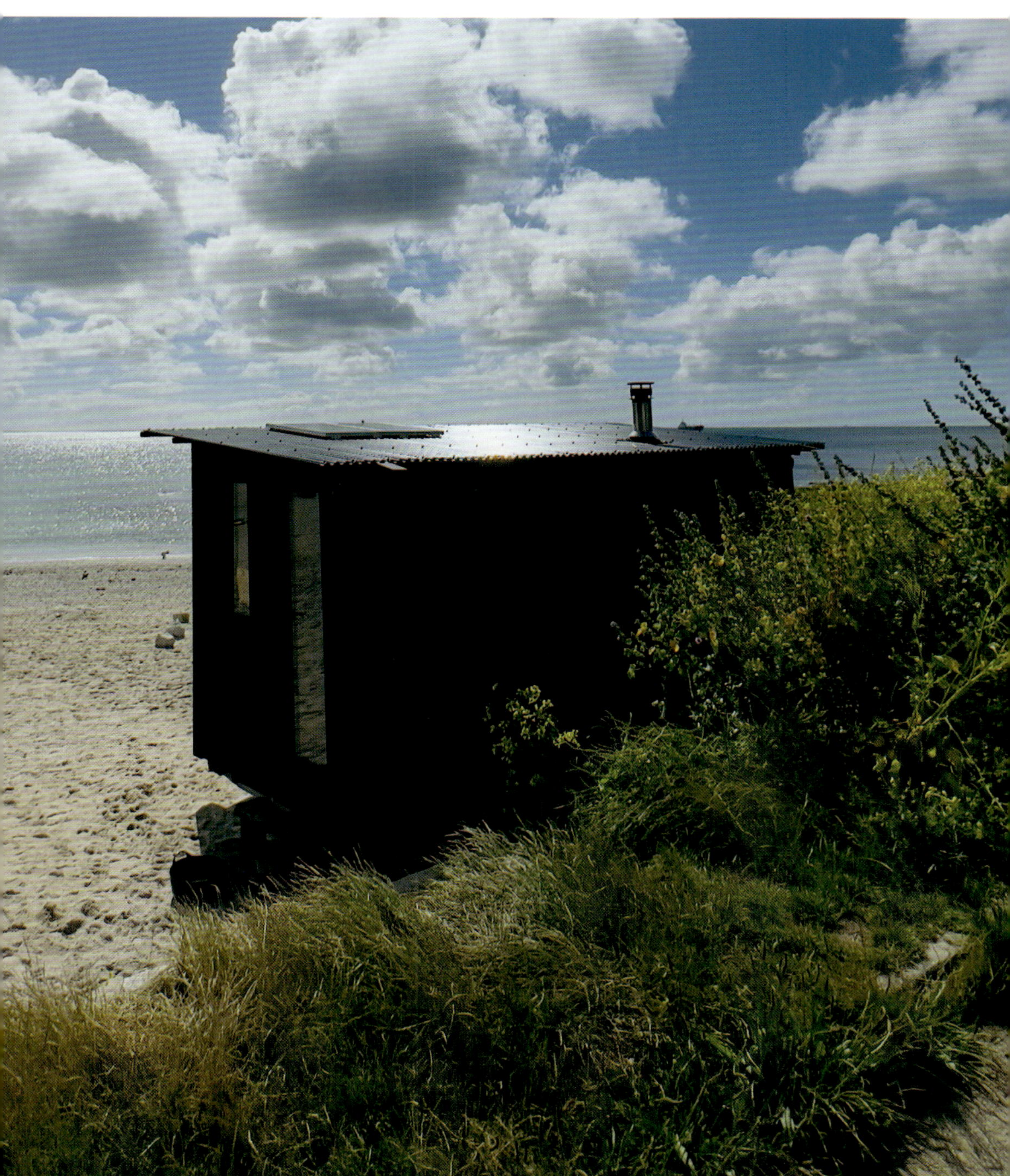

Kiln Sauna

04

Saunassa

NEWQUAY ❦ CORNWALL

Saunassa Nordic Spa is an urban contrast therapy centre tucked behind Newquay's busiest thoroughfare. It was co-founded by local lifeboat crew and lifeguard Zoey Cotton, who returned home to Cornwall after ten years working in hospitality in Canada, and carpenter Derry Smith. The venue offers a 12-person sauna, three ice baths, wood-fired hot tubs and hot showers. It also runs a programme of events and rituals. Zoey and Derry know that contrast therapy and the impact and simplicity of putting the phone away and meeting new people can improve our mental health. To this end, the spa is dedicated to its community and works with many local charities.

saunassa.co.uk

Ice bath 50.4133, -5.0756

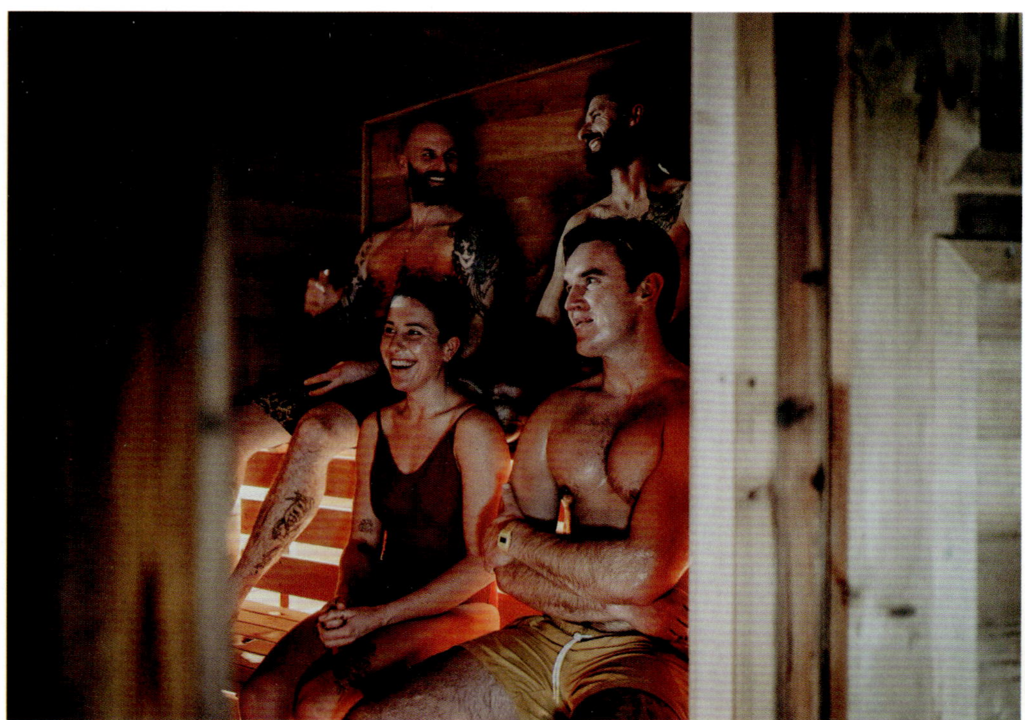

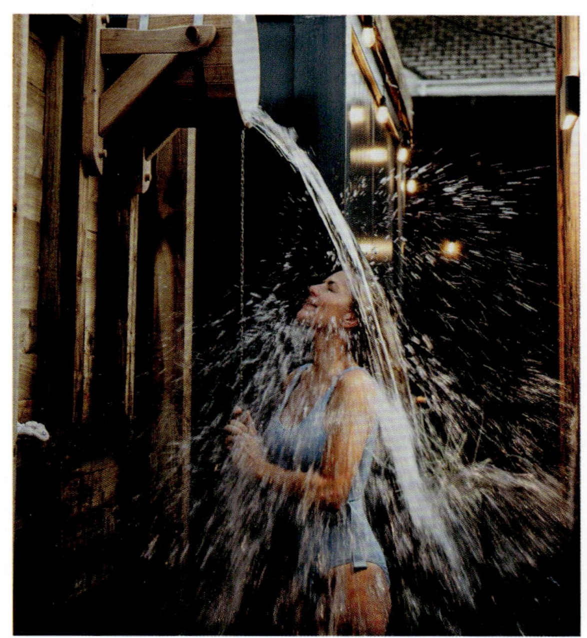

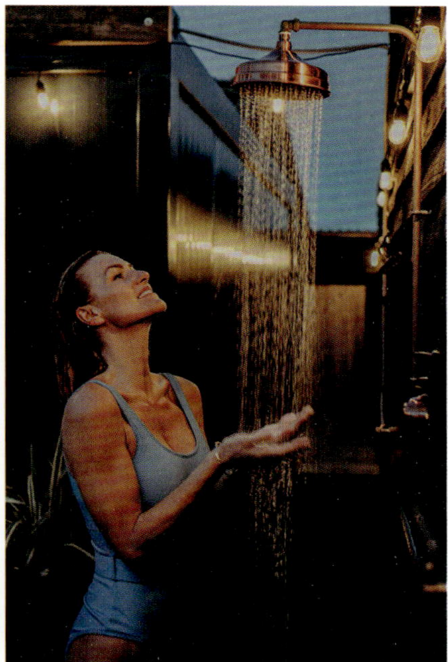

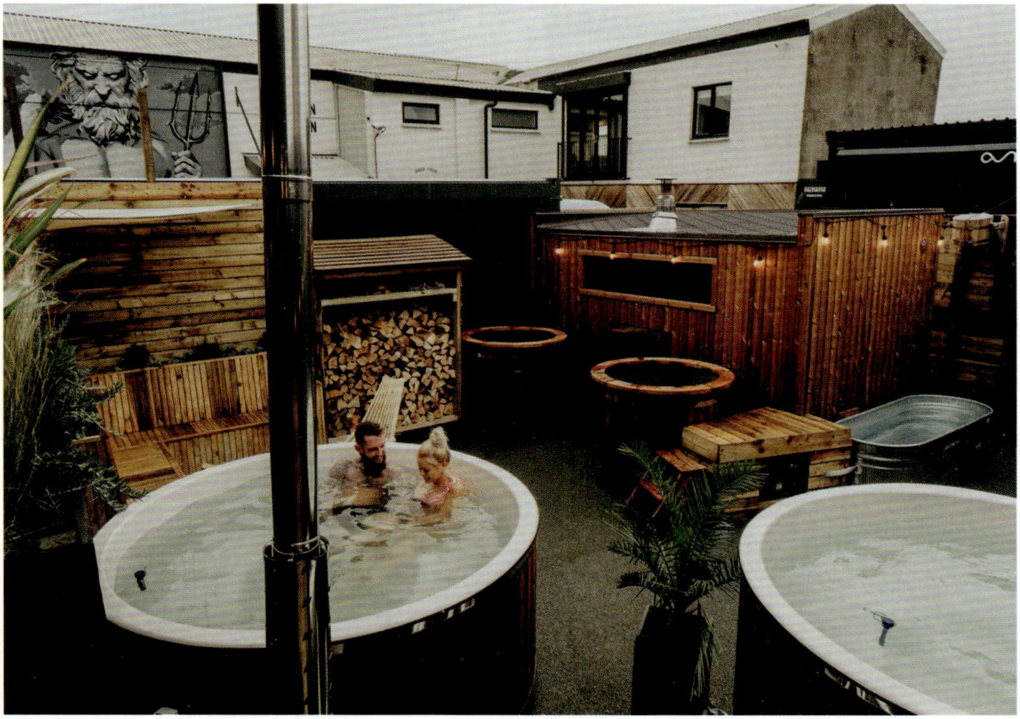

05

Olla Hiki Sauna

NEWQUAY ❦ CORNWALL

Who says British summers are not for sauna? On 21 June, the day after a glorious solstice, I was one of a handful of bathers packed into a small trailer on a cliff overlooking the wide rollers of Watergate Bay. It was 12°C, pouring with rain, and, undeterred, a lone surfer was bobbing through the swell. The trailer was shaking, in part due to the howling wind outside, in part because we were beating ourselves with whisks made of birch, oak and elderflower. As we were guided through a nature-based ritual, typical of Latvia and Lithuania, we whisked ourselves and then each other, gently at first, on the back, the feet, the shoulders.

'Olla Hiki' means 'to have a sweat' in Finnish. Sarah, our host at Olla Hiki, is German and grew up with sauna. She likes to experiment and invites a range of practitioners and hosts a variety of events, from Irish storytelling and sound baths to full moon saunas, and she has quite a following. Olla Hiki is a mobile sauna, and at various times can be found at Bedruthan Steps, Newquay Harbour and Watergate Bay.

ollahikisauna.co.uk · Sea/bucket/hose
50.4437, -5.0387 Watergate Bay
50.4173, -5.0874 Newquay Harbour

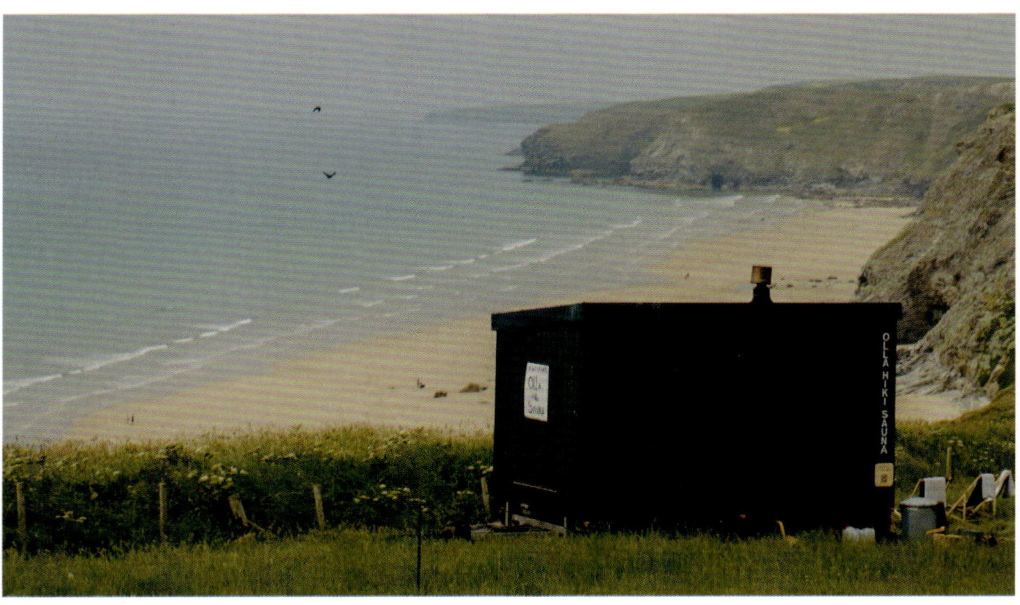

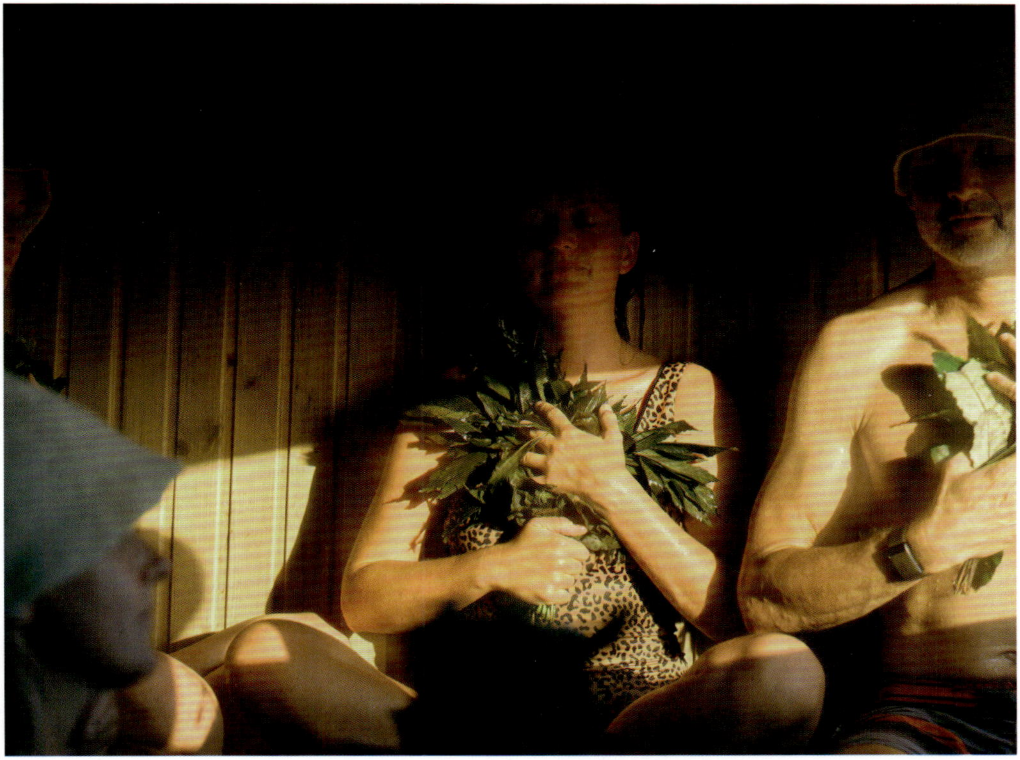

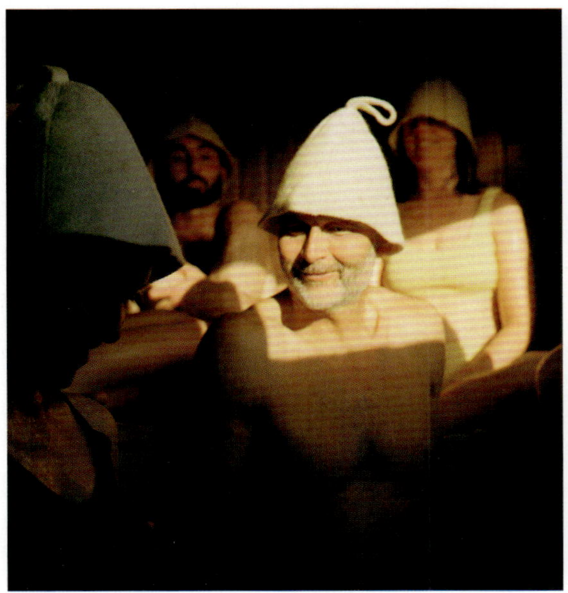

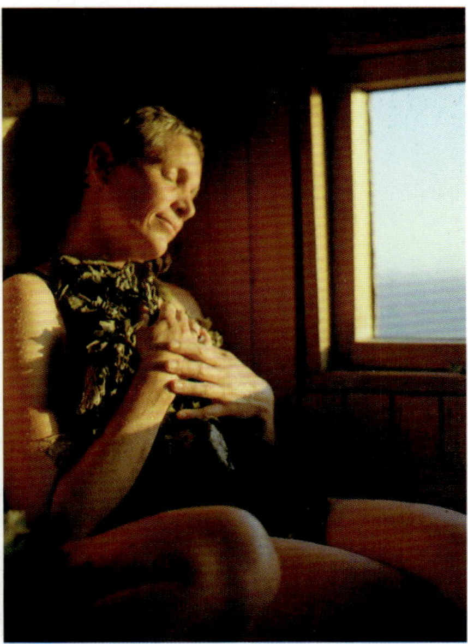

Watergate Bay

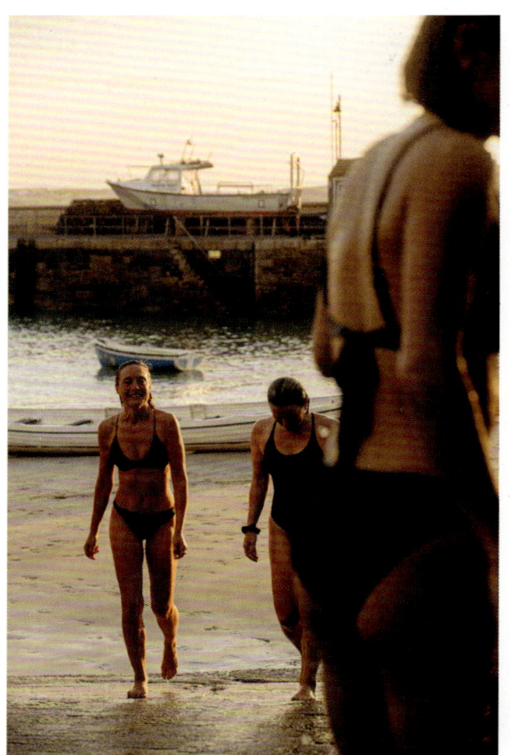

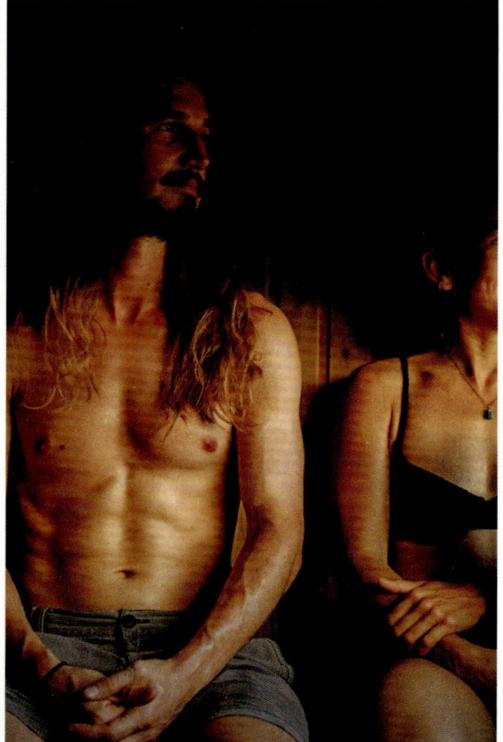

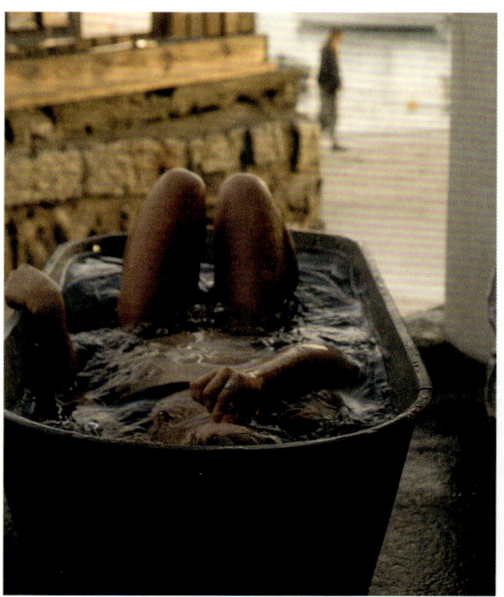

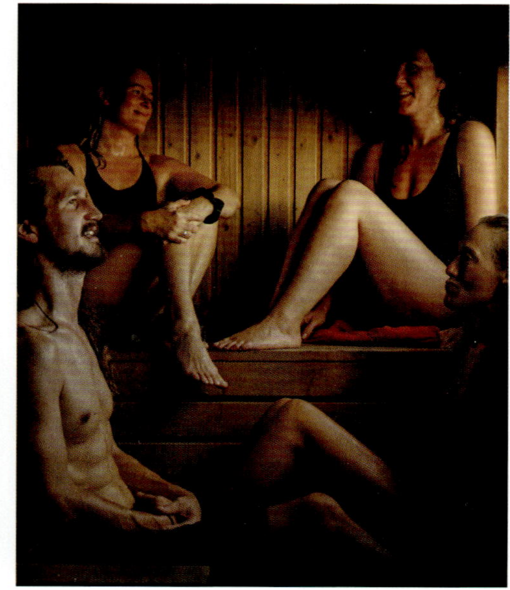

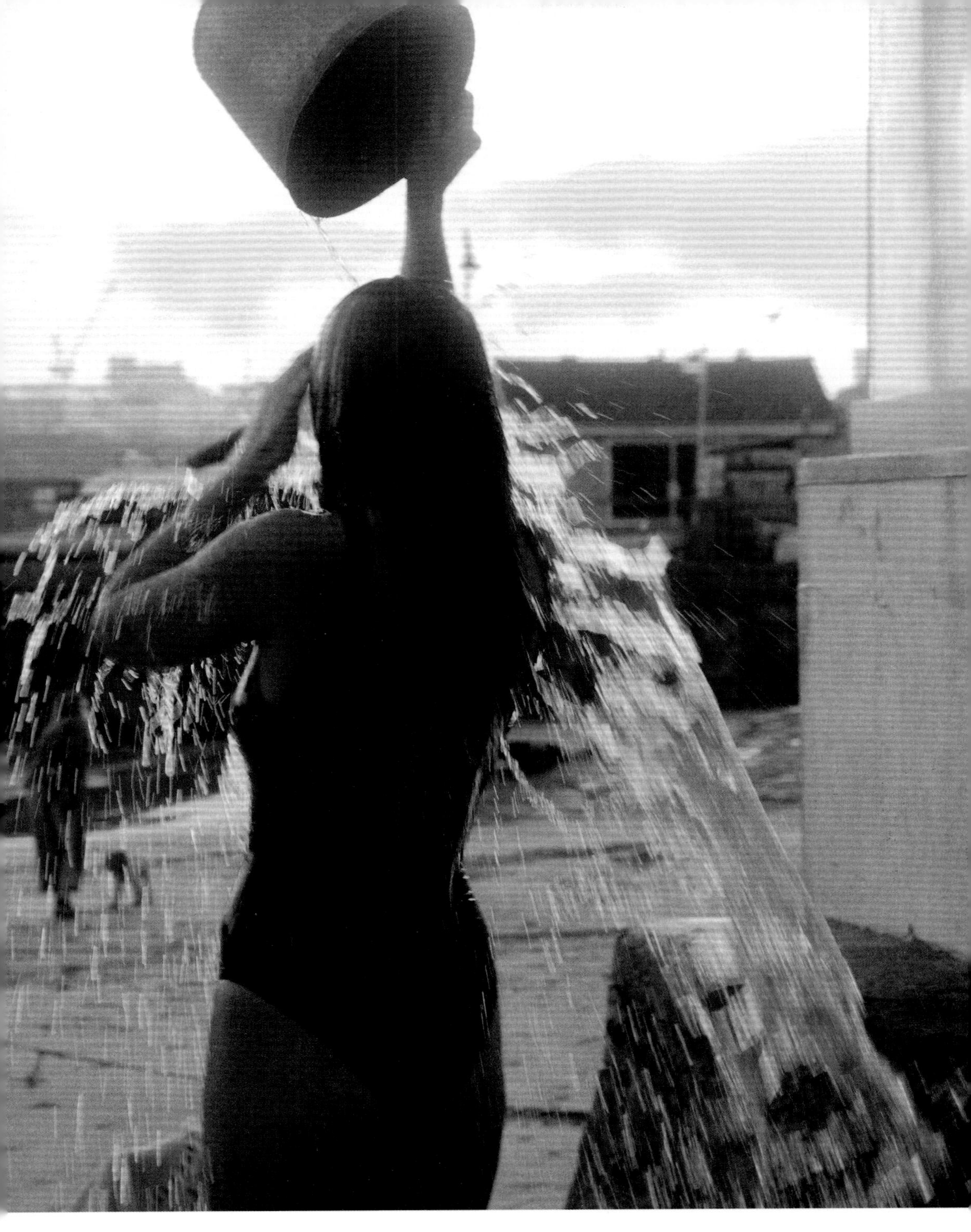

Olla Hiki Sauna Newquay Harbour

06

The Wildwood Spa

MAWGAN PORTH ❦ CORNWALL

The Wildwood Spa is big news for the UK sauna scene, its centrepiece Roundhouse Sauna being both a novel design and the UK's first event sauna in a natural, woodland setting. Crafted by one of the UK sauna scene's pioneering companies, Cornish spa owner and builder, Kernow Springs, the five-metre diameter space hosts up to 35 people for social gatherings, rituals and next-level steam adventures, and is run by the team behind Water & Stone. Tucked away in a secluded glade amongst the mixed woodlands of The Park Cornwall, a few minutes' walk from Mawgan Porth beach and a five-minute drive from Cornwall Airport Newquay, The Wildwood Spa also offers individuals and groups an outdoor pool, traditional copper, tin and brass ice baths, wood-fired hot tubs, a fire pit, drench bucket and outdoor hot showers. A holistic therapy and retreat village consisting of timber-clad yurts with log burners makes this a top sauna event destination, drawing practitioners and enthusiasts alike.

thewildwoodspa.com
Ice baths/wood-fired hot tubs/swimming pools/showers 50.4652, -5.0256

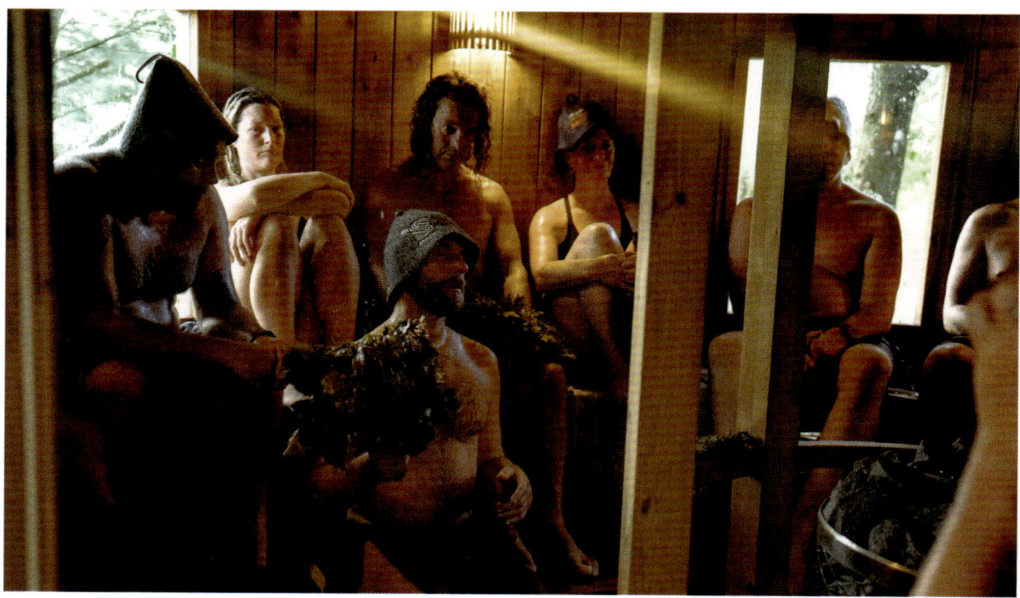

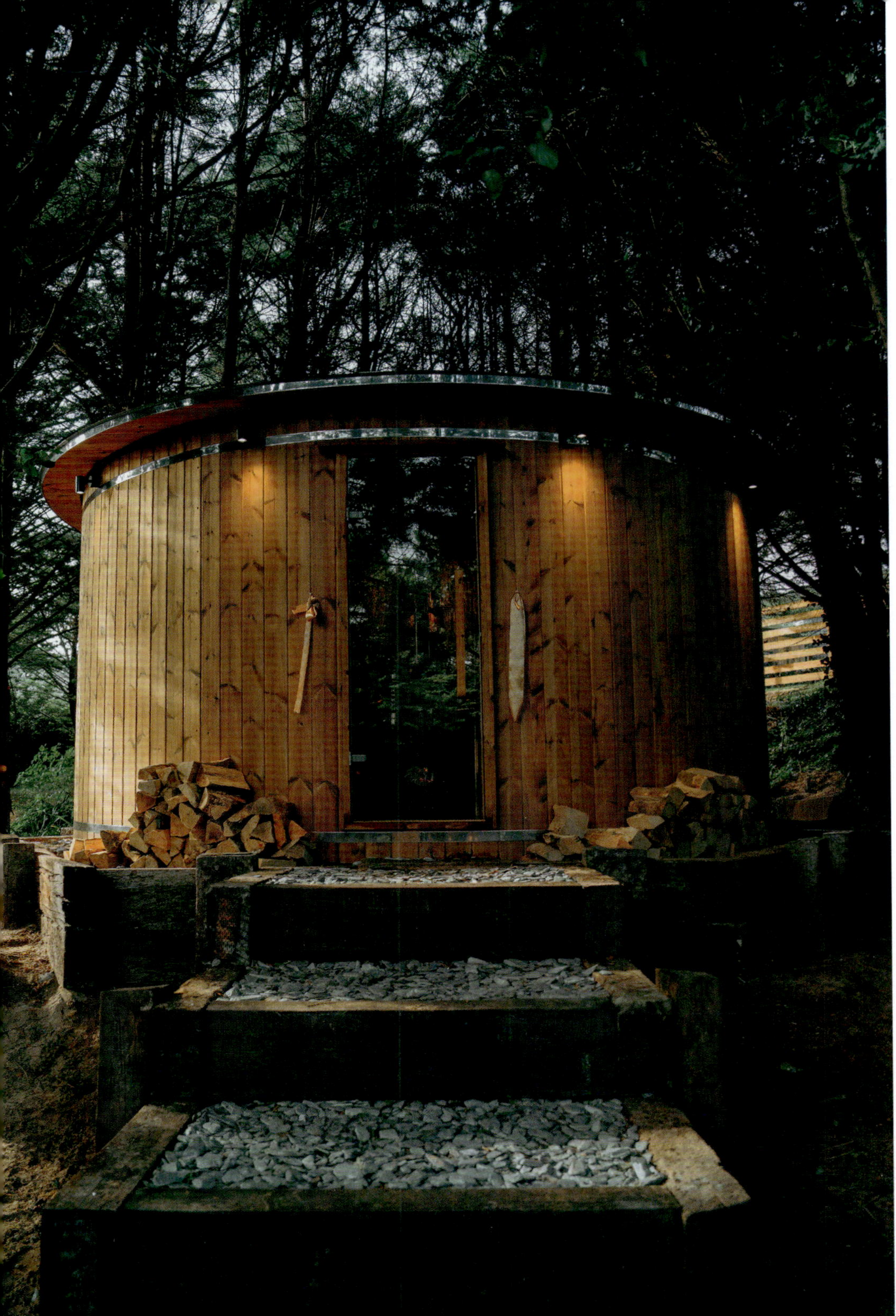

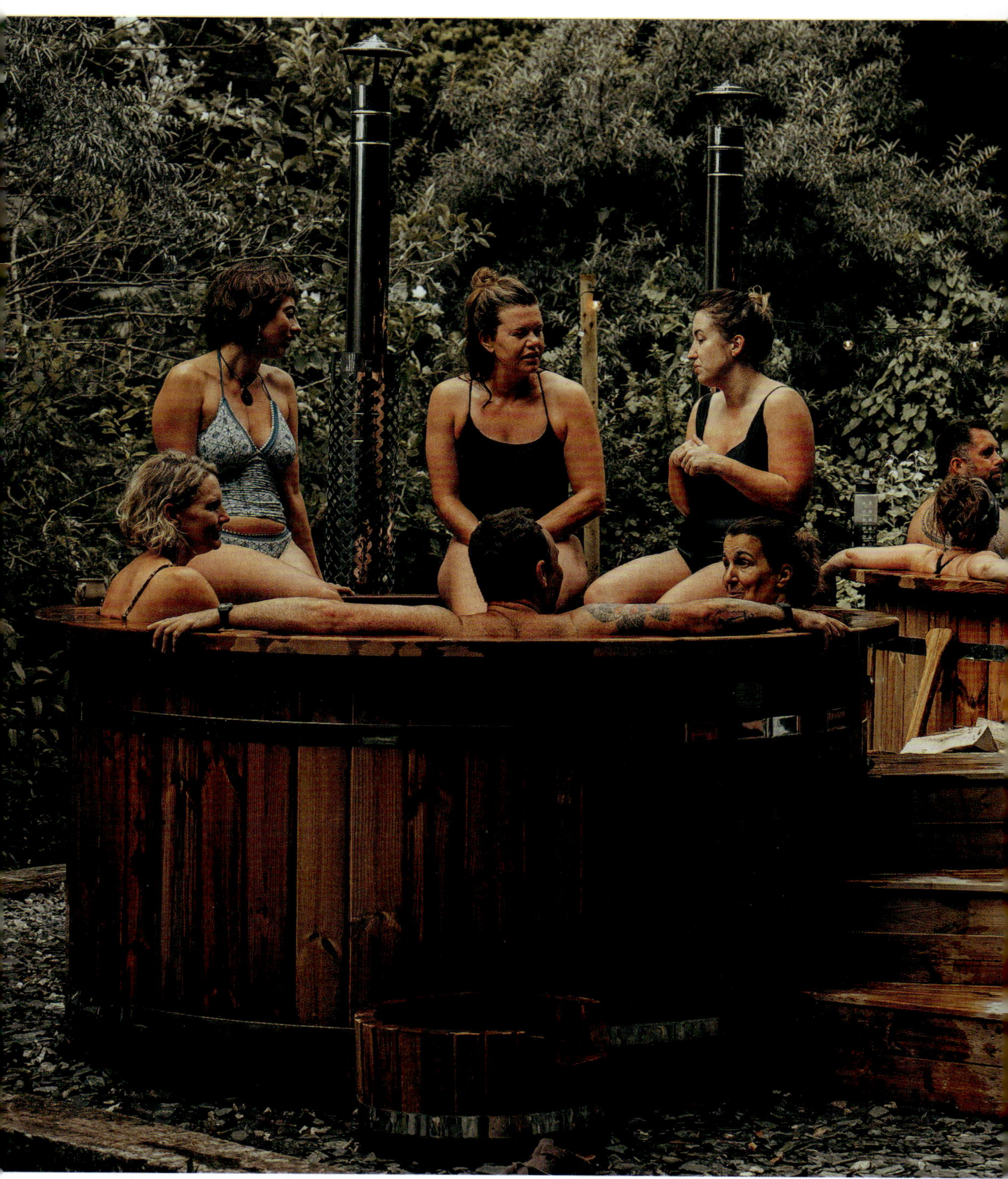

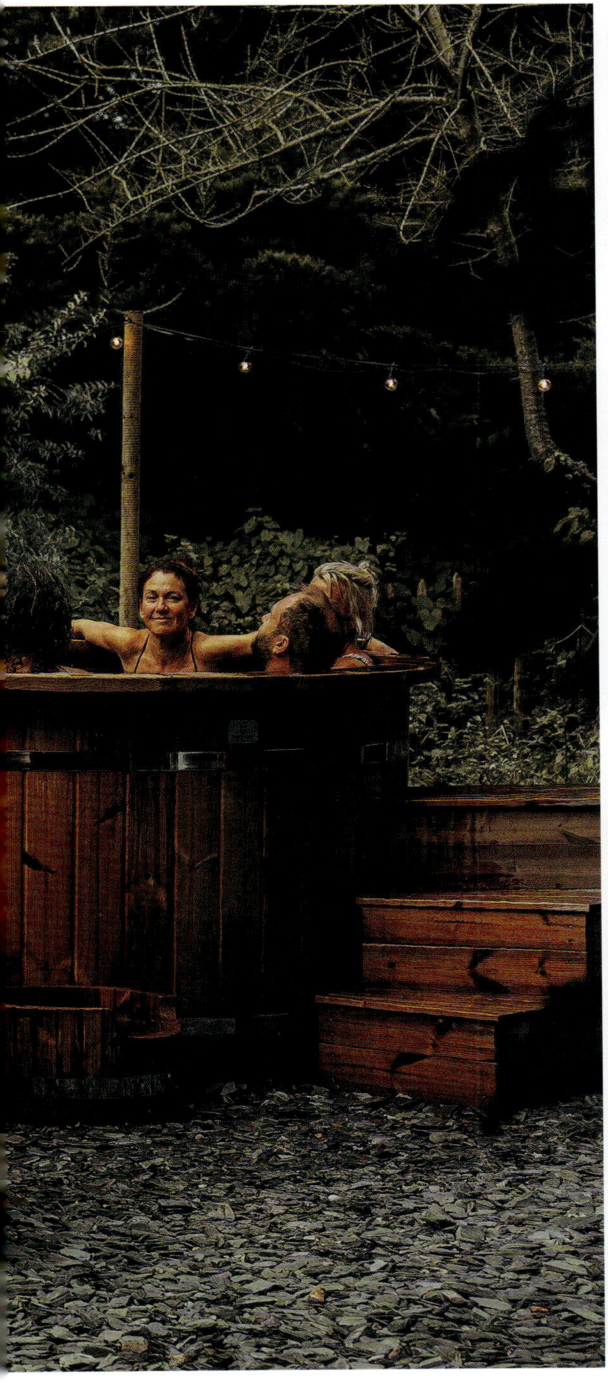

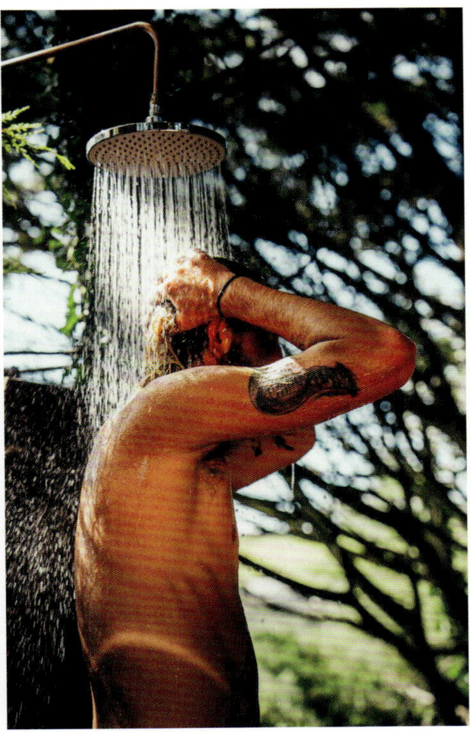

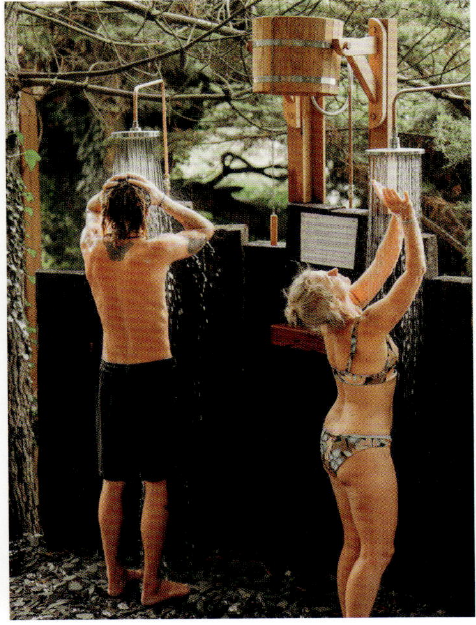

07

Steamy Wonders

TRENARREN ❦ CORNWALL

Tucked away at Trenarren House on the south coast of Cornwall is Steamy Wonders. This bespoke sauna was created by founder and host Jez Tozer, designer Sam Ludgate, and a team of local craftsmen and helpers. Conjured from reclaimed cedar and local Douglas fir, it has a tiered bench layout to honour different heat tolerances, which ensures that people of all ages can enjoy it, and is a great space for pirtis training and workshops.

Guests can wander through the three acres of private gardens and woodlands in between rounds and enjoy the stunning sea views from the sauna veranda. Steamy Wonders also hosts monthly sauna camps, where guests can come for two or three nights to hang out with a host of international sauna aficionados and enjoy plant-based food, foraging walks, wild swimming, and yoga around daily saunas. An original Victorian roll-top bath acts as the cold plunge, and there is a cold outdoor shower and toilet, which make it a completely self-contained set-up. It's open for private hire and hosts weekly community sessions, including a clothing-optional session every Friday night.

➔ steamywonders.as.me
❄ Ice bath ⚲ 50.3074, -4.7639

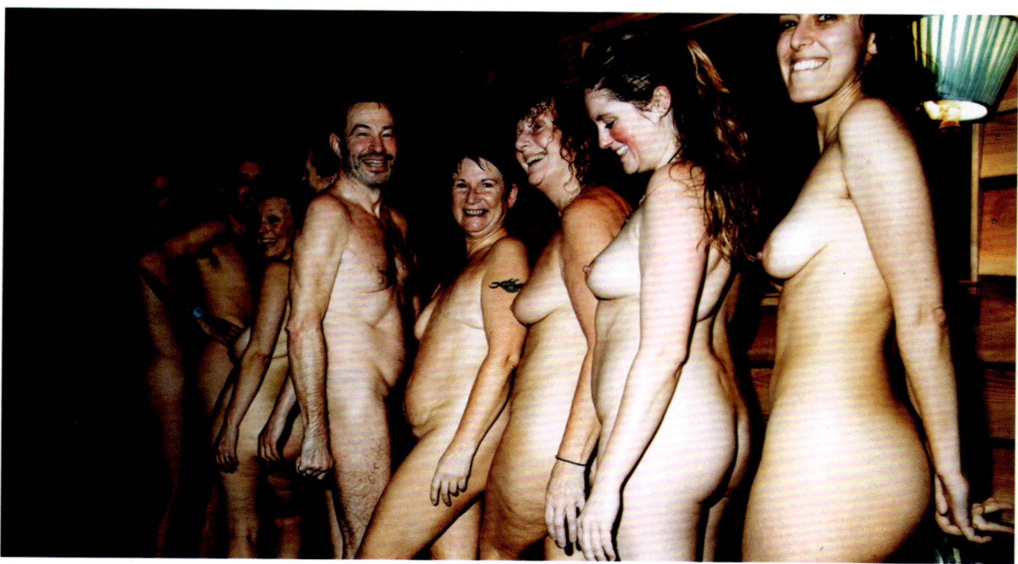

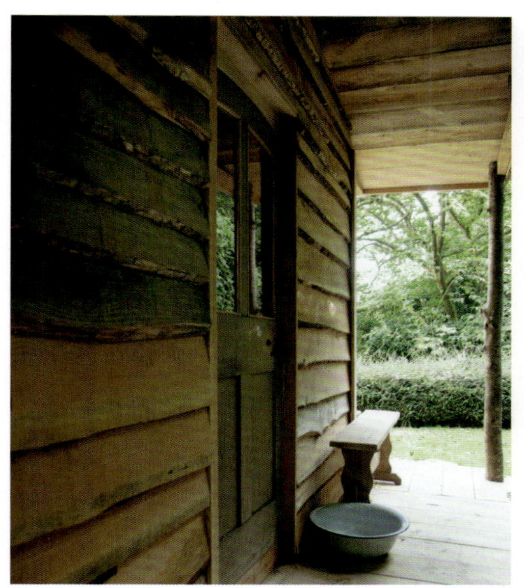

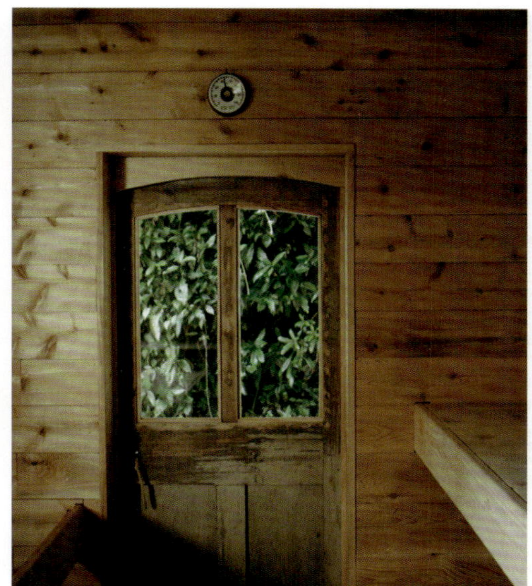

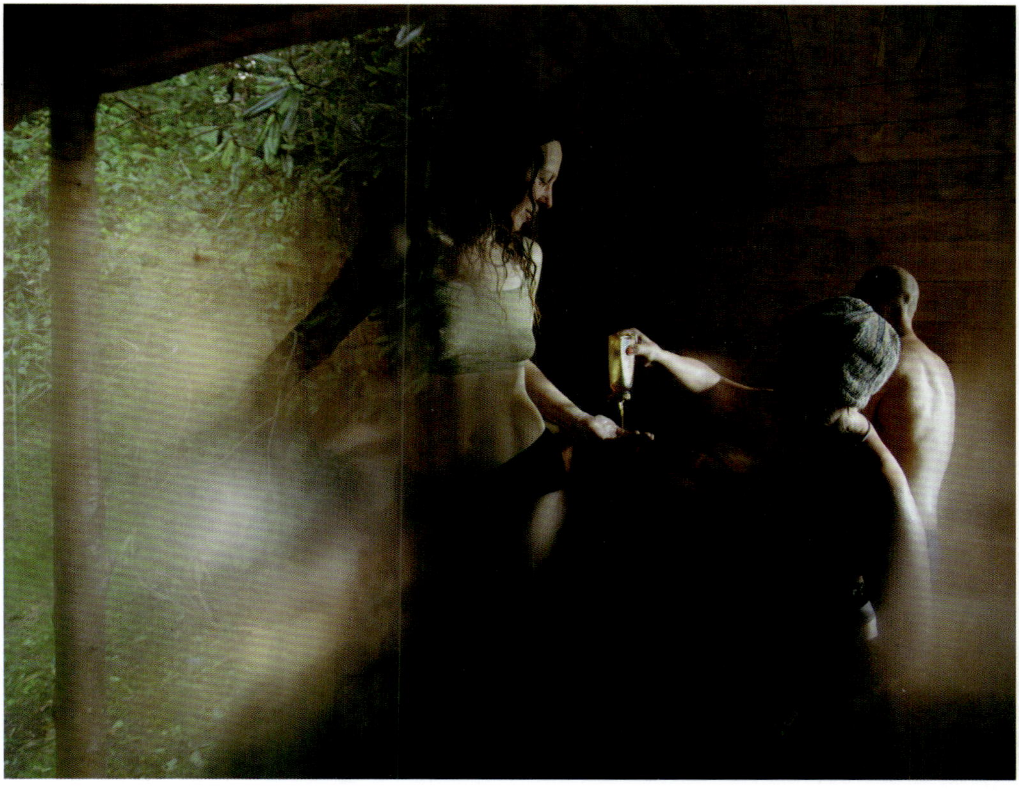

08

Escape to the Sauna

HAYLE ❦ CORNWALL

A qualified beach lifeguard and open-water swim coach, Jem Wallis has all the right skills to be a beach sauna operator. He knows the tides, currents, swells and perils of many of the beaches around Cornwall, and his barrel saunas can be found in Hayle and Falmouth.

Prior to setting up his saunas, Jem was in charge of welfare and safeguarding at a large secondary school through the pandemic – a role that resulted in burnout and left him frustrated. 'We were really good at raising awareness of mental health issues and wellbeing, but offered no solutions.' The water has always been his church, and he started taking groups of people into the cold water as part of a social prescribing scheme offered through GP surgeries across Cornwall. Most people were completely turned off by the idea, so he added sauna as a route to rally them into the water. He now works with two schools who also socially prescribe cold swimming and sauna for their students at Carlyon Bay.

At Hayle, panoramic views stretch across tidal waters towards Lelant and St Uny's church, and the sauna offers stunning sunsets at high tide. A second sauna sits just steps from Maenporth Beach near Falmouth. Ice baths and cold plunges offer an alternative to the sea, and it's here you can see the sun rise.

escape-unplugged.co.uk
ice bath/ cold plunge/sea
50.1908 -5.430 Hayle
50.1249 -5.0942 Maenporth

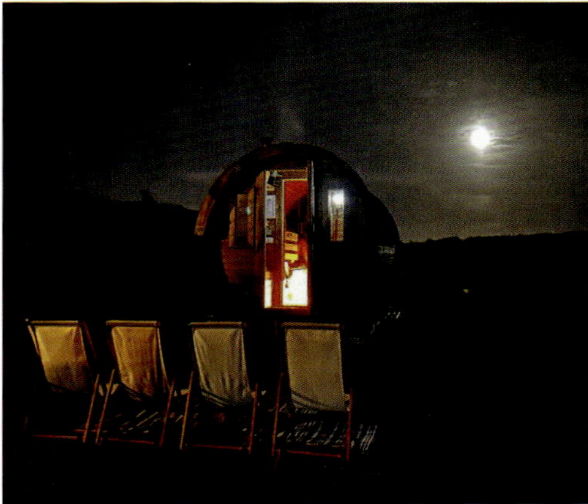

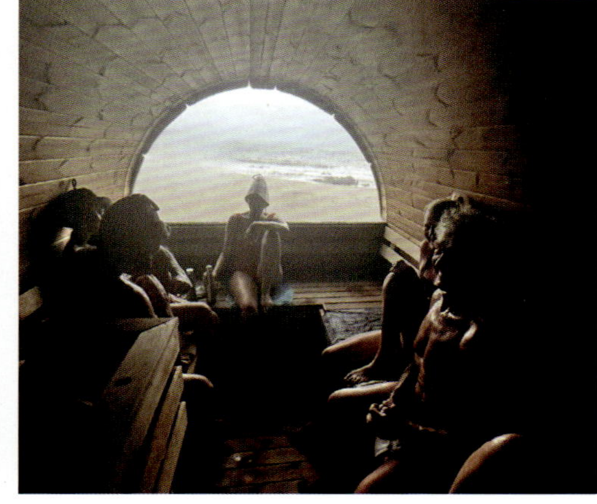

09

Saunas by the Sea

POLZEATH & HARLYN BAY ❦ CORNWALL

I heard about a sauna near Polzeath from a bather in Lowestoft – quite the other end of the country. It's on a little hidden cove called Baby Bay, next to the popular beach at Polzeath. She said she walked round to it from Polzeath at low tide, had her sauna and swam back. It sounded like a magical spot.

How different it was on the day of my visit in June; waves were crashing onto the white sand, and only a few brave bathers were cooling off knee-deep in thick surf. No one would be swimming to Polzeath unless they had a death wish. The alternative approach to it is a scramble down a cliff path – there's no road access. That the sauna is there at all is because Baby Bay is, in part, privately owned, and Saunas by the Sea, aka Steve, Henry and Luke, are friendly with the owner. The sauna (a hefty trailer) has almost washed away in a tidal surge in the past, and sometimes you step out and the sea is at your feet. For a fully immersive beach sauna experience, there's nowhere better, not least because there's a shower, and separate horseboxes for changing, shelter and storage.

They also have a spot on Harlyn Bay, on the other side of the estuary, behind Padstow, and their latest venture is a Wild Spa in Polzeath. Surfers head in droves to this area to ride the waves as the small, sheltered beaches offer surf all year round. It's no surprise that the open-air Wild Spa is focused on muscle recovery; but there are also performance-focused activities, such as HIIT classes, ice baths for those who prefer the controlled environment of the cold plunge to the sea, and two saunas which hold ten people each. Set back from the road on what used to be a mini-golf course, there is also a boules court, firepits and a wild garden, making it a refreshing change from beachside activities of old.

- saunasbythesea.co.uk
- Sea/cold plunge/shower
- 50.5803, -4.9173 Baby Bay
- 50.5397, -4.9949 Harlyn Bay
- 50.5725, -4.9159 Polzeath Wild Spa

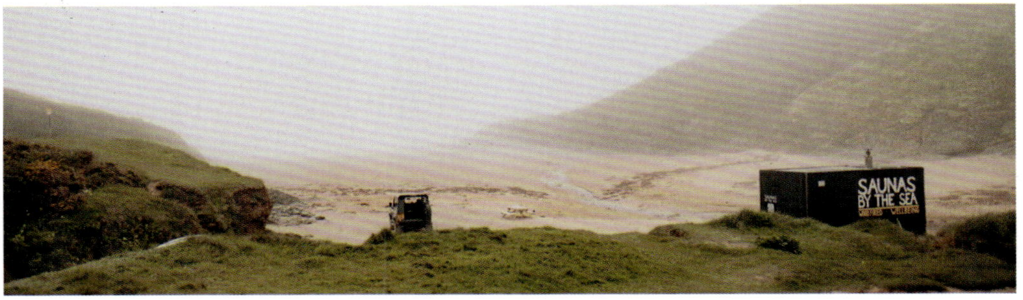

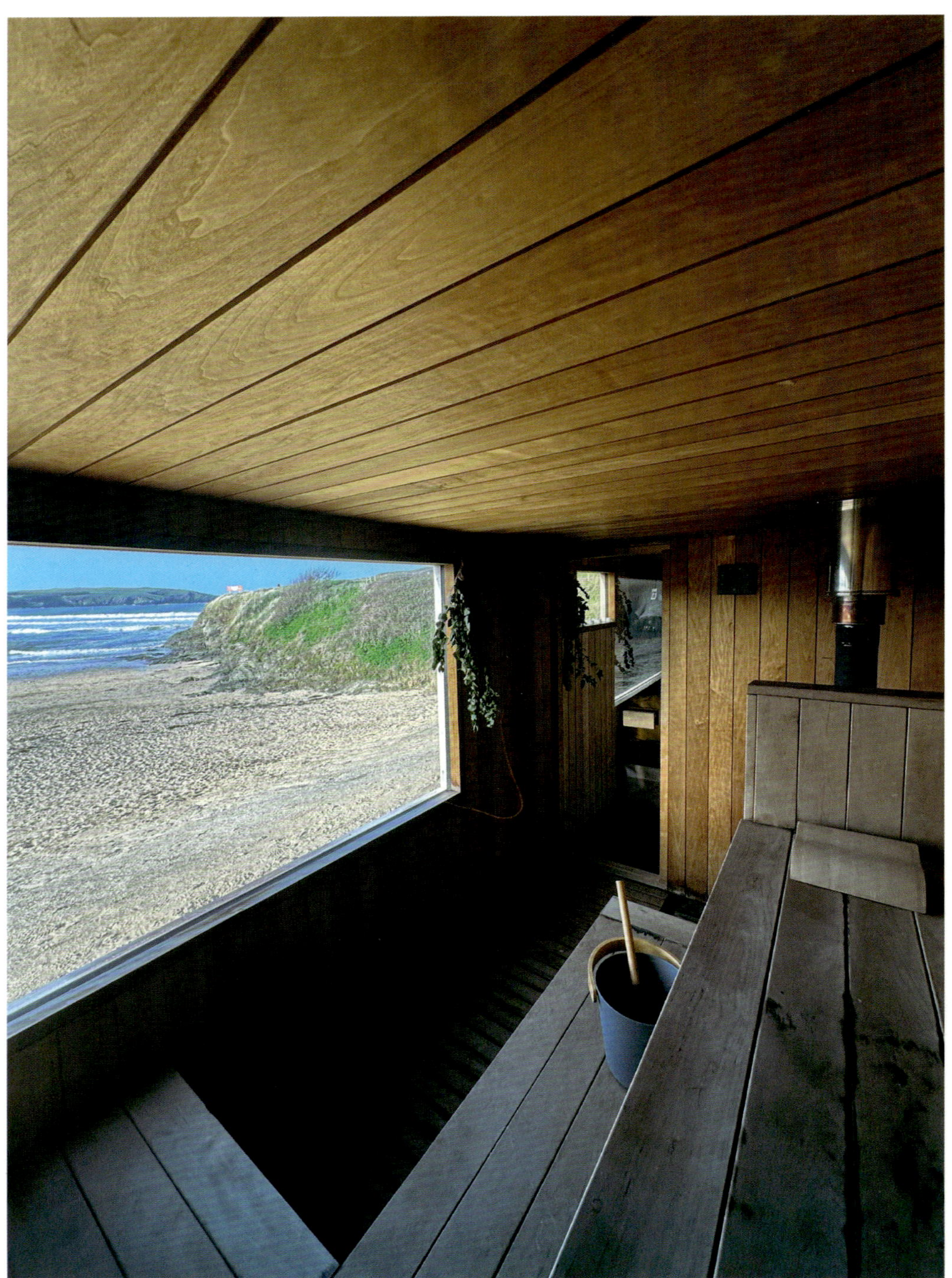

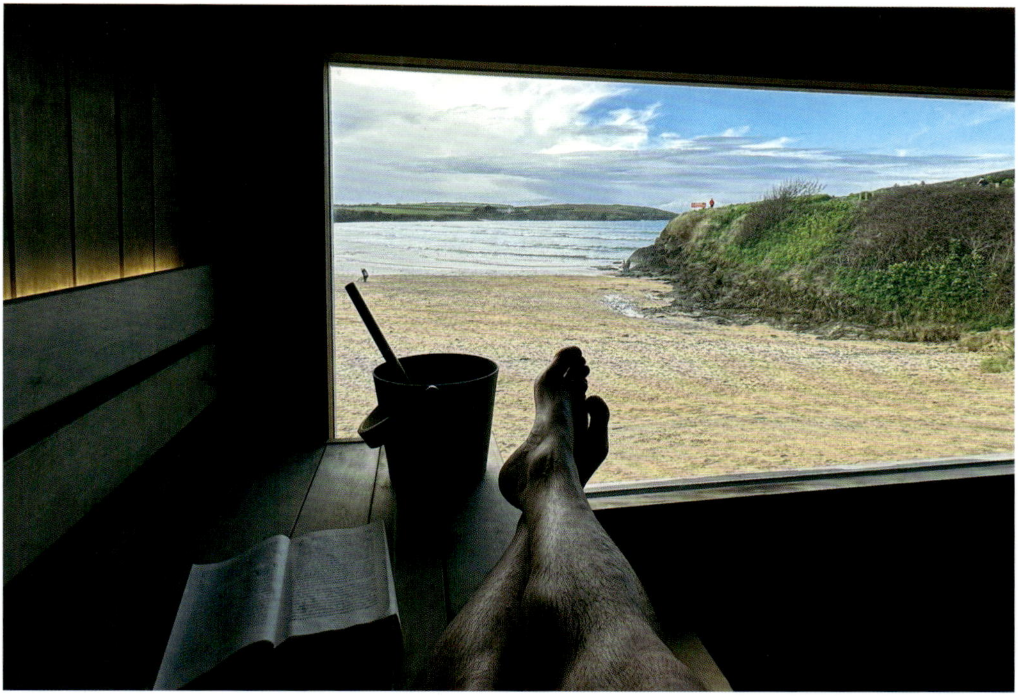

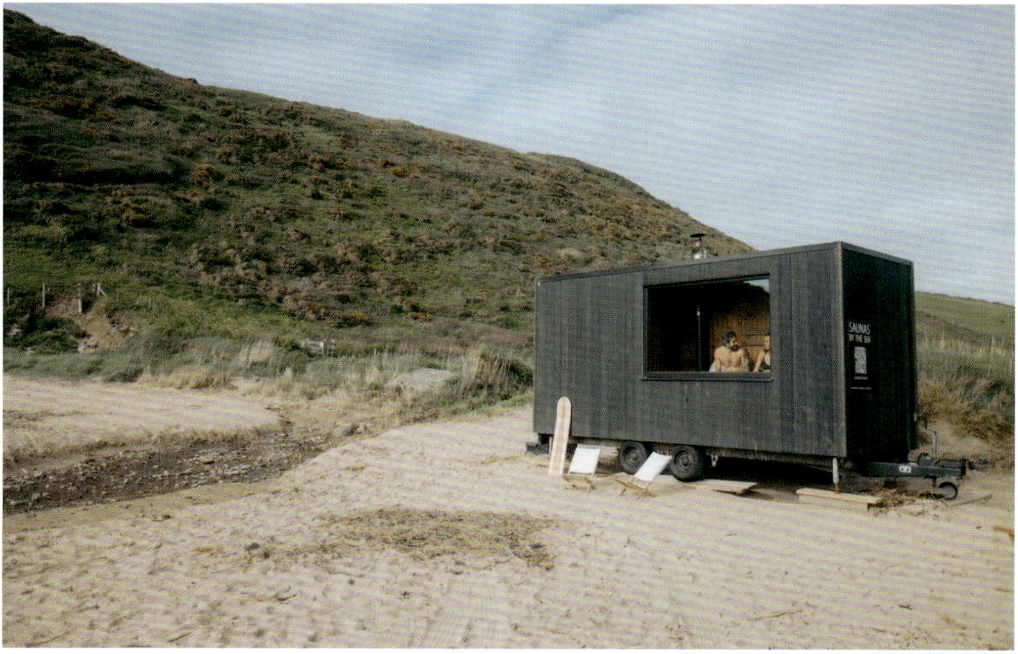

Saunas by the Sea

10

Kernow Springs Nordic Spa

WADEBRIDGE ❦ CORNWALL

In the southwest, where sauna is booming, a new spa model has been taking shape – the contrast therapy centre. It typically includes sauna, cold plunge, ice bath, hot tubs, showers – all those elements needed to indulge in a little thermotherapy. Kernow Springs Nordic Spa in Wadebridge is one such concept. Tucked away behind a first-floor bar in Saltbox, a hip foodie hangout made from shipping containers in Wadebridge, it's inspired by those no-frills Scandinavian day spas, such as Salt in Oslo.

Despite the bustle of the bar, a hot tub for 12, a softly lit sauna, along with showers, spotlessly clean changing rooms and a vanity area, quickly dissolve the world outside. Founder Martin Dean ran saunas and hot tubs at festivals for a decade, after learning his trade building traditional boats with Cornish Crabbers; Nordic Spa has something of that alternative, festival vibe.

➔ kernowsprings.co.uk/nordic-spa
❄ Cold plunge ⚲ 50.5184, -4.8383

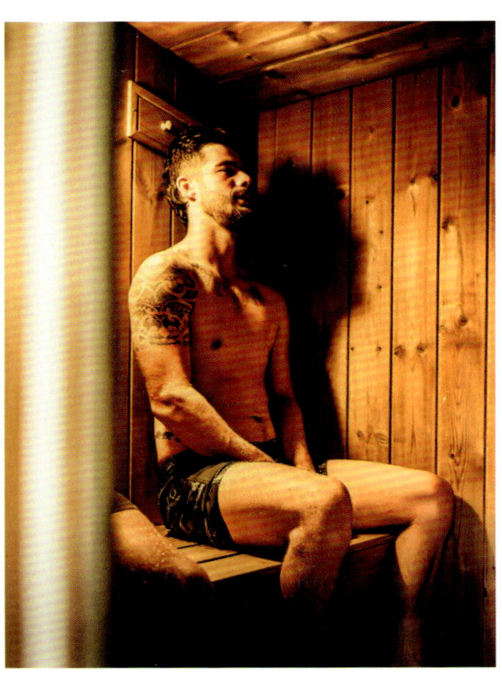

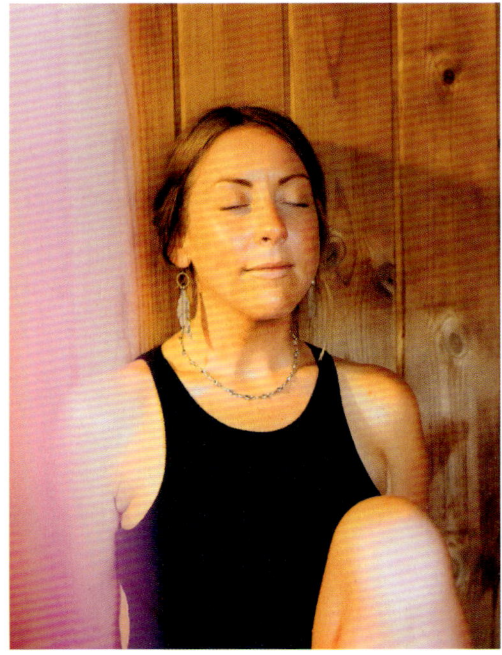

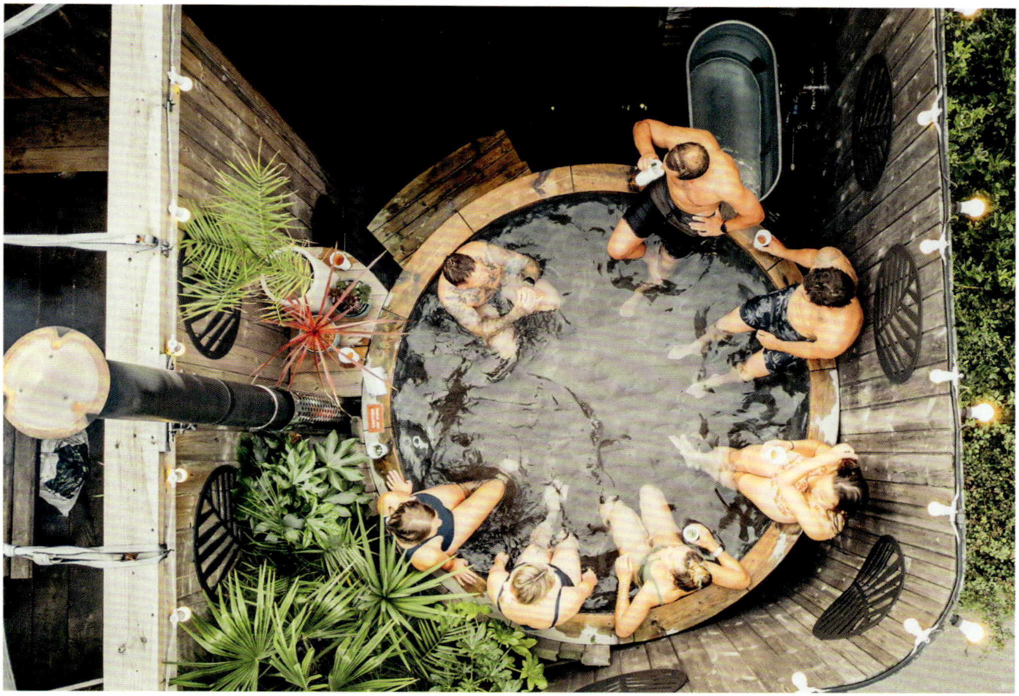

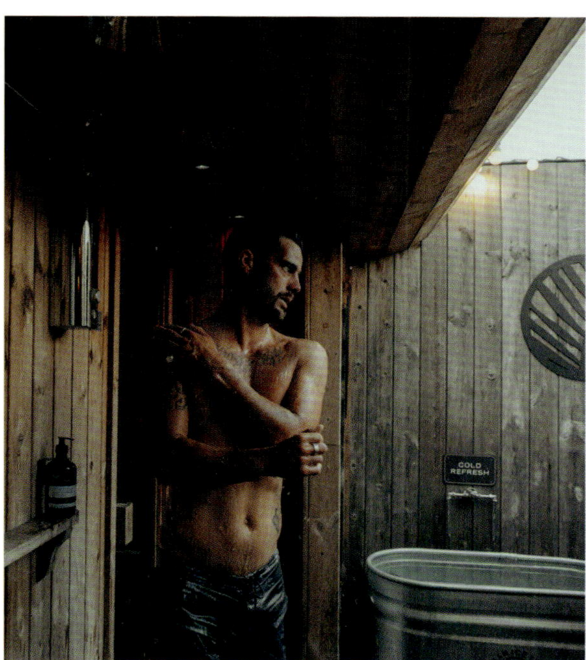
COLD
REFRESH

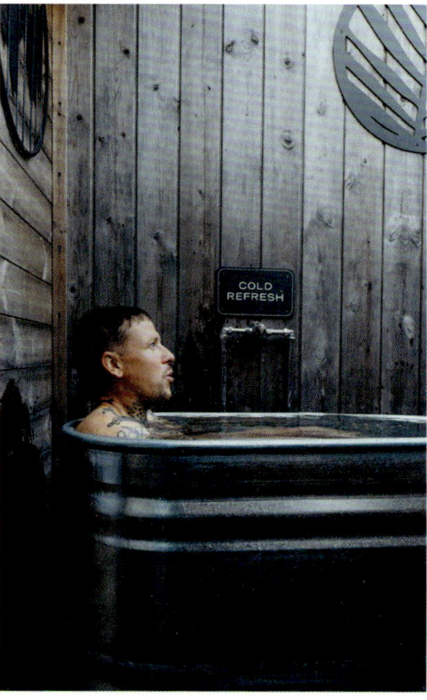
COLD
REFRESH

11

Motts

MENHENIOT ❦ CORNWALL

All summer Jess Sneyd and Jo Baskott park their horsebox sauna in Mount Edgcumbe Park, an idyllic 864-acre park that forms part of Mount Edgcumbe House Estate. Picnickers, walkers, cyclists, swimmers and tourists come and enjoy the waterfront gardens, park and Grade II listed stately home, and Motts sits on grassy spot between a beach and a duck pond adorned with lily pads. The sauna, which Jess built with her stepdad, holds 5-6 and the clear waters of the sea breaking on the rocky shore, offers an idyllic setting with views across to Plymouth. A great way to arrive at the sauna is by boat or SUP from the historic Royal William Yard in Plymouth.

In the winter, the sauna spends six months at Millendreath Beach, a sandy cove just east of the busy fishing town of Looe. Situated in the shelter of the cliff and next to a café, it's set up for the winter months with a warm area for changing, cold plunge and outside shower. Both locations offer great opportunities to connect with the elements, and space to slow down relax.

In addition to the mobile sauna, Jess runs a sister sauna all year round on the outskirts of picturesque village Menheniot. This secluded rural setting sits close to the River Seaton, which is great for cold dips and a swoosh in the stream. The bespoke sauna seats 8-10 and there's no need to rush off; guests can relax around the fire, drink tea, enjoy food and special collaborations with other wellness practitioners.

motts-sauna.com Sea/cold plunge/stream
50.4298 -4.4091 Menheniot
50.3614 -4.4368 Millendreath

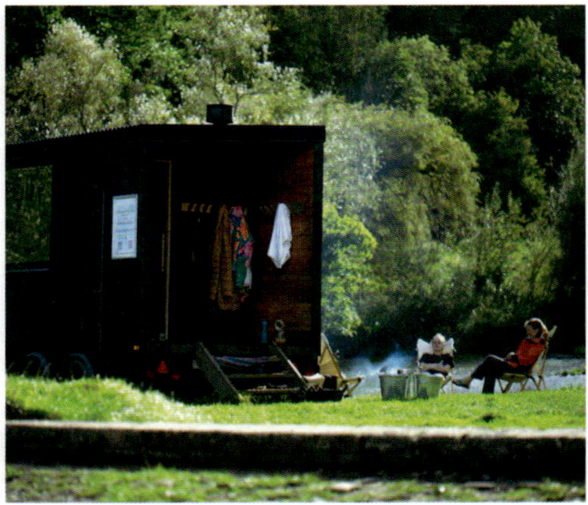

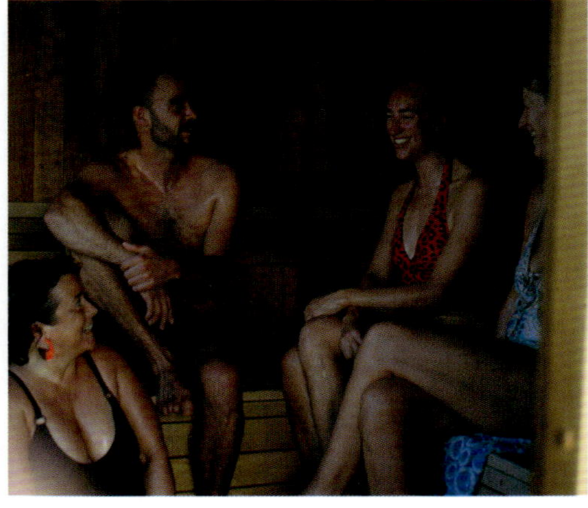

12

Ocean Soul Sauna

BUDE ❦ CORNWALL

Ocean Soul sauna at Crooklets Beach in Bude was Cornwall's first sauna 'pilot' to open on council-owned land. It sits right in front of the Bude Life Saving Club and is a buzzing spot, popular with hikers on the South West Coast Path, surfers, paddle-boarders and swimmers who come to enjoy the Bude Sea Pool. Ocean Soul founder Lorna Townsend is a trained sauna master and her eight-person sauna is a popular place to gather and watch the sunset. Lorna also collaborates with local practitioners to host yoga, meditation, soundbaths and full moon events.

oceansoulsauna.co.uk

Sea/bath 50.8358, -4.5533

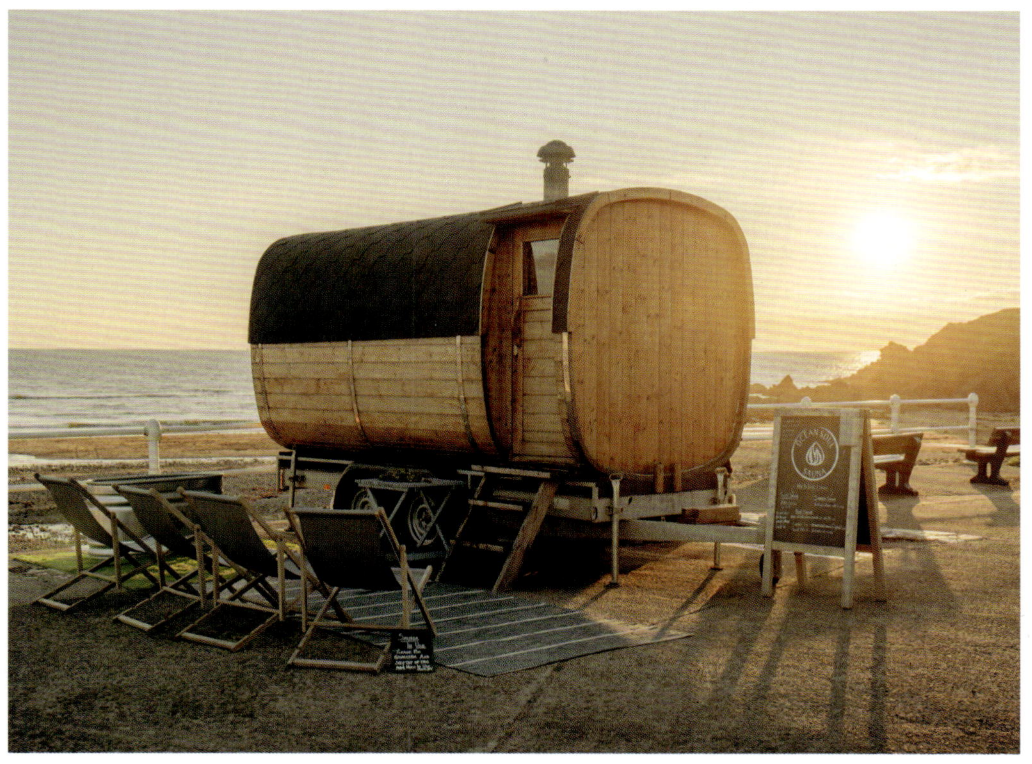

13

Lit Sauna & Space

MAKER HEIGHTS ❦ CORNWALL

This is the kind of multi-purpose space founder Lara Kramer would like to go to herself. A sauna, two cold plunges, a cold shower, toilets, changing rooms, and a cosy indoor room in which to eat, do yoga, or work make it a comfortable sauna experience. What sets Lit apart is its inclusivity, being one of the few saunas that welcome under-16s, making it an attractive choice for parents seeking a family-friendly session.

But it's not just parents who will visit. Lit is the latest addition to Maker Heights, a former military site on a windswept headland outside Plymouth, and a thriving creative hub. Derelict garrison buildings from the 18th century have been repurposed over the years into cafés and bars, creative workspaces, and venues for live gigs and exercise classes. The site's 12 hectares of grassland stretch across Rame Head, one of Cornwall's Areas of Outstanding Natural Beauty, and are home to Maker Camp, a 350-person campsite with glamping bow geodomes available from Wilderme. The campers love Lit too.

Toilets and changing rooms are located in the Grade II listed garrison buildings, with the adjoining indoor space doubling up as a wellbeing hub, hosting reflexology, coaching and massage, as well as a comfortable place for sauna-goers to relax and have a cup of tea after their sauna. It is also perfectly equipped to host sauna & dinner soirées and has regular yoga & sauna pop-ups.

Lara's background as a health coach contributes to the vision of fostering collaborations and community engagement, reflecting the vibrant and evolving sauna culture in the south-west region. Lit Sauna & Space is a promising addition to the sauna scene, offering a blend of relaxation, creativity and communal spirit in a stunning coastal setting.

➔ litsaunaandspace.com
❄ Cold plunge. ⚲ 50.3425, -4.1999

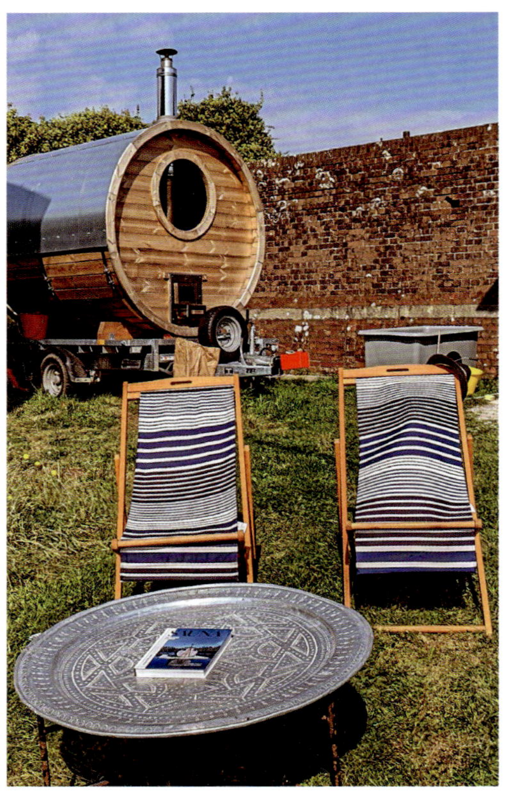

14

Hálogi

BRIXHAM & PLYMOUTH ❦ DEVON

Hálogi means 'high flame' in Old Norse, and the Nordics have been a huge inspiration for Ross, the founder of this horsebox sauna in Plymouth. His day job is located in the North Sea, where he works as a saturation diver and lives in a small, pressurised chamber for three weeks at a time. When he's on dry land, he heads straight to the sauna.

Ross built Hálogi himself as a side hustle and took it to Shoalstone Sea Pool in Brixham. It proved so popular that Royal William Yard in Plymouth invited him to set up in its grand grounds too. The yard had significant military prowess in the 1800s and now has one of the UK's largest collections of Grade I listed buildings. Hálogi and its three ice baths are perched on The Lookout with views over Plymouth Sound. From there, you can head down to Firestone Bay and its tidal pool, which are popular year-round swimming spots.

→ halogico.com ❄ Ice baths/sea
📍 50.4010, -3.499 Brixham
📍 50.3626, -4.1631 Plymouth

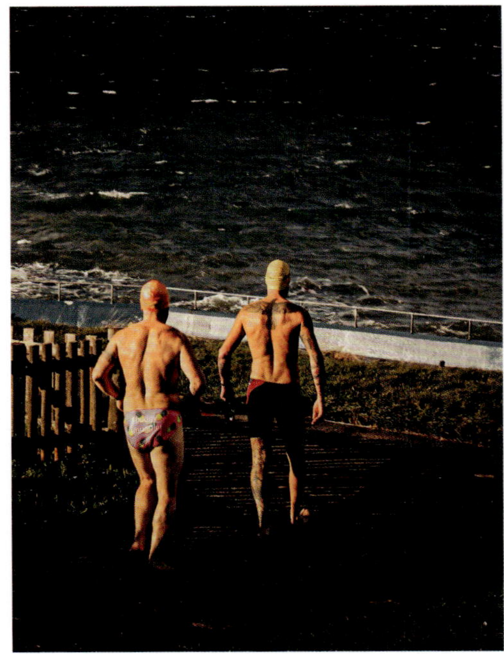

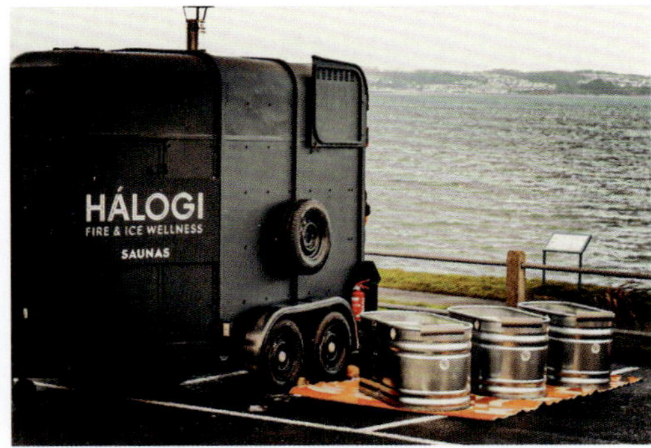

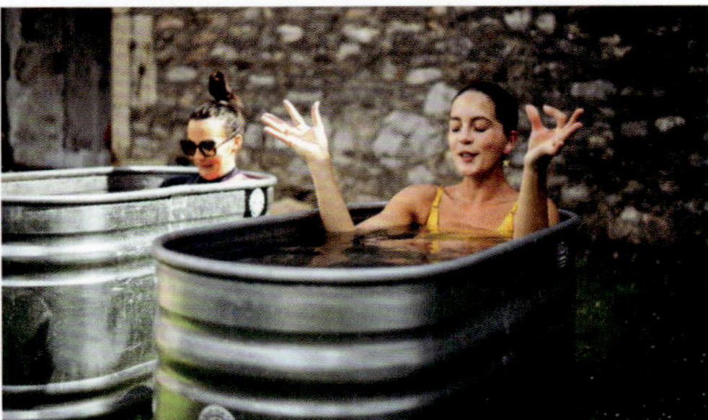

15

The Somewhere Sauna

MOTHECOMBE ❦ DEVON

Like many a carpenter, Columb Thompson has built his sauna in a passionate, ad hoc manner, often using up bits of leftover wood that he has in his workshop. The Somewhere Sauna, which sits in a forest clearing above Mothecombe Beach, is the culmination of many years of experimenting with eco-structures (including his own home). The larch-clad exterior is blackened in the Japanese style, while inside the benches are a mixture of local woods – plum, oak, ash, beech, chestnut, elm, holly. They have been tested for their thermal qualities – 'I didn't want to import wood,' Columb explains. 'The sauna is a bit shonky and not super streamlined, but it has character.'

This character is so much loved by the locals that they won't let him take it on the road as he had originally planned. A cold plunge looks down to Mothecombe Beach, a 15-minute walk away, and a fire pit, changing room, shower and resident weasel add to the fairy-tale setup.

There's a strong creative community around Somewhere (a recent workshop involved making sauna hats with wool from local sheep). A sleaker sister sauna opened in Dartington in spring and Columb is raising funds to create the CIC Somewhere Community Sauna in Ashburton.

- thesomewheresauna.com
- Cold plunge/shower
- 50.3132, -3.9514 Mothecombe
- 50.4479, -3.7117 Dartington

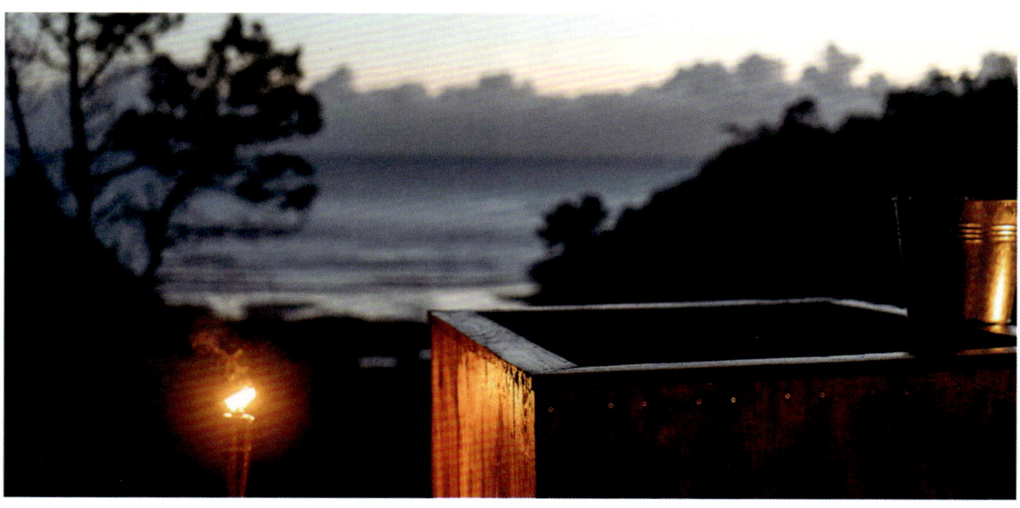

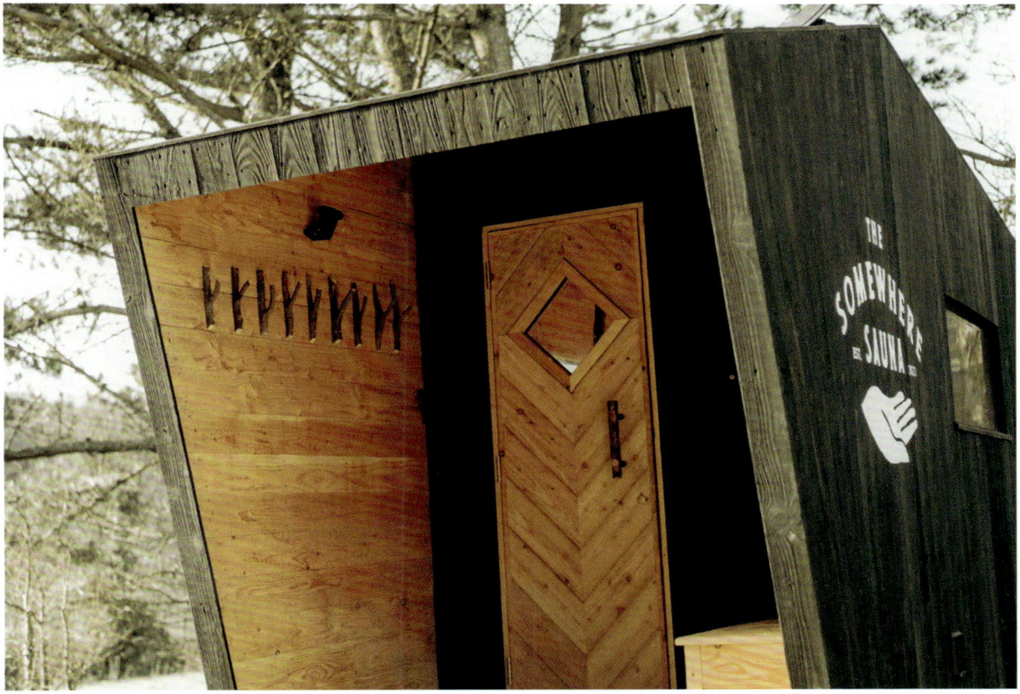

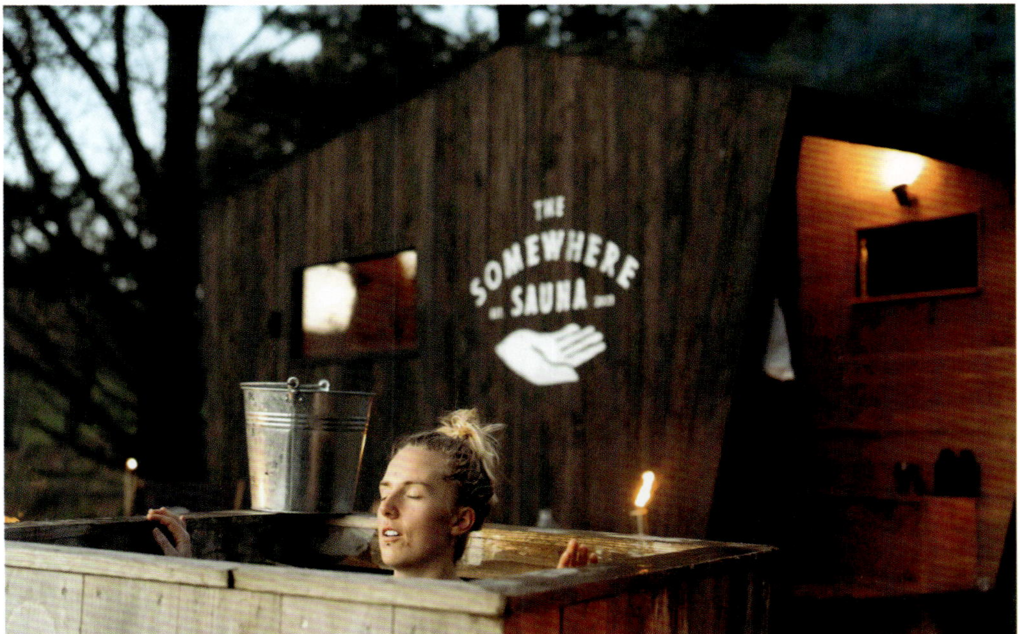

16

Devon Sauna Hub

TEIGNMOUTH ❦ DEVON

Fed up with the local authority saying no to her, Sara Dance bought a tent sauna and started doing pop-up saunas on private land next to the River Teign. Eventually, the council granted Sara, who is a level 2 Wim Hof instructor and a thermalist teacher, a permanent spot on the prominent beachfront at Teignmouth where she runs Devon Community Sauna. The pop-up tents operate at Fishcombe Cove and the River Teign and regularly come to London to the shores of the swimming lake at Beckenham Place Park.

devonsaunahub.co.uk
River/sea 50.5453, -3.4938

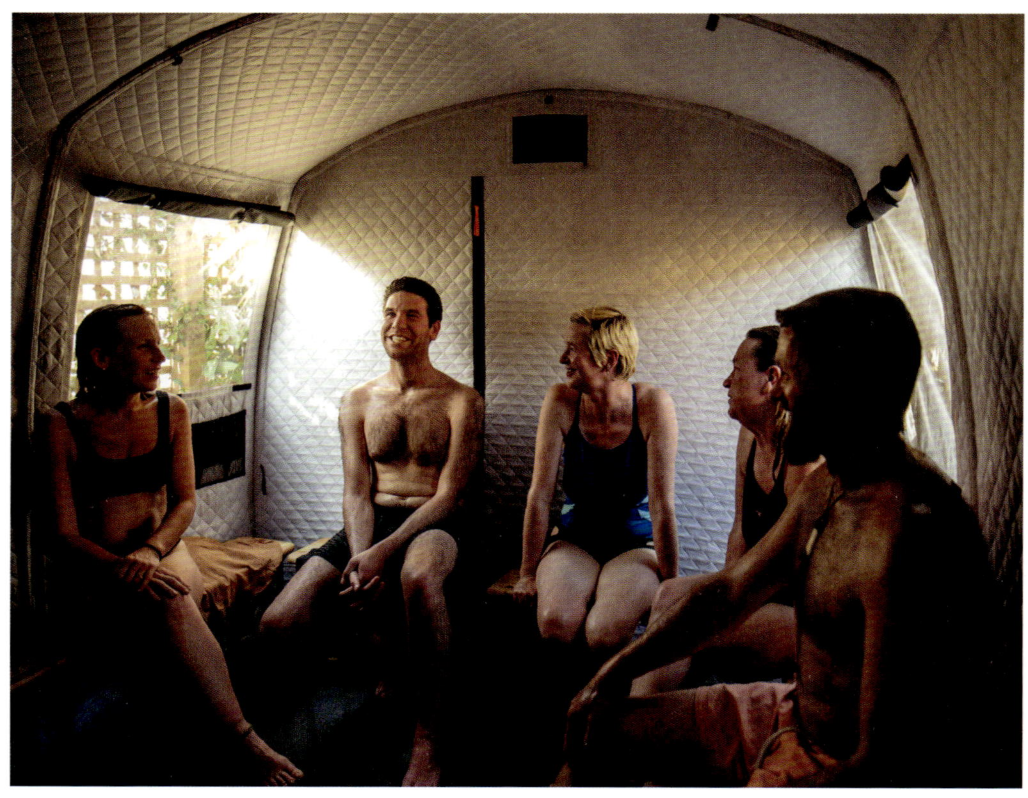

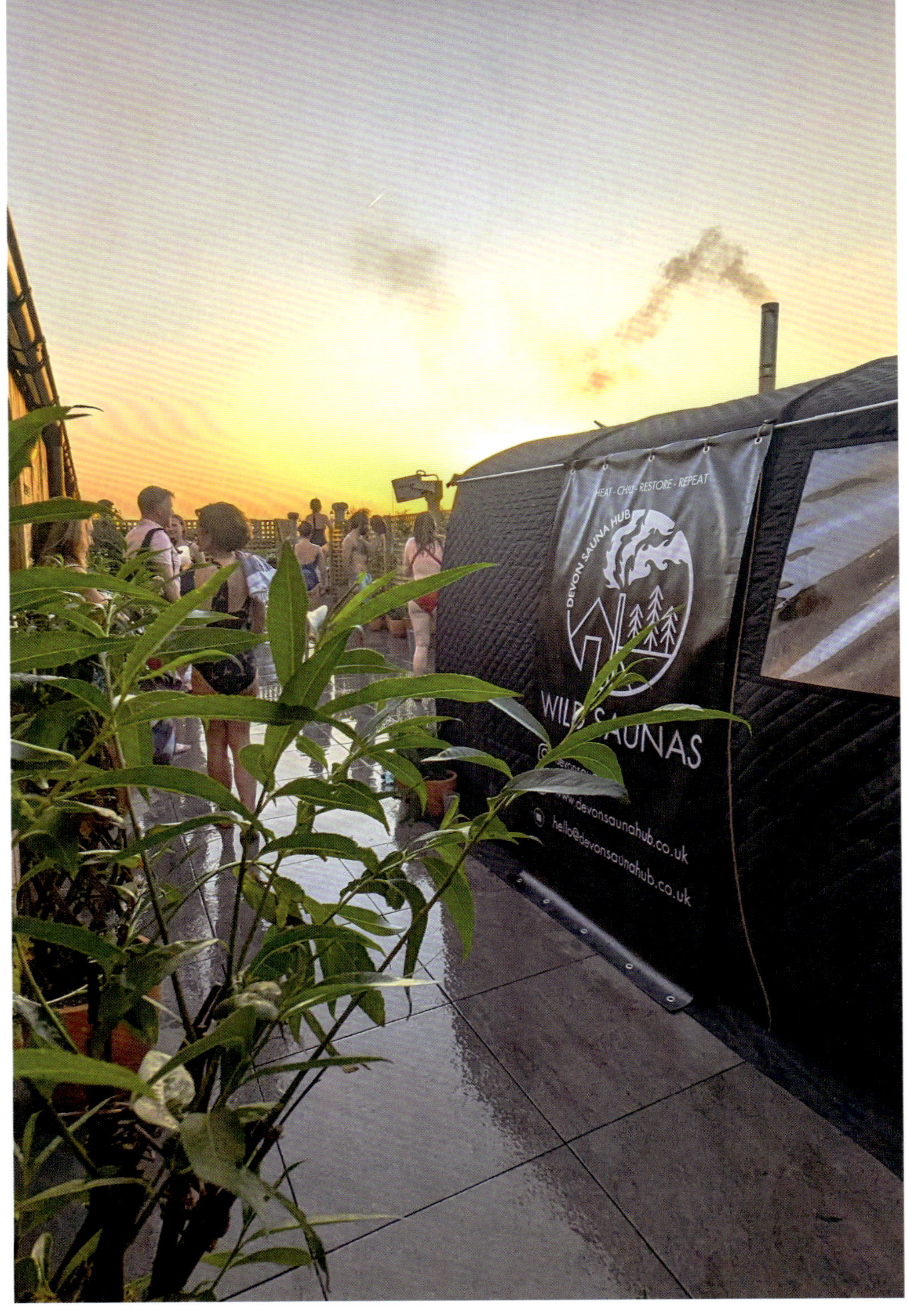
HEAT - CHILL - RESTORE - REPEAT
DEVON SAUNA HUB
hello@devonsaunahub.co.uk

17

Shoreline Sauna

LYME REGIS ❦ DORSET

Despite its 1950s pastel colours and retro look, Shoreline Sauna is easy to miss as it's tucked away by the kayaks and paddleboards on the main beach at Lyme Regis. A calm and sheltered spot all year round means that a bucket of cold water is a fresher plunge option than the balmy sea in summer.

Former customer Louise Roberts loved it so much she bought it and has now tapped into a whole new local community she never knew was there.

shorelinesauna.co.uk
Sea/bucket/bath 50.7212, -2.9386

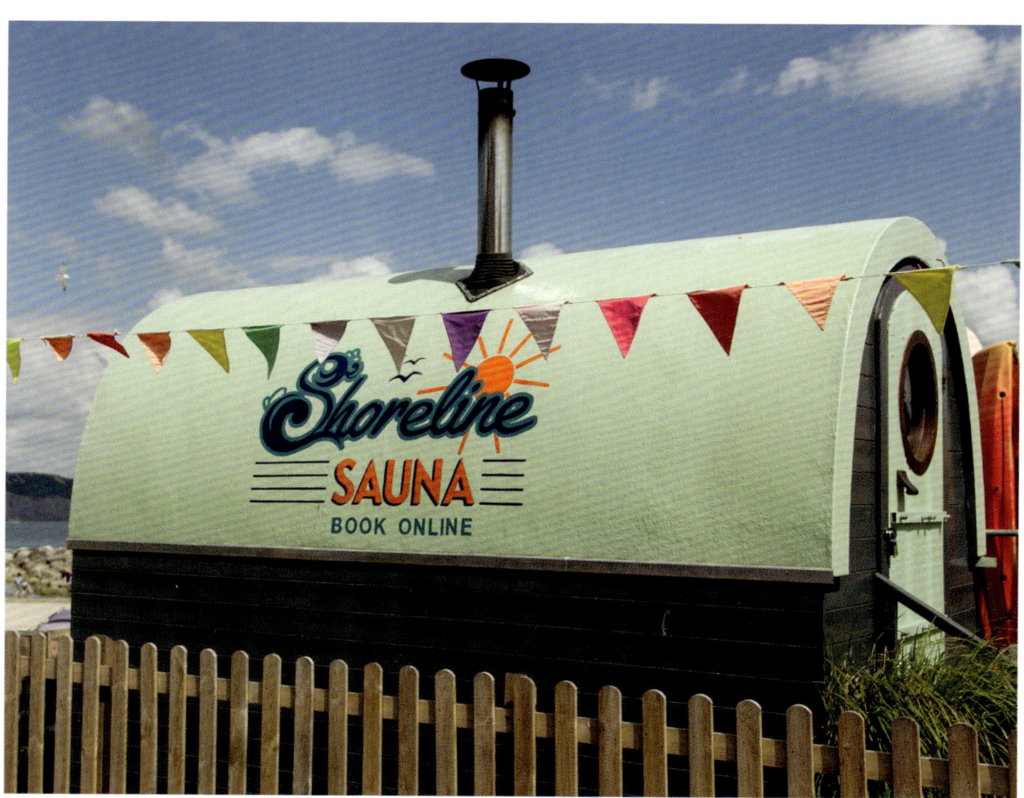

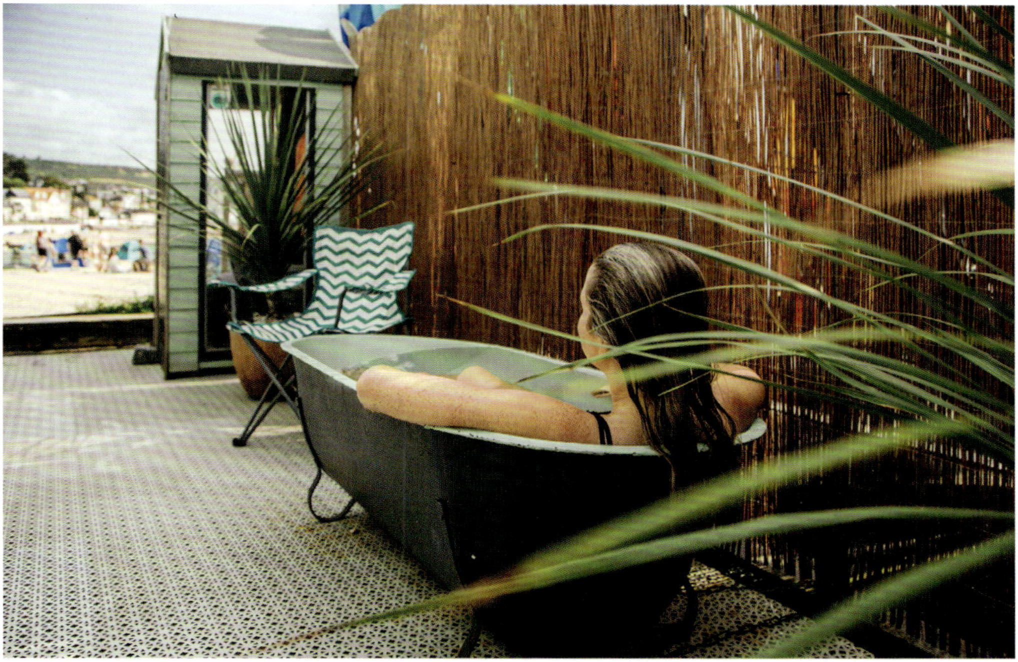

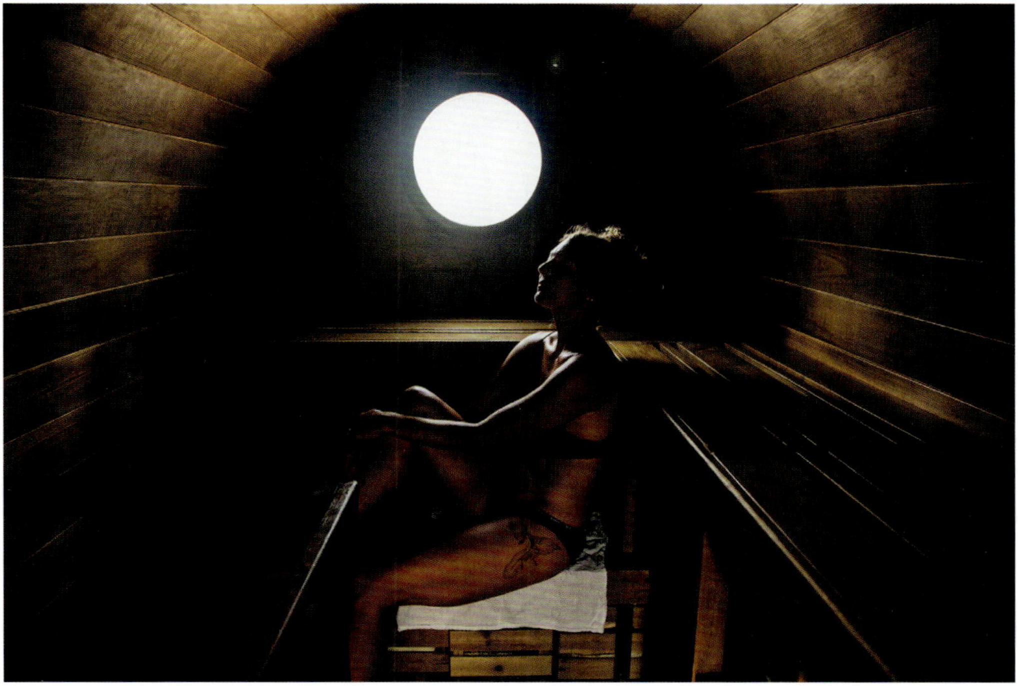

18

Seaside Sauna Haus

SEATOWN ✤ DORSET

Seaside Sauna Haus sits just above the waves at Seatown Beach, yet another fossil-rich spot on the Jurassic Coast. Its founder, Sarah Higgins, is one of the OG beach box pioneers. She crowdfunded £5,000 for her sauna side hustle and a NatWest Bank business scheme put in the rest – and in 2020, she opened the sauna doors. At the time, Sarah had to operate within Covid-19 lockdown restrictions, offering saunas to bubbles and private groups of six. Nevertheless, her enterprise took off, and four years later, she was given a 10-year lease. The sauna, along with the Anchor Inn, is now a fixture on the beach and offers both communal sessions and private hire, and Sarah also runs a popular sauna club. She used to be a social worker at HMP Portland, a line of work that also encouraged people to be seen for who they are and to reduce isolation and stigma.

seasidesaunahaus.co.uk
Sea 50.7223, -2.8228

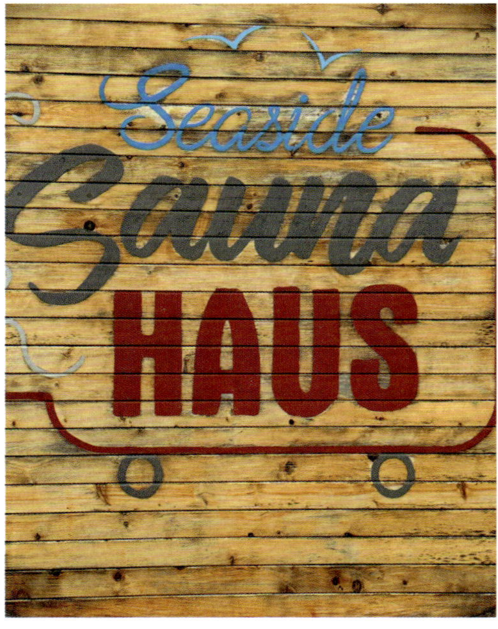

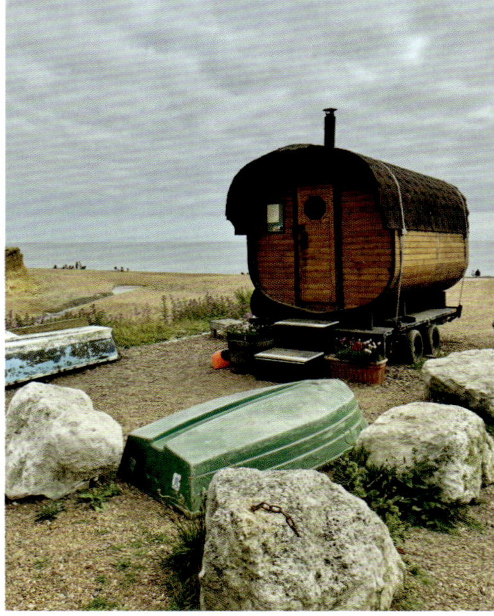

19

The Island Sauna

PORTLAND ❦ DORSET

There are not many saunas where you can see helicopters landing, dolphins feeding off moorings, old castles, a harbour and the Jurassic Coast all in one view, but The Island Sauna takes in all these sights. Sitting in a car park at Black Barge on the Isle of Portland, the sauna benefits from the sheltered clean waters of Portland harbour, which, when it was completed in 1872 for the British Navy, was the largest man-made harbour in the world. The Navy moved out in 1995, and the island is now home to the British Olympic sailing team and draws outdoorsy types who are into water sports.

'This part of town was absolutely wild in its time,' says The Island Sauna founder Emma Carter. 'The castle area was thick with sailors and ladies of the night.' People are still clearly intrigued by the area's past, as sauna rituals involving Portland folklore and tales of the sea, stone and seals are hugely popular. Events, rituals, clubs and bespoke saunas are all on offer here.

theislandsauna.co.uk
Sea 50.5677, -2.4477

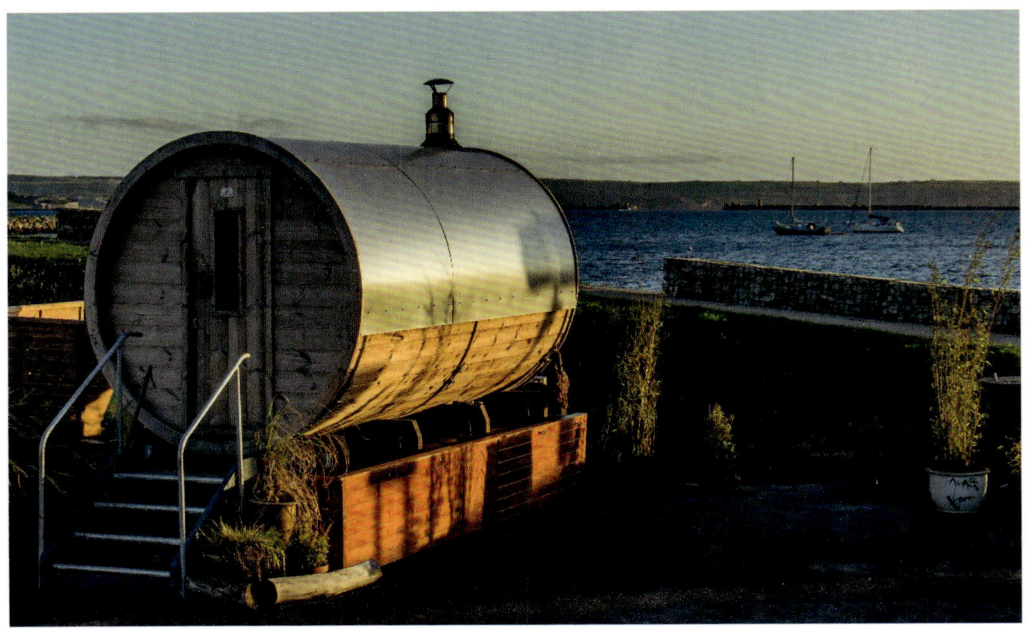

20

Revive Wild Sauna

PORTLAND & WEYMOUTH ❦ DORSET

It was a heated race to get the first floating sauna in the UK, and Revive Wild Sauna were the winners. The six-person barrel sauna at Portland Marina migrated off its temporary trailer location and onto a permanent floating pontoon in the autumn of 2024, and others are sure to follow. It sits next to a large, decked area with ladders into the sea and offers a plunge bath for those who don't fancy the salty option.

Portland Marina is the perfect spot; it sits behind its own breakwater so is accessible in all weather, and onshore facilities include the Salt pub-restaurant, free parking and toilets. Opening on the water was a dream come true for Katy and Alex who operate Revive saunas at various locations around Dorset, among them Bowleaze Cove in Weymouth. Both saunas draw local swim and community groups, and Bowleaze offers a subsidised mid-week wellbeing evening aimed at anyone having a tough week who thinks a sauna, cold plunge and company might help.

➡ revivewildsauna.co.uk
❄ Sea/cold plunge 📍 50.6364, -2.4230

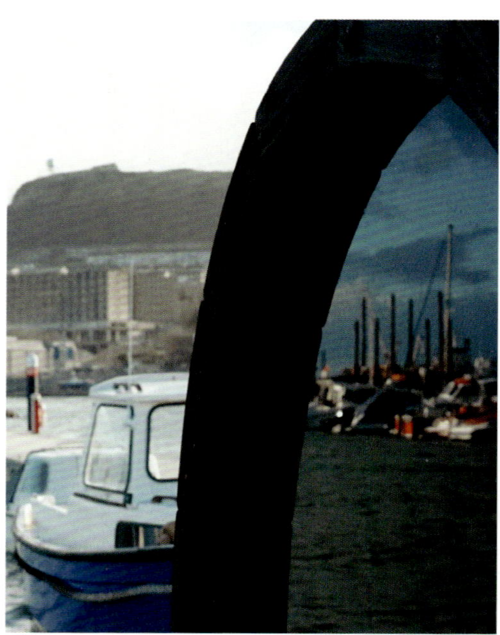

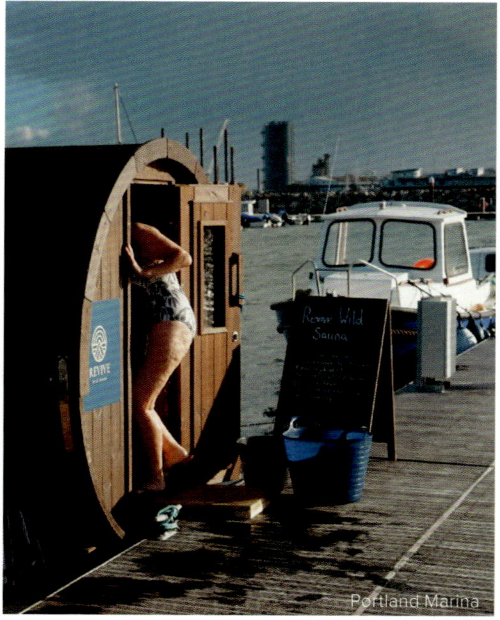

Portland Marina

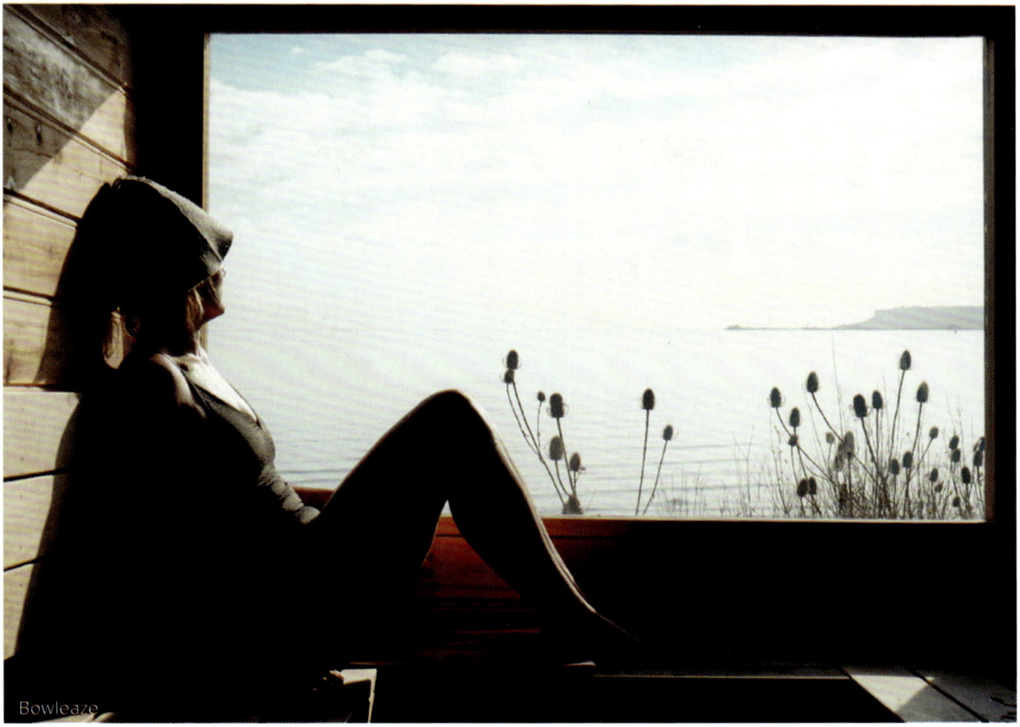

Bowleaze

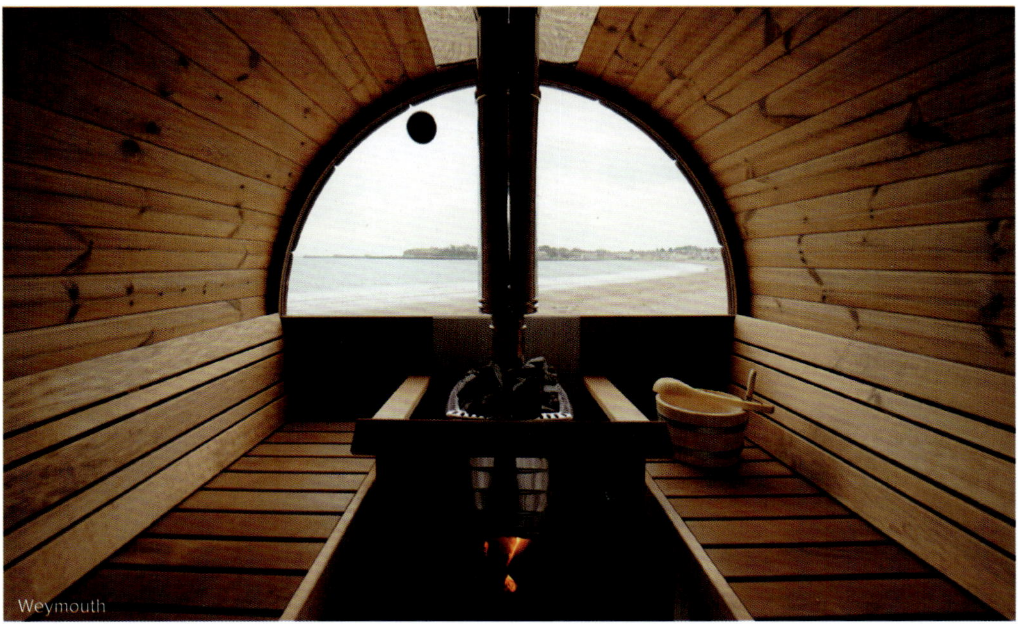

Weymouth

21

The Forest Sauna

WAREHAM ❦ DORSET

Nestled in an idyllic forest clearing, the setting of Happy River Retreat in Wareham on the Isle of Purbeck, the Forest Sauna certainly lives up to its name. When you arrive at Happy River you wouldn't know it was there; so tucked away is it. You pass a giant yurt, two cabins, a shepherd's hut and a Maker's Studio before signs pinned to trees guide you to the sauna.

It's everything a forest sauna should be: quiet, secluded and surrounded by birdsong. A back gate opens onto 15 square miles of lush forest, and walkers and mountain bikers are among those who come to bathe.

'Everything we do is about putting health back into your own hands, whether that's mental health, body health, soul health,' says Rachel Bright, who founded Happy River with her partner Robbie. The retreat is largely built from reclaimed materials, with conscious living, sustainability and connection with nature in mind. A biomass boiler heats the whole site, and guests stay in cabins and lodges surrounded by organic food gardens and an orchard.

The sauna is now a regular part of the yoga, meditation, breathwork and nutrition courses on offer at Happy River. But you don't have to be staying there to use it: in the summer, there are pop-up events involving meditation, massage or stargazing; early bird groups can book Sauna and Breakfast; and regular sauna and plunge enthusiasts can join the Forest Sauna Club, which gives members a guaranteed sauna slot every week.

➔ theforestsauna.com
❄ Tub plunges/shower 📍 50.7072, -2.1389

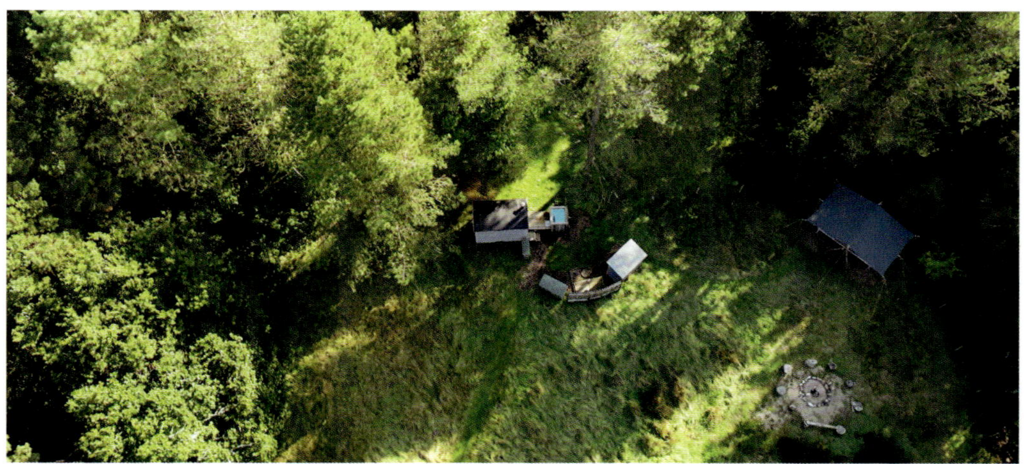

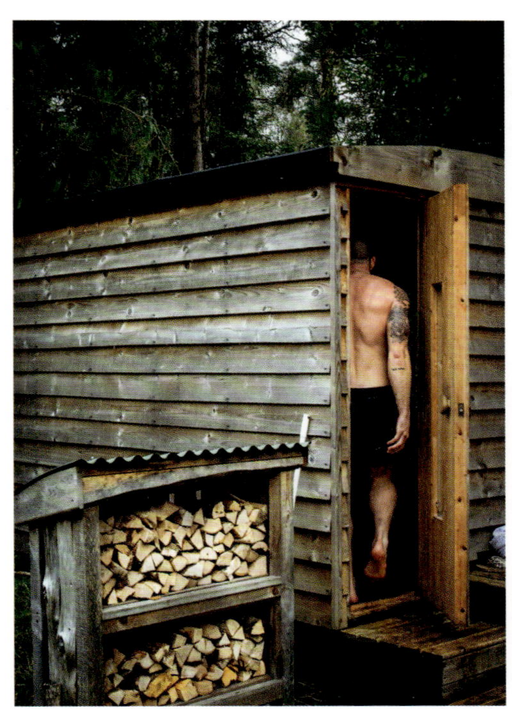
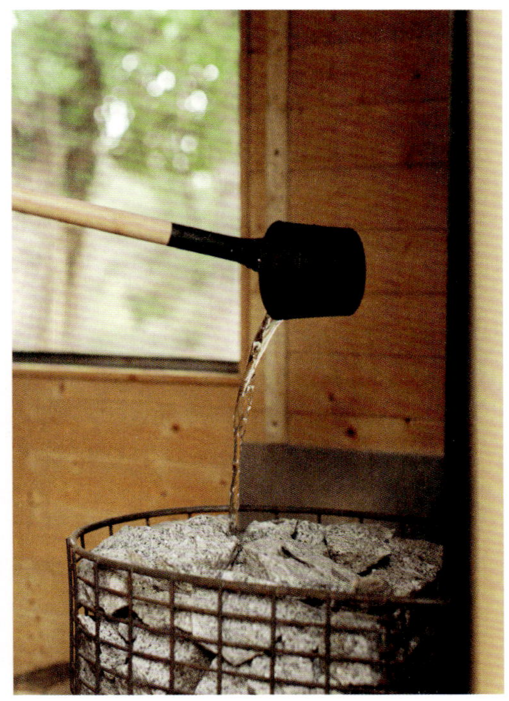
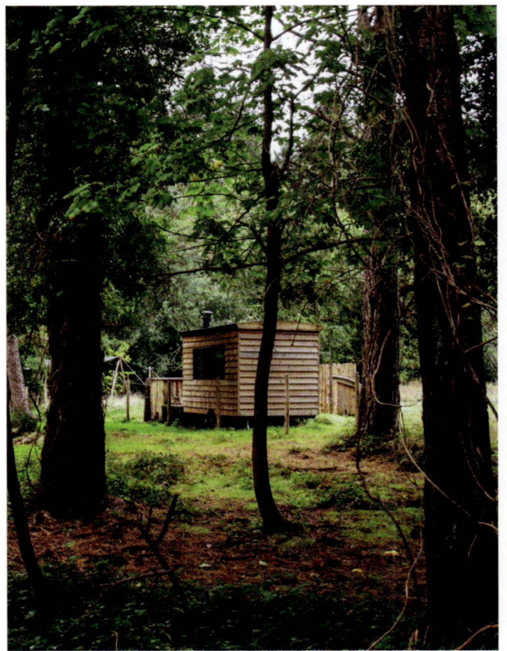
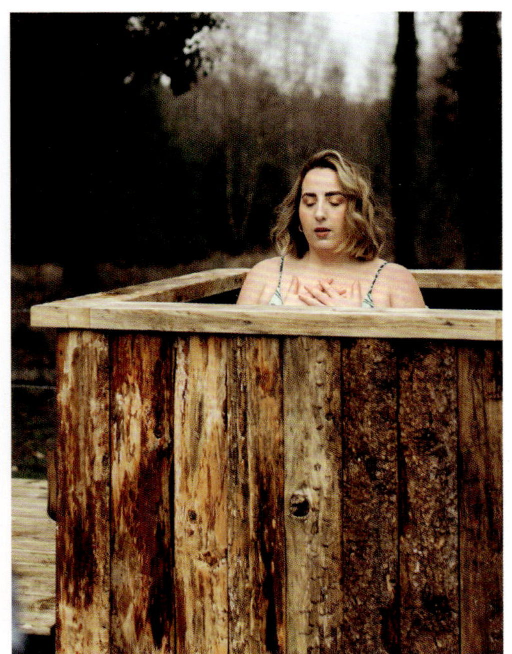

22

Studland Sauna Hut

SWANAGE ❦ DORSET

Studland Watersports has been running on Knoll Beach for 24 years, so there's not much its owners Tracey and Paul don't know about the tides, temperatures and people who come to relax and play on this iconic Dorset spot. Two saunas that echo the rustic aesthetics of Studland's famous beach huts nestle among the water-sport equipment – paddleboards, kayaks, windsurfs, dinghies, pedalos and more are all on offer. The National Trust owns all of Studland Bay, including Knoll Beach. While the bay is popular in every season, rough seas and bad weather meant that the water-sports business slowed down in winter; now, their two saunas have brought it to life all year round.

The first sauna appeared in 2020 as a Christmas pop-up. The sea swimmers loved it, especially at dawn when the sun rises over the sea and Old Harry Rocks take shape in the soft morning light. It was so popular that a second sauna quickly followed, built from wood reclaimed from the former Middle Beach Café, a much-loved beach spot that had to be pulled down before it fell into the sea due to coastal erosion. One sauna operates at 90°C, the other around 100°C; one accommodates six bathers, the other ten. While booking is recommended, occasionally you can walk up and the saunas will also be opened on request.

NB: Neighbouring Studland Beach may be one of the most famous naturist beaches in Britain, but, for now, swimwear in the sauna is mandatory.

studlandwatersports.co.uk
Sea 50.6515, -1.9532

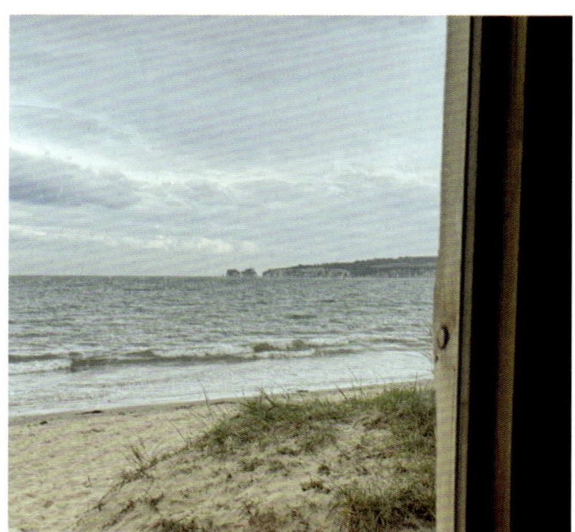

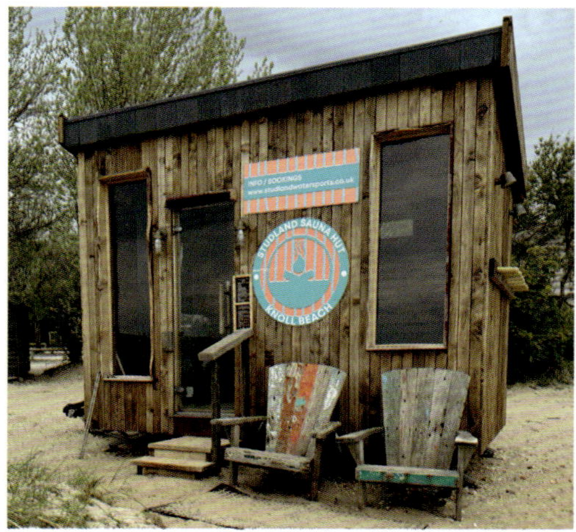

23

The Saltwater Sauna

SANDBANKS & CHRISTCHURCH ❦ DORSET

'As hard as getting tickets for Glastonbury' is how one local describes booking a session at The Saltwater Sauna in Sandbanks. This early adopter opened in lockdown and hasn't looked back. In 2024, it won best design at the inaugural British Sauna Society Awards for its striking aesthetics created by Heartwood Saunas, and its resident sauna therapist, Jane Witt, also scooped the prize for best sauna practitioner.

Despite the accolades, Saltwater's founders, Arlene and Sam, are not resting on their laurels, rather, they are determined to bring authentic, high-quality sauna to the UK. As a cold swimmer, surfer and most importantly, a Finn, sauna is part of Arlene's DNA. She runs sauna retreats to Finland, but they have also opened a local sister Saltwater Sauna at Avon Beach in Christchurch. Avon offers two seven-seater saunas with a view of the Isle of Wight and changing rooms. Meanwhile, there are bigger, better plans for Sandbanks, and a new location at Lulworth Cove is in the pipeline.

- thesaltwatersauna.com
- Sea/shower
- 50.6901, -1.9361 Sandbanks
- 50.7300, -1.7334 Avon Beach, Christchurch

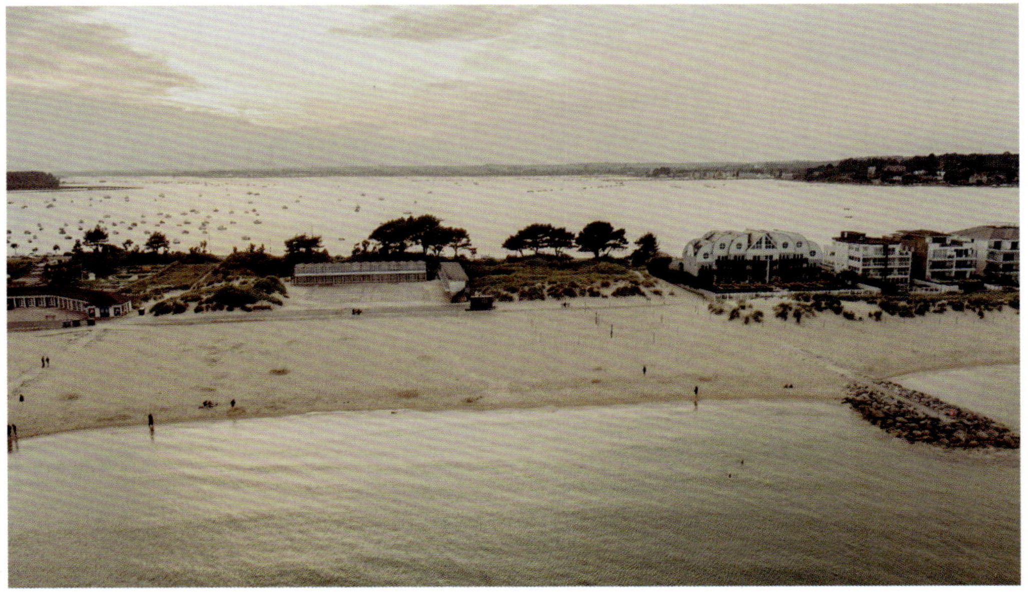

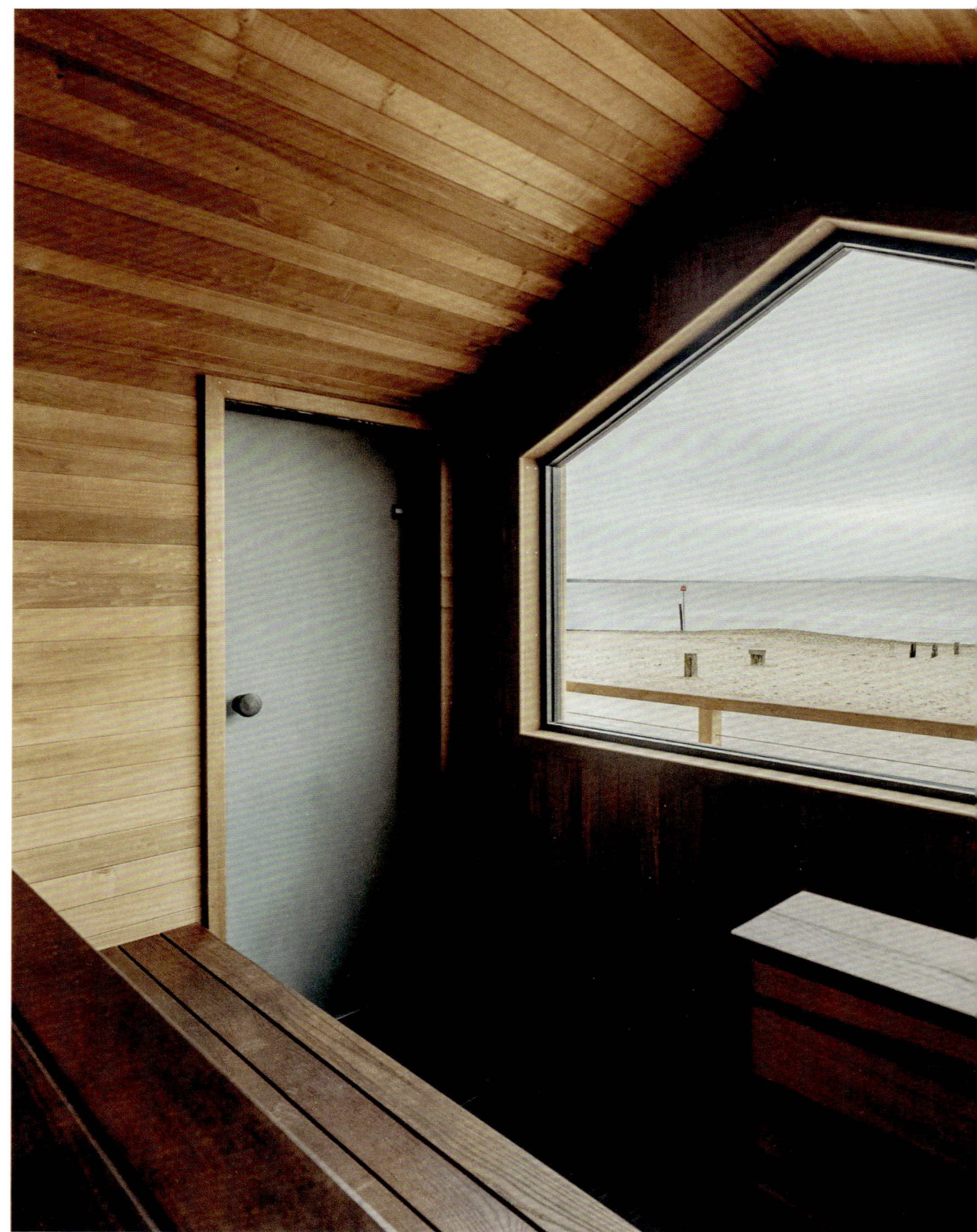

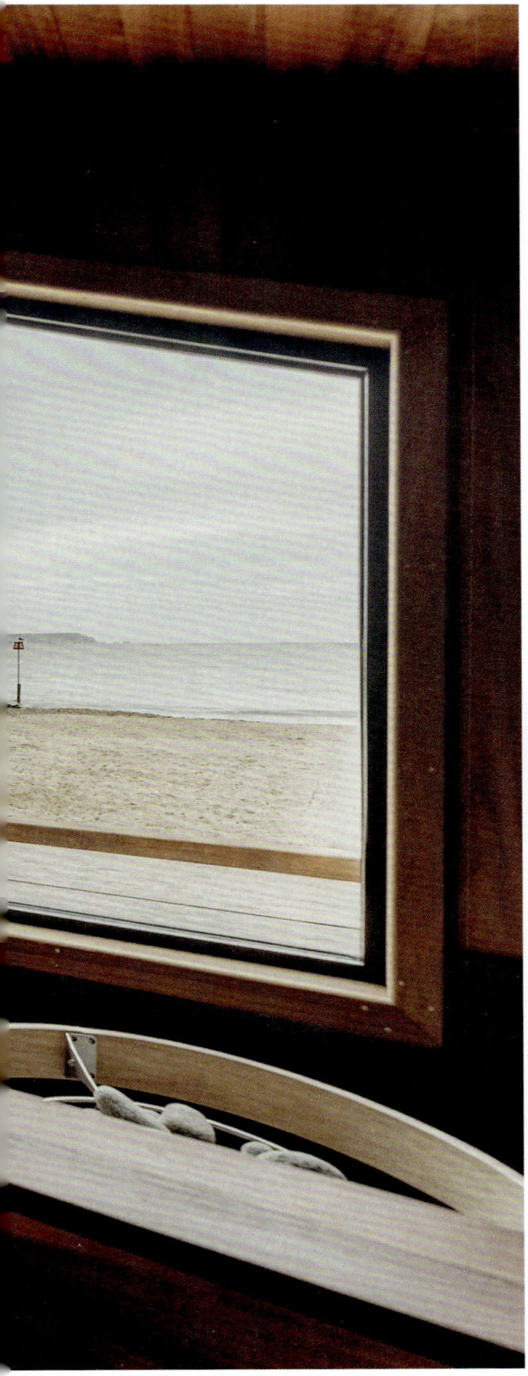

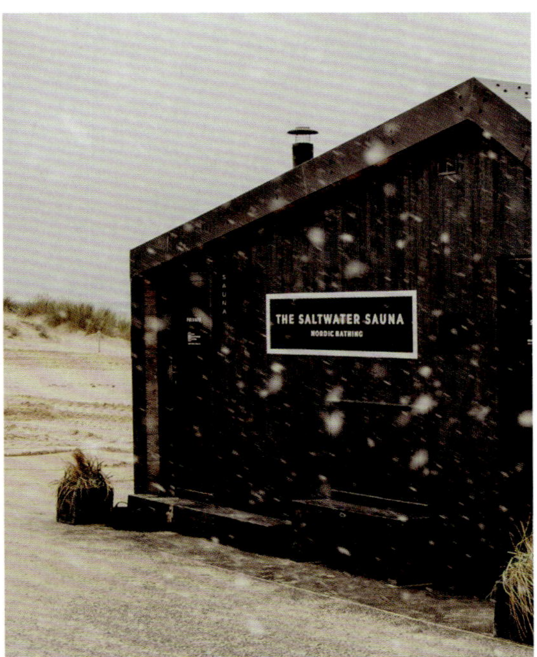

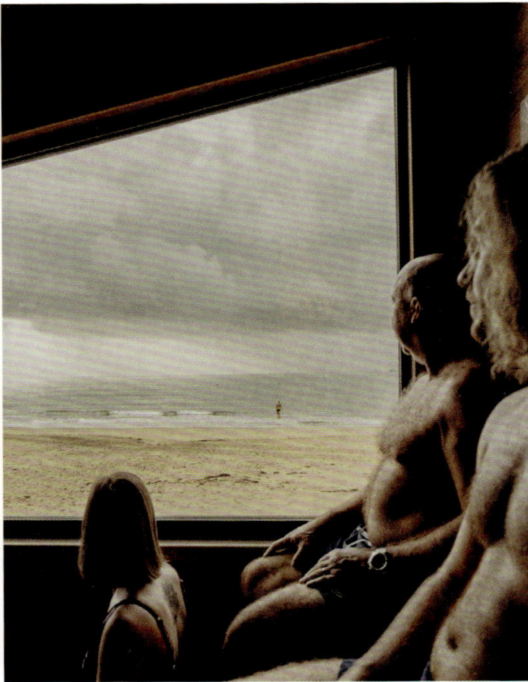

The Saltwater Sauna

24

Orchard Sauna

BEDMINSTER ❦ BRISTOL

When Bristol resident and winter swimmer Greg Moody saw saunas popping up on beaches, he left his corporate tech job behind and opened Orchard Sauna in Bristol. Located at Windmill Hill City Farm, a ten-minute walk from Bristol harbour, the sauna is surrounded by sheep and goats and sits in a beautiful city oasis. Greg imported an eight-seat barrel sauna from Lithuania and built his own cold plunge, hot and cold showers and changing rooms. Determined to overcome the challenges posed by tightening clean air restrictions, he chose an emission-free electric heater powered by a generator running on recycled vegetable oil. Windmill Hill City Farm is a charity and has a big following. The sauna hosts mostly communal and silent sauna sessions, though there are a limited number of private or group slots.

➔ orchardsauna.co.uk

❄ Cold plunge/shower 📍 51.4420, -2.5937

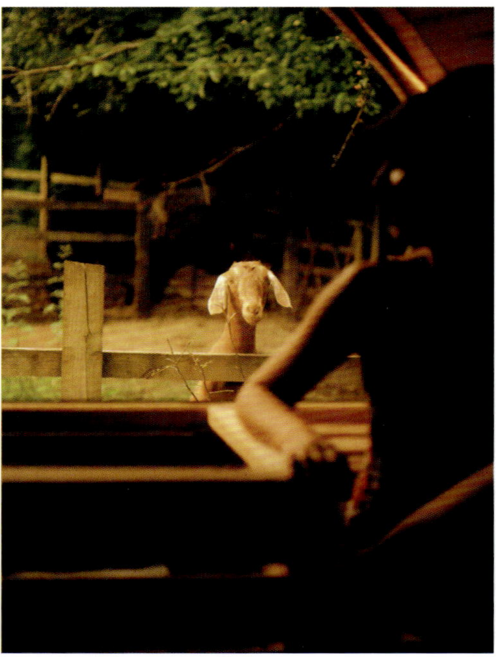

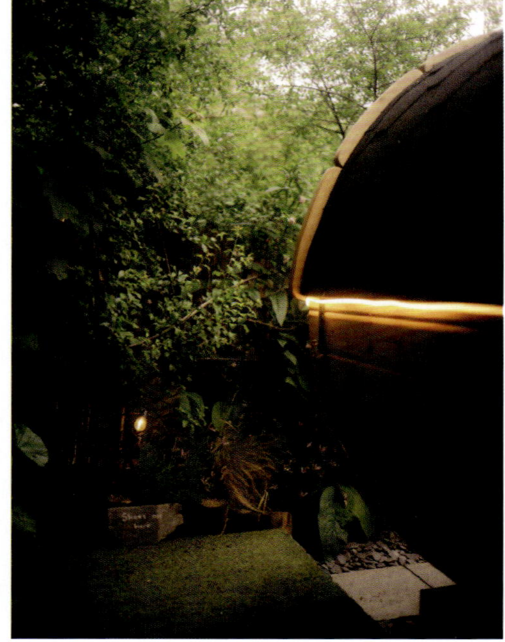

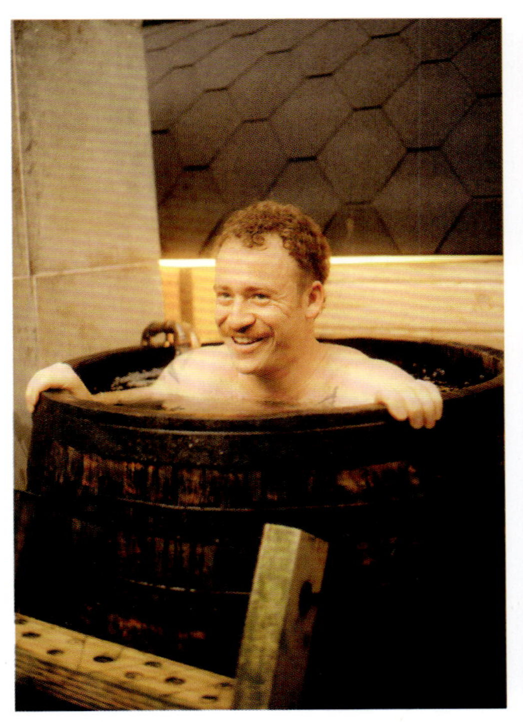

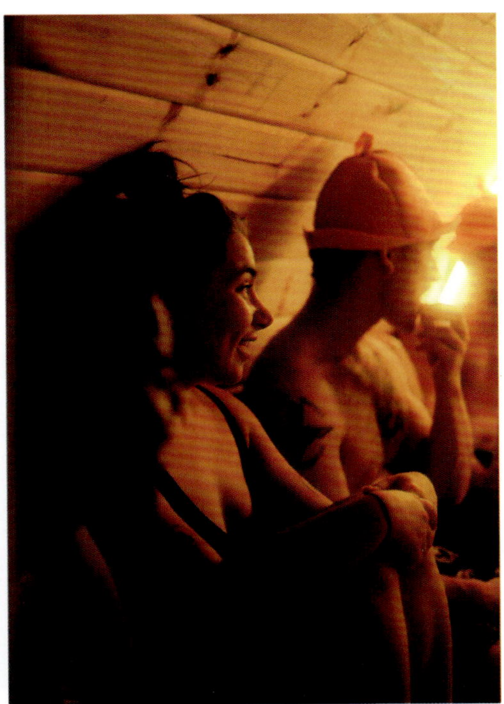

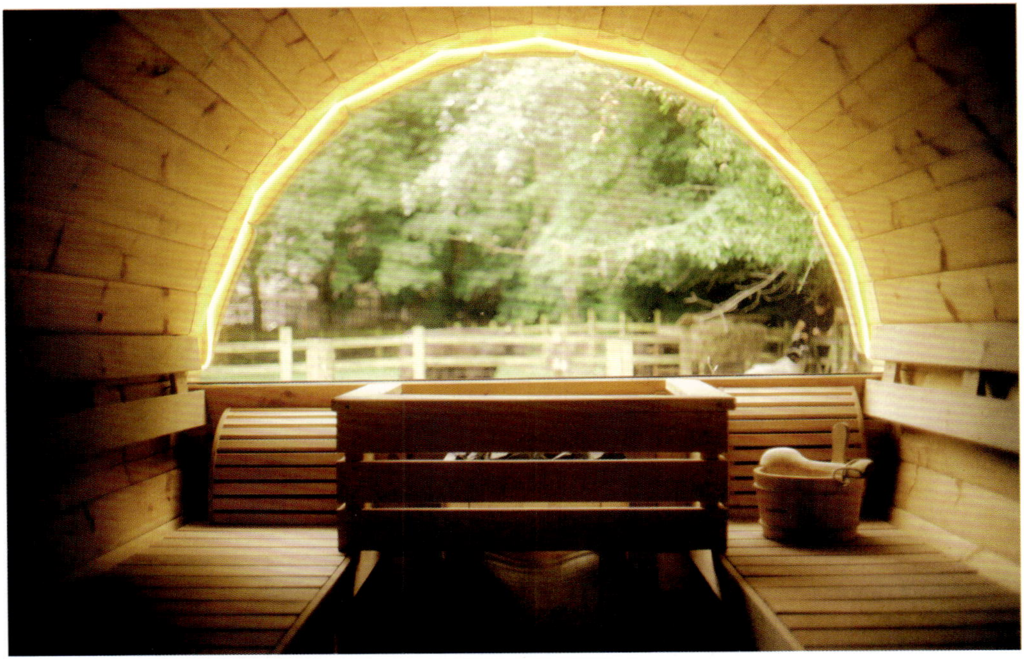

25

Bristol Community Sauna

BRISLINGTON ❦ BRISTOL

Nestled behind St Anne's House, a 1950s office block turned community hub in the heart of Bristol, you find a leafy oasis that is home to Bristol Community Sauna. A selection of electric saunas and cold plunges occupy a small but growing footprint in the back garden.

Copper-piped showers adorn the back wall of the primary sauna, which was designed with step-free access and extra wide doors with accessibility in mind.

As Bristol Community Sauna continues to grow, the key focus remains affordability and inclusivity. At £10 (£5 for members) per session, the goal is that sauna and plunge sessions become a part of visitors' weekly routine rather than a rare indulgence. The 75-minute sessions provide ample time for several rounds of contrast therapy, recuperation and stillness.

St Anne's House is owned and occupied by Bricks, a charity set up to support creative and social local enterprise initiatives, and Bristol Community Sauna is the latest addition to this thriving community hub. Other occupants include Bristol Cooperative Gym (one of the only member-owned gyms in the UK), a theatre rehearsal space, art studios, a pottery space, exhibition and therapy rooms, community-focused activities, and a community café. Two rooms are rented to GPs who plan to socially prescribe sauna for good health.

Bristol Community Sauna is a member of the newly launched Community Sauna Network. To date, the network has funded more than five sauna start-ups; it assists with costs and advises on operational aspects. Hot on the heels of Hackney, Bristol is certain to become a major sauna hub in the South West.

→ bristolcommunitysauna.org

❄ Cold plunge/shower 📍 51.4527, -2.5478

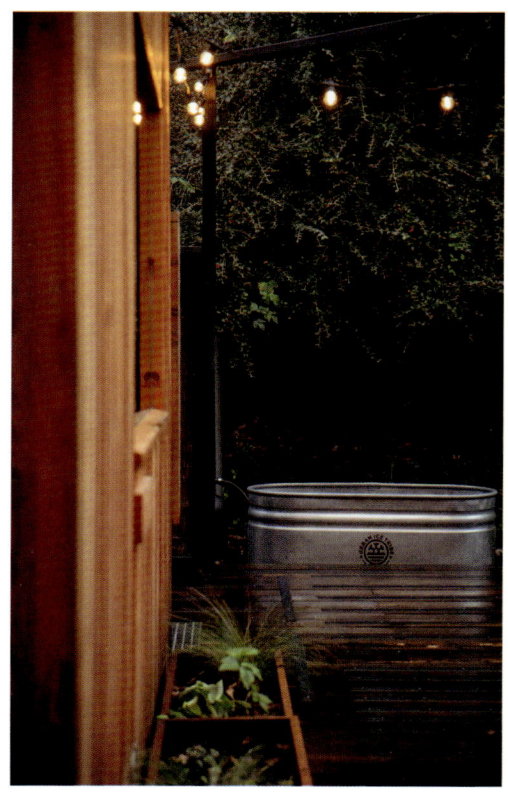

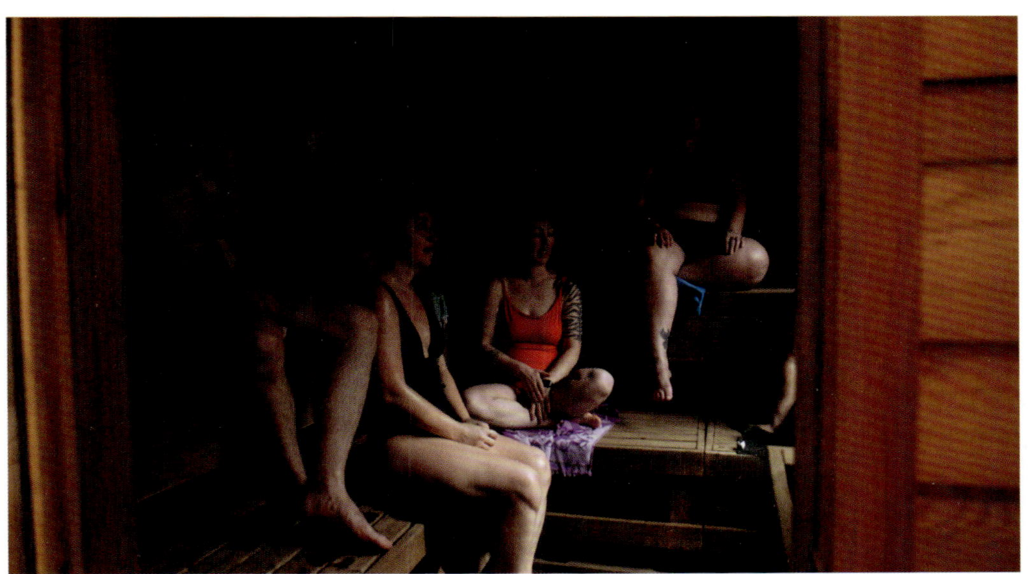

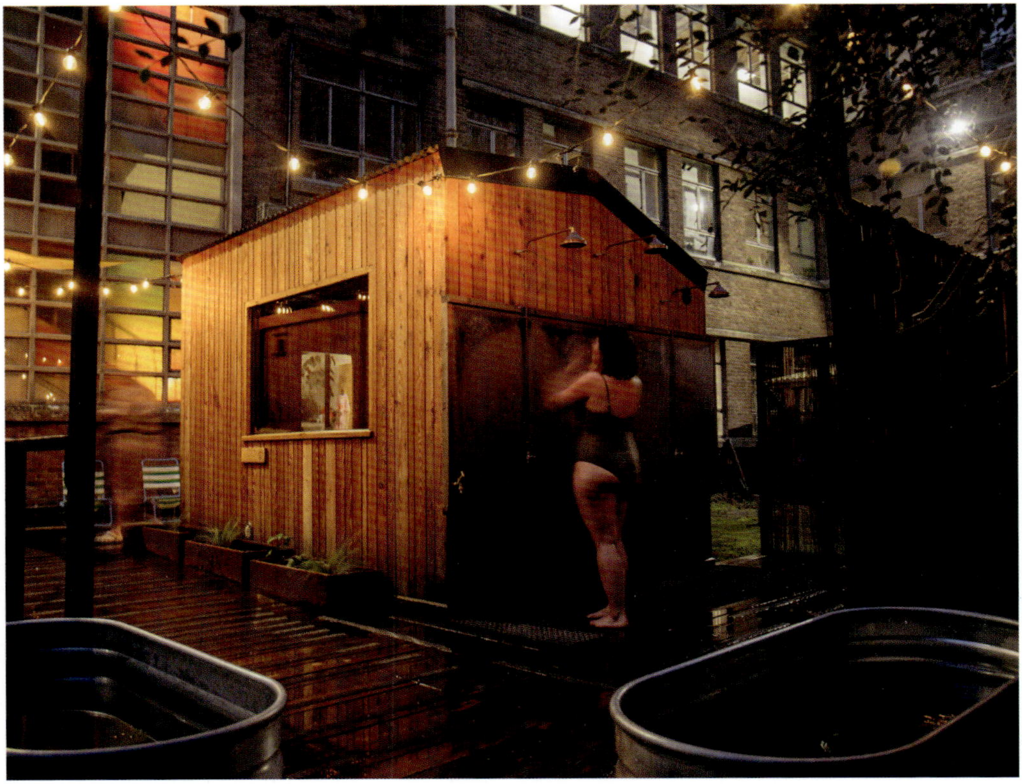

26

Campwell

WINSLEY ❦ WILTSHIRE

Tim Bowles is the fifth generation of Bowles at Campwell Farm in Somerset. Farming proper never really appealed to him, but as a nature lover, he found himself drawn to sharing his rural idyll, so he set up Campwell as an off-grid eco-camp. As co-founder of Ice-breakers, a men's health cold-swimming group operating in several locations, including Bath, Bristol, Brighton and London, Tim got into sauna on the beaches. He quickly became addicted.

Wellness has always been a part of his mission at Campwell Farm, and a large wood-fired sauna with contrasting ice dip and cold showers was an obvious addition to the site's facilities. Set away from the road and car park, the wild spa has a gentle, bucolic, luxury feel – with a generous changing area and outdoor space for relaxation.

There is now a second woodland sauna at Tim's sister eco-camp at Campwell Woods, which is available for camp guests during spring and summer and for private bookings out of season. Both saunas were built by Sauna Craft, and are available for private bookings, community sessions, silent sauna and women-only sessions.

campwell.co.uk

Cold plunge/shower 51.3492, -2.2915

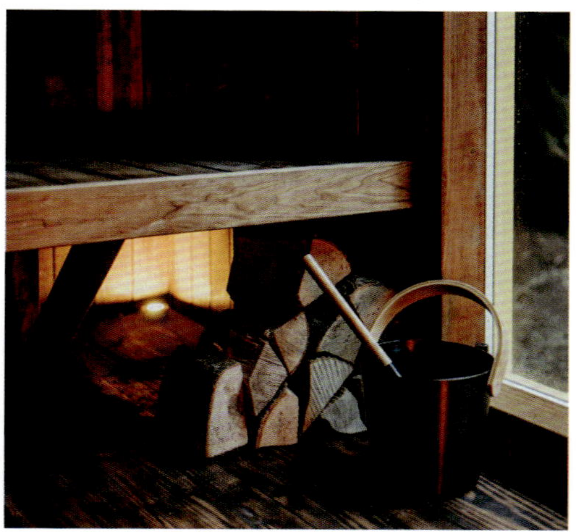

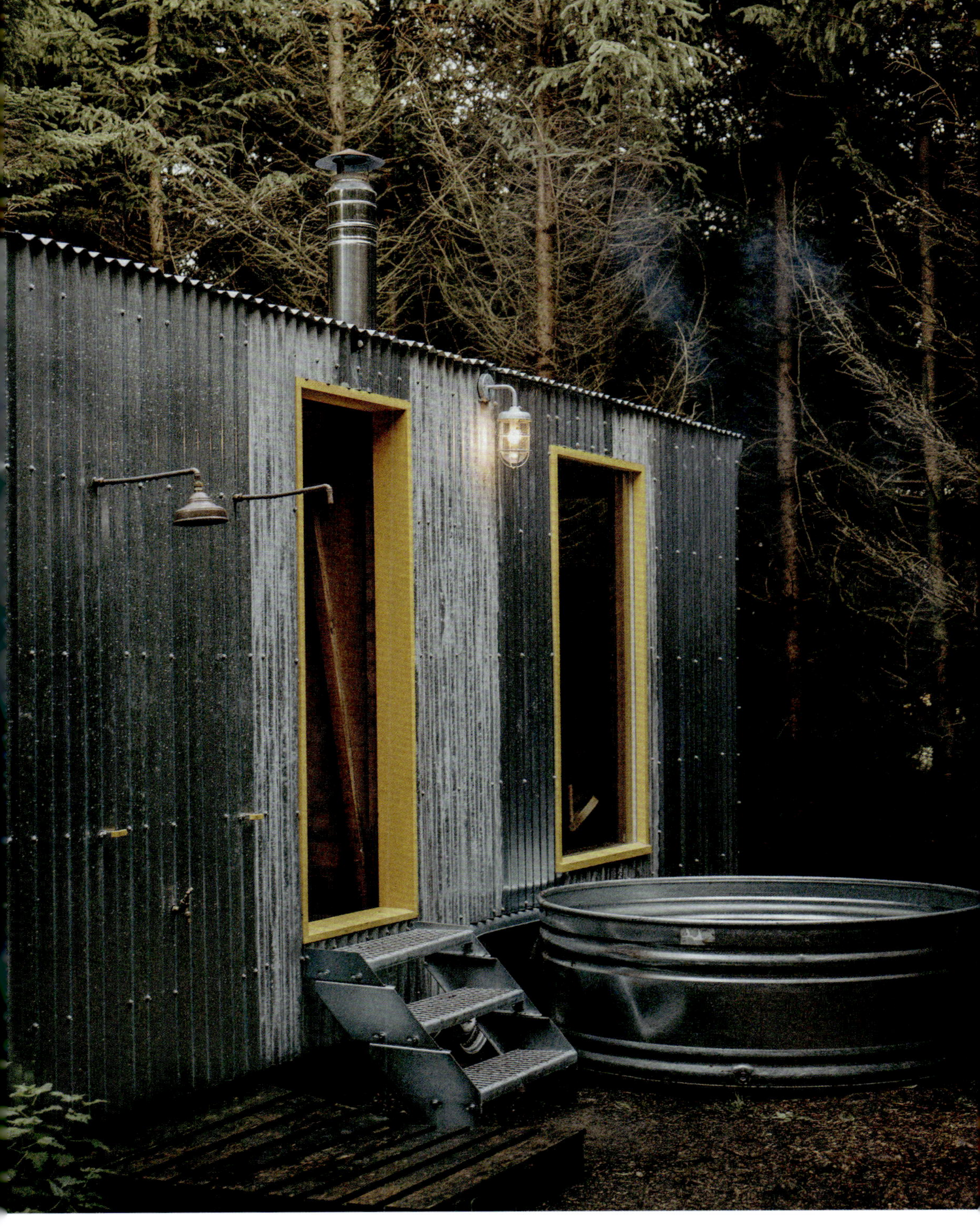

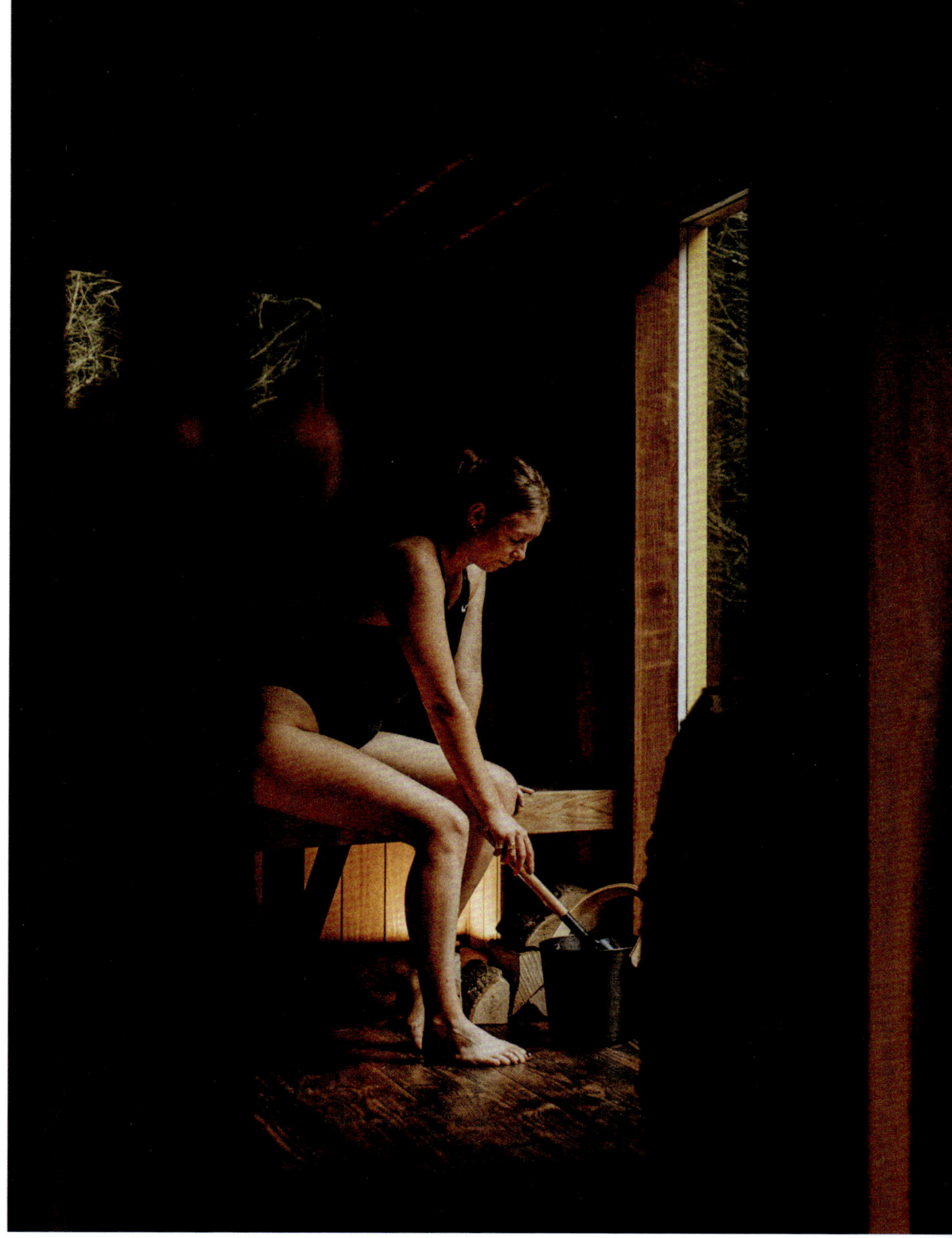

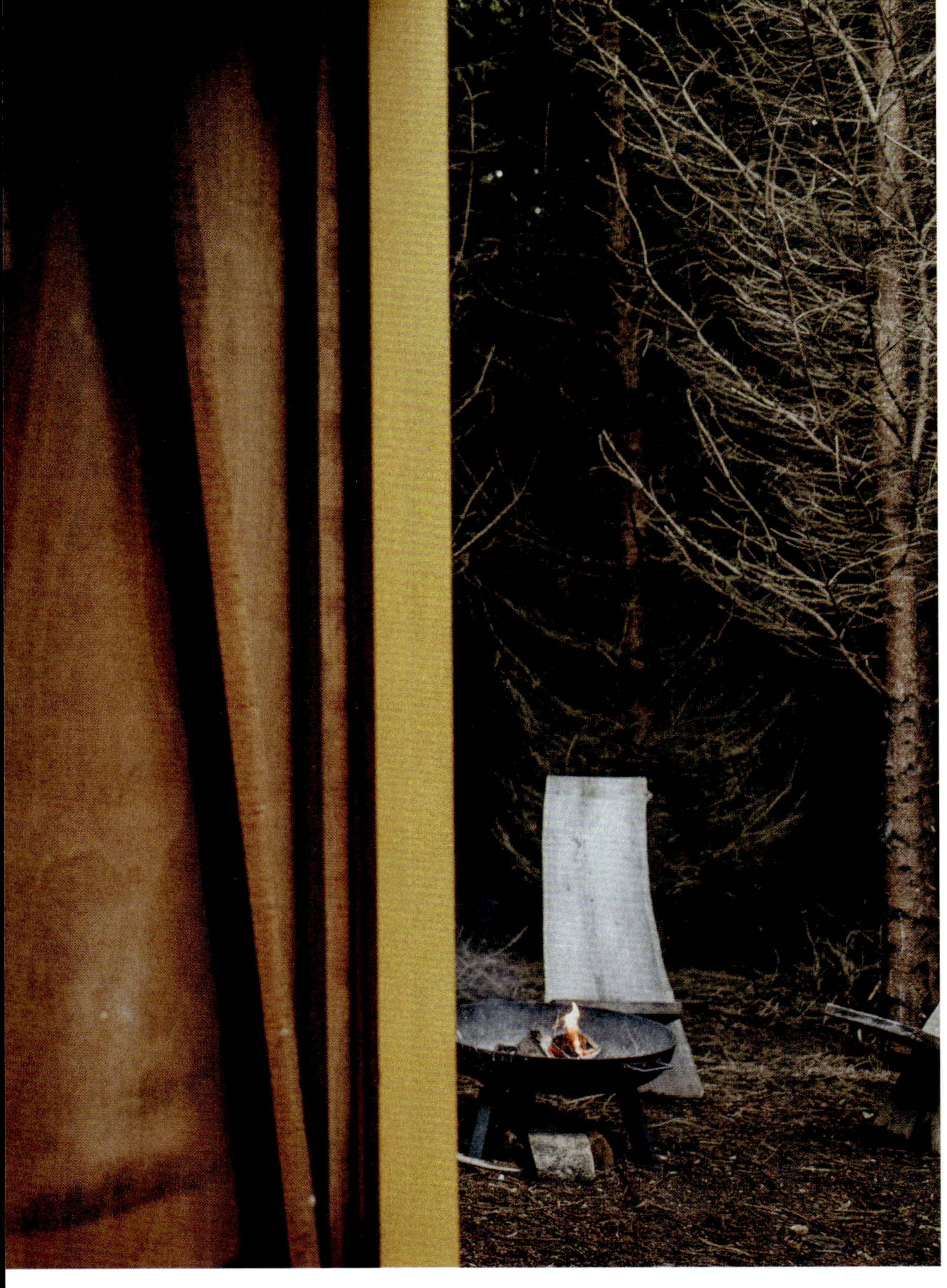

27

Scenic Sauna

NORTHLEACH ❦ GLOUCESTERSHIRE

Taking its cues from forest bathing, Scenic Sauna sits among tall conifers and overlooks the rolling fields of the Cotswolds. A sauna, temperature-controlled ice bath, relaxation areas and changing rooms, as well as weekly yoga and breathwork classes, allow for a nature hit and contrast therapy.

The focus here is very much on health. Founder Jamie Christopherson is a trained Wim Hof instructor, and his wife, Olivia Burgess, is an osteopath and yoga teacher. Both have suffered from serious autoimmune issues (see *Jamie's Story* overleaf), and recovered using many of the treatments now on offer at Scenic Sauna. Their health journeys inform the spa's ethos, and they welcome everyone from those with poor mental health and autoimmune issues to addiction groups and athletes.

scenicsauna.co.uk
Ice bath 51.8162, -1.8608

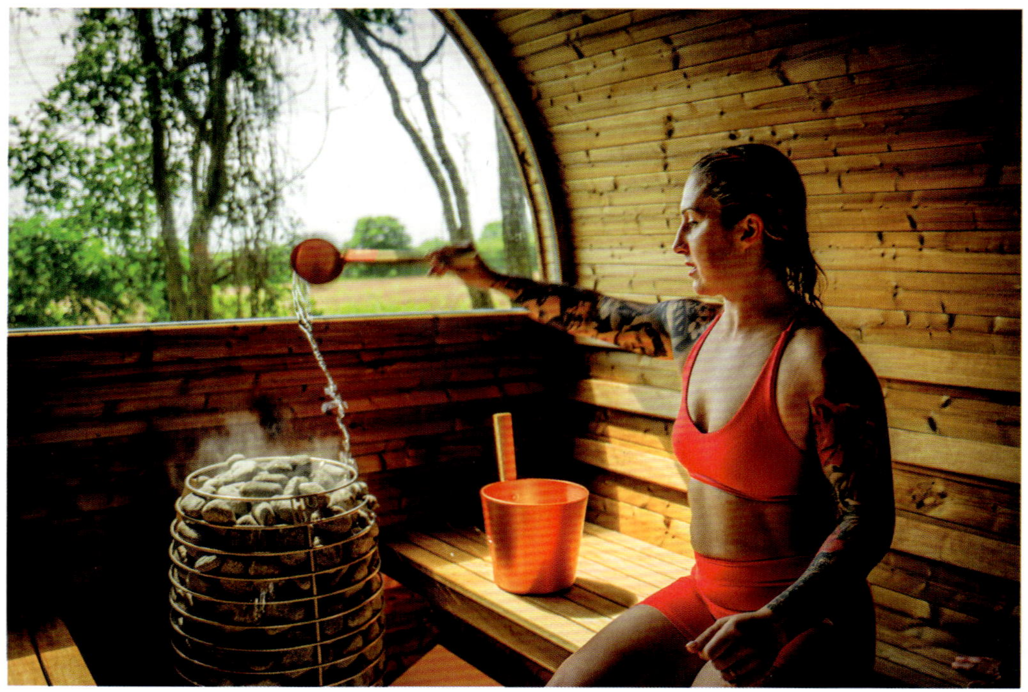

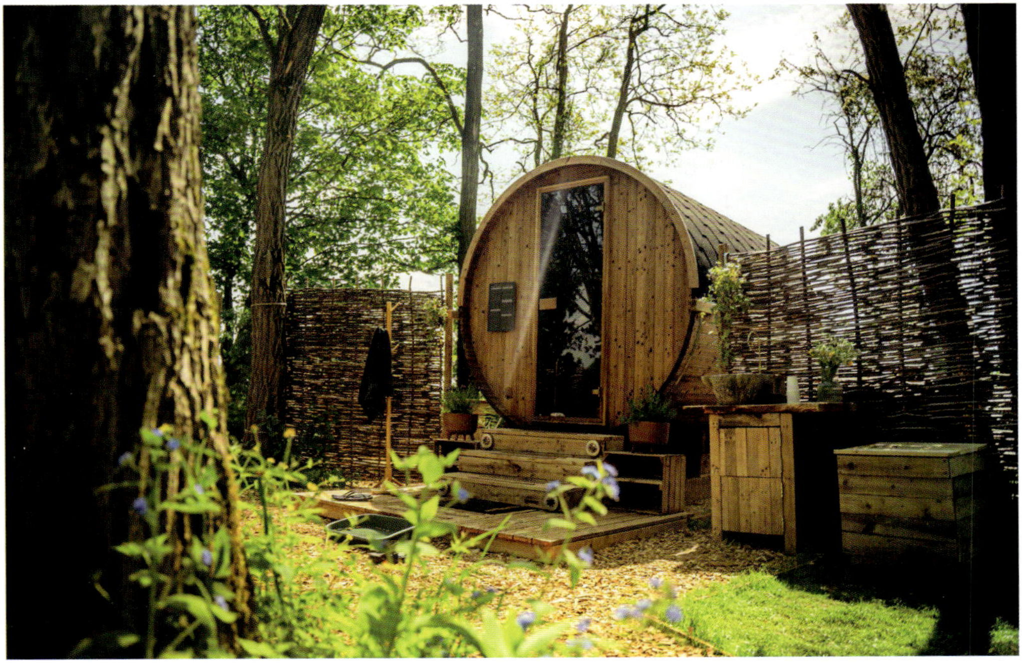

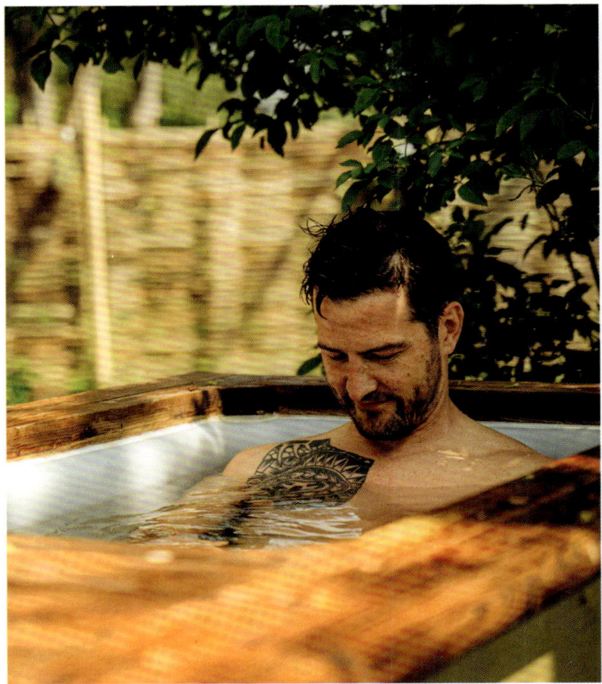

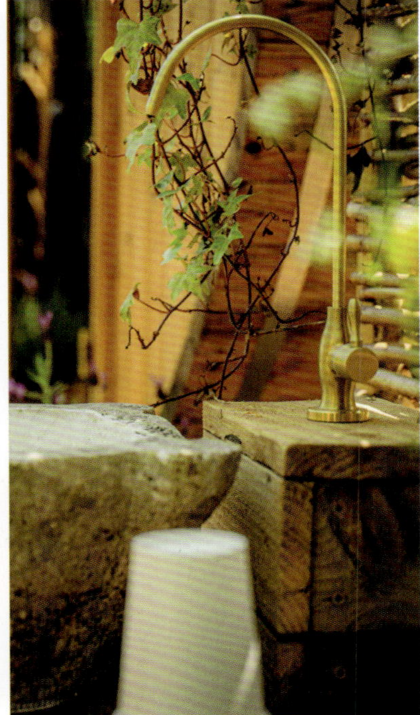

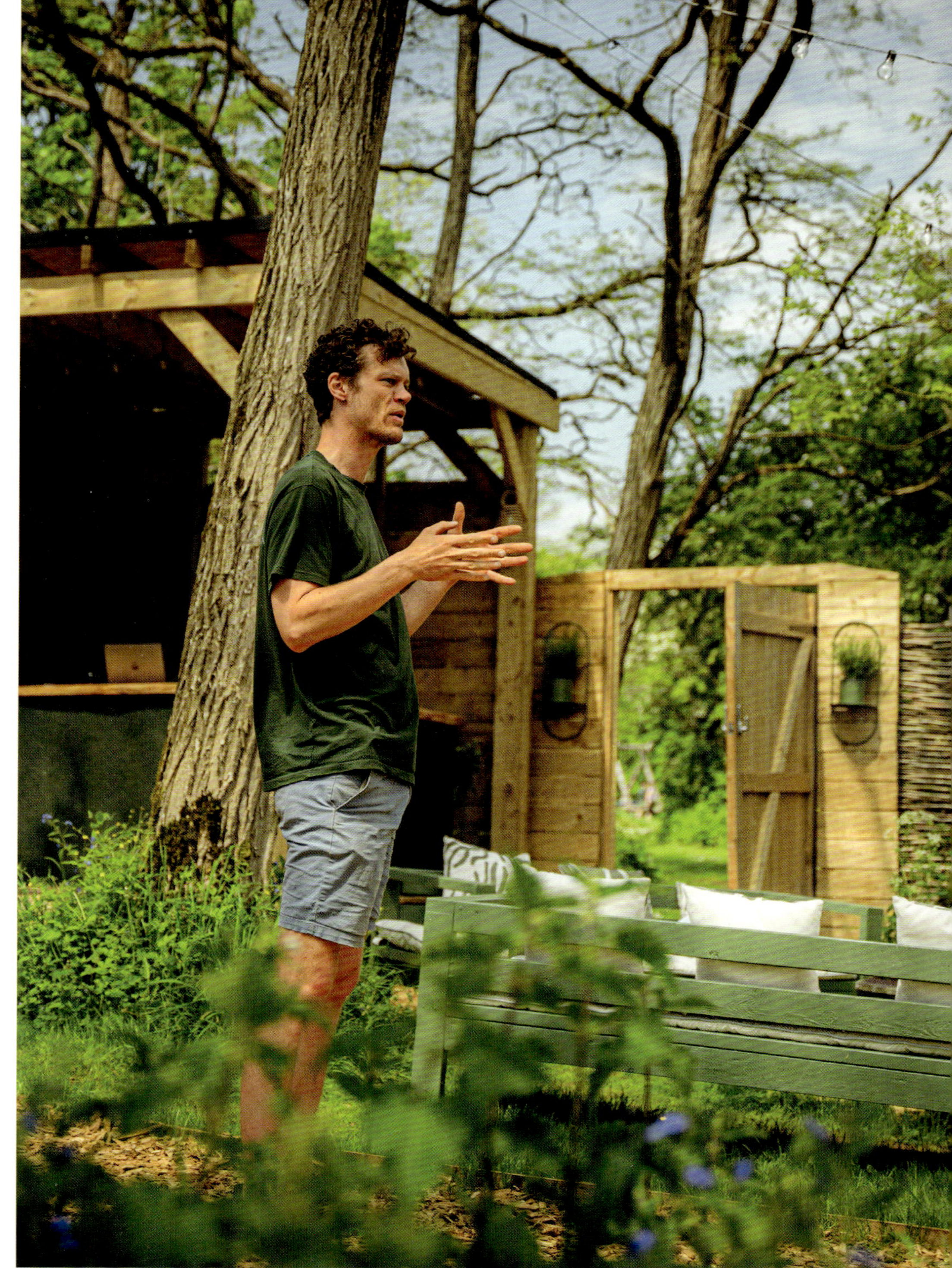

Jamie's Story

In 2024, Jamie Christopherson co-founded Scenic Sauna, a woodland wild spa in the Cotswolds. Over a sauna and an ice bath, he recounts his remarkable story from full-body paralysis to recovery.

'When I was 21, I developed Guillain-Barré Syndrome or GBS – a condition where the immune system attacks the nervous system, resulting in paralysis. Around 80 per cent of people recover, around 20 per cent might stay severely paralysed and 5 per cent may die. I was lying in a ward, and I had no feeling or movement from the waist down; the doctors told me there was no known cause and no known cure. When the left side of my face also became paralysed, I had a crisis of self. I thought, "Now I'm not me anymore. I'm worthless." In that state, I made a choice to stop living in what I thought I was and instead live in the future of what I was going to be. I decided I was going to be the most well I had ever been.

'I was moved to a neurological rehabilitation facility, where I embarked on a programme of nutritional, physiological and occupational therapy; I had to try and teach myself to move again, to stand and balance. They had me making breakfast, sitting at a computer, other normal things that you'd have to do in life, to re-establish the neural pathways needed to recover and achieve my goal. You have to work at it, to reignite those pathways, otherwise your ability to fire those signals diminishes.

'Once I was discharged, I could walk – but it was conscious, not natural, behaviour. Physical and mental fatigue meant I could do maybe one thing a day, like walk to the fridge, before having to rest for a few hours. Seven years later, with nutrition, exercise, and meditation, I was on half the dose of medication I left the hospital with, and I could do three things in a day before it was all too much. But then my progress stopped.

'I came across a video of a man in his sixties in the US with GBS who was sitting in an ice bath and practising the Wim Hof Method®. He said he no longer took medication, he had energy and felt great.

'I'd never had an ice bath or swum in cold water. I cried when I first went in; the pain in the nerves of my lower legs was horrendous. But after a year of ice baths and practising the Wim Hof Method breathing technique and meditation daily, along with everything else I was doing, I was able to come off *all* medication and even started running half marathons. I have not taken my medication since.

'I became evangelical about the practice. I went to Poland to learn to teach the Wim Hof Method. At the training centre, there was a barrel sauna and a tub filled with ice water, and I learned about the combined benefits of doing hot and cold therapy.

American practitioner Dr Joe Dispenza uses neuroscience to track and report on what happens in the brain when we heal ourselves. He speaks about the black space we go into when we are deep in meditation or focus – about mind and body coherence. I found that space in the sauna! I hadn't found that in the ice; the cold is an exercise in divorcing yourself from your body's pain and the tendency to panic. But in the sauna, because I was there for so long, chanting and humming with 30 other people, I felt that space.

'The combination of hot and cold can take me into that space where I can visualise the future I want – and my body can follow. For me, it was revolutionary.'

28

Hot Haus

LA VALLETTE ❦ GUERNSEY

Since 1865, the La Vallette bathing pools in St Peter Port have provided safe, free sea swimming to everyone on the island of Guernsey – everyone, including eminent visitors such as the writer Victor Hugo and painter Pierre-Auguste Renoir. After years of neglect, in 2019, the pools were renovated and provided with new toilets, a café and an award-winning design. They are enjoyed by the thousands of wild swimmers who also congregate on Guernsey's 22 swimming beaches.

Among these swimmers is Kirstie Allen, founder of Hot Haus sauna. A former health and fitness consultant, Kirstie had worked in St Alban's where she used sauna for cardiovascular treatment. She got into cold-water swimming when she moved to Guernsey. She was granted a seven-year lease at La Vallette, and runs Hot Haus from a grassy verge opposite the pools. Views stretch to the tiny islands of Sark and Herm, and even Jersey on a good day. Private and community sessions are available, and Kirstie offers local mental health charities free sessions.

➔ hothaus.gg
Sea pools 49.4477, -2.5307

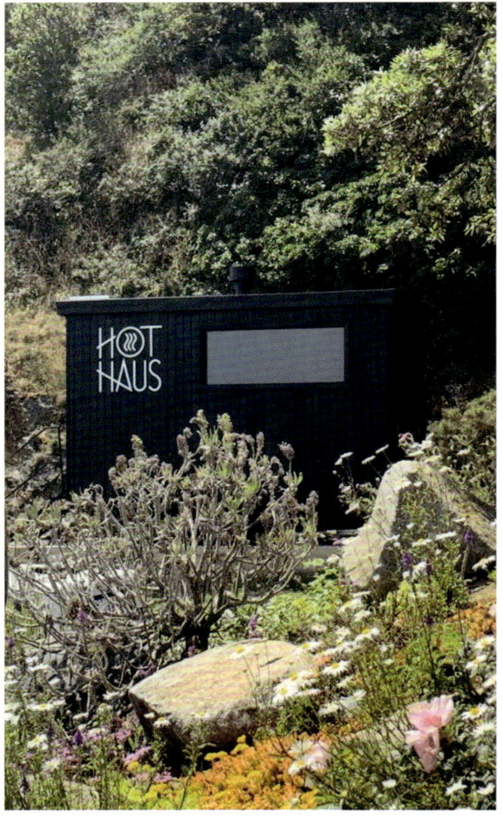

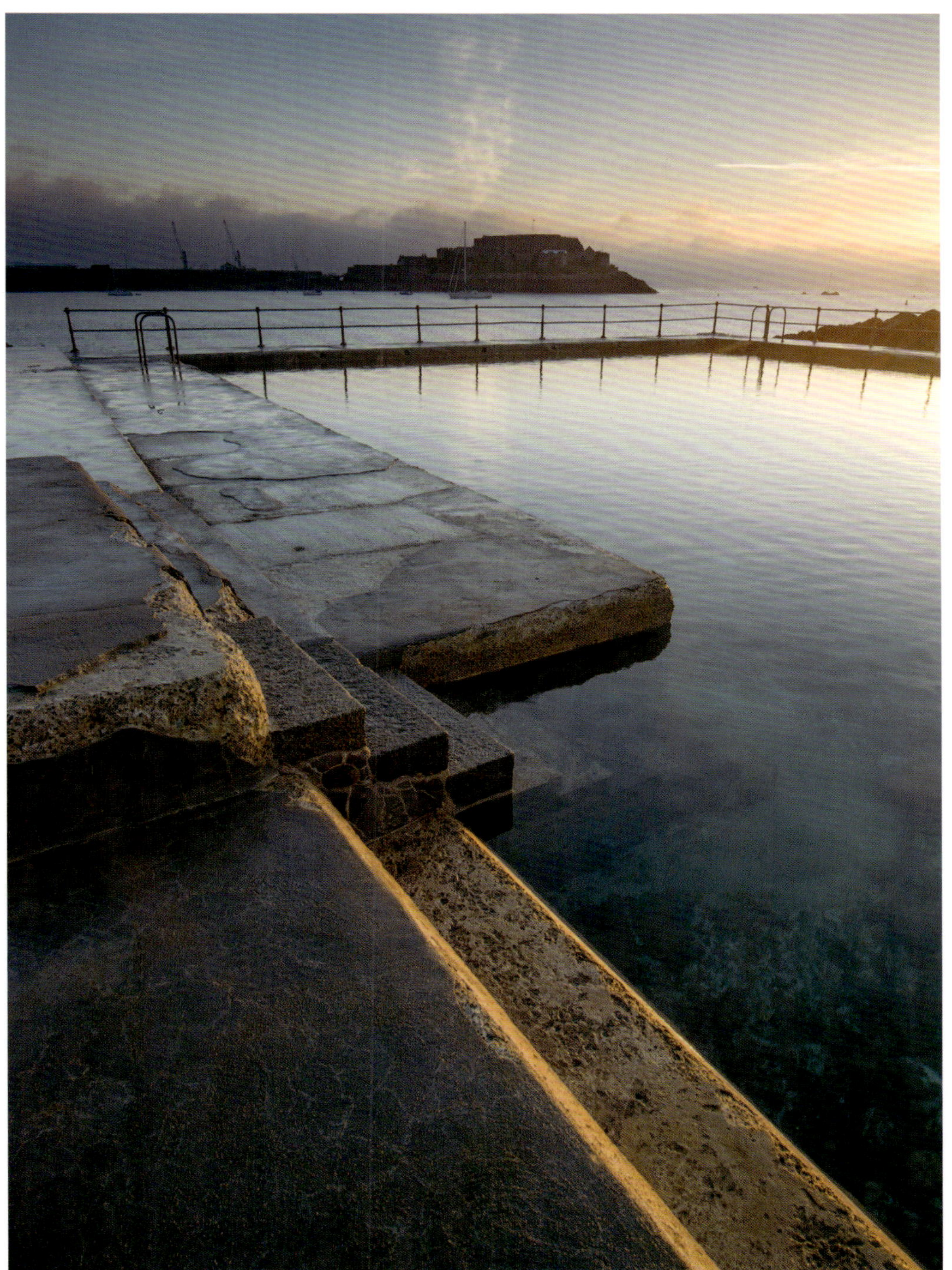

29

Sauna Society

ST CATHERINE'S ⚘ JERSEY

Jersey has the second largest tidal movement in the world, which means that at low tide it can be a 600-metre walk to the sea. This is why Sauna Society's location on the slipway at St Catherine's Bay is perfect – it's a one-minute walk to the water at low tide, and at high tide it's still easy and safe to get in. Founder Cole McLean got into sauna for post-exercise recovery; finding gym saunas to be below par, he went to the mainland and bought a wood-fired version from Wild Hut. Now Sauna Society has become just that – a society – where new arrivals to the island find friends, elderly ladies regularly meet for chats, and business deals are done. It's so popular, Cole is now planning a 'social wellness club' at the beach, with two saunas, six ice baths, seating and coffee. 'It's a healthy alternative to boozy nights out,' he says. 'I think it's the future.'

saunasociety.co.uk

Sea/shower/cold plunge 49.2242, -2.0203

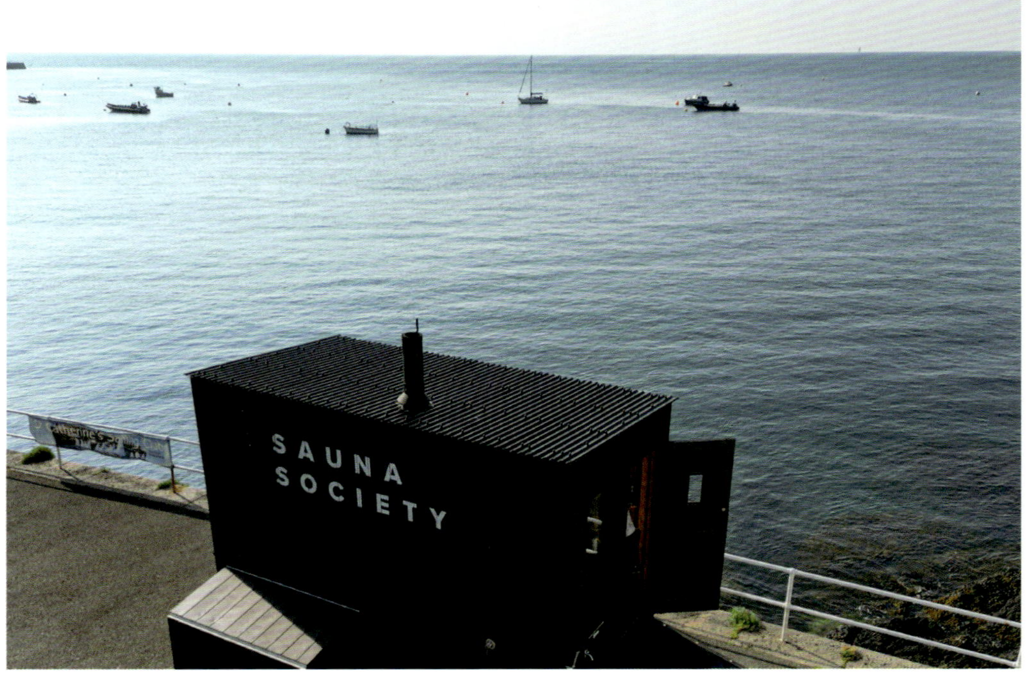

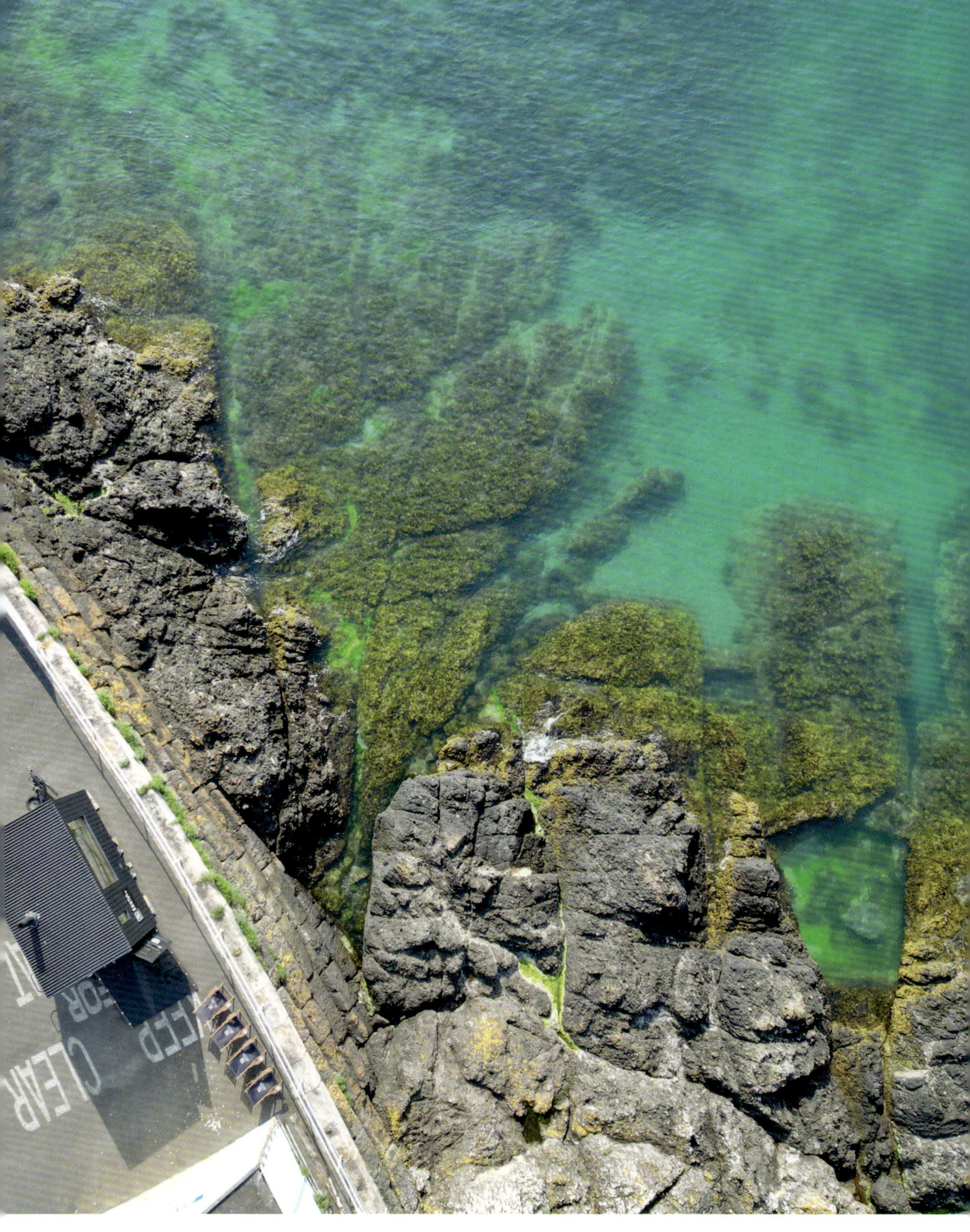
CLEAR

More

30 Adventure Scilly

ST MARY'S ❦ SCILLY ISLES

Nick and Bryony Lishman have brought a sauna to the Scilly Isles. They run the local Mincarlo guesthouse and Adventure Scilly, which provides sea swimming, trail running and a lot more. The sauna has easy access to the sea and a great view across Mincarlo Strand. Drench buckets are on hand for those who don't fancy the sea.

adventurescilly.co.uk
Sea/bucket 49.9166, -6.3117

31 Rising Embers Sauna

NEWLYN ❦ CORNWALL

Rising Embers sauna sits on Newlyn Green outside the Newlyn Art Gallery in Penzance. It has a community buzz, and women who've never even worn a swimsuit before rub shoulders with dawn swimmers and beach yogis. High tide is best for a swim, and a bucket provides a cool off at low tide.

Instagram.com/rising_embers_sauna
Sea/barrel/bucket. 50.1079, -5.5484

32 Dala Sauna

REDRUTH ❦ CORNWALL

Lee Malkin and Mati Ringrose offer informal three-hour sessions at full and new moons. You have to walk into their valley alongside a stream and cross a footbridge to find the sauna. There is a wonderful overhead coal scuttle water shower and an old bath cold plunge.

instagram.com/dala_sauna
Shower/bath 50.2325, -5.2474

33 Scorrier House

REDRUTH ❦ CORNWALL

Scorrier House is an events venue for weddings, festivals and corporate events, but the sauna (made from recycled woods from the estate) and pool can be booked by private groups for two-hour sessions. There is a shower next to the sauna.

scorrierhouse.co.uk
Shower/swimming pool 50.2497, -5.1923

34 Blackpool Sands Sauna

DARTMOUTH ❦ DEVON

A barrel sauna for four (five or six people can be accomodated for private bookings) with running water, changing rooms and water sports galore on stunning Blackpool Sands beach.

Seakayakdevon.co.uk/blackpool-sands-sauna
Sea/hose 50.3200, -3.6082

35 Sea Sauna

SAUNTON ❦ DEVON

This 12-man barrel sauna can be found on Saunton Beach every weekend, and runs communal sessions alongside surfing, sea swimming and yoga on this popular beach. The sauna is also available for private hire sessions throughout the week by appointment.

seasauna.co.uk
Sea 51.1172, -4.2213

36 South West Saunas

STAVERTON ❦ DEVON

After a long, gruelling search, Jake Rocking and Yussef Robinson finally found a spot for their wood-fired eight-seat sauna at Meadowfields Campsite in Staverton. Metal cold plunges, showers and changing rooms, sauna hats and free electrolytes complete the set up, and they collaborate with local practitioners to host aufguss, and sauna and massage sessions.

southwestsaunas.com
metal baths from Urban Ice Tribe
50.4588 -3.7366

37 Saunair

CULMSTOCK ✽ DEVON

Saunair mobile sauna has been popping up on beaches and at events since 2021. It is run by engineer Joni Sedgwick, and has been used at naturist events and even by the England Rugby team at training sessions. Two 100-year-old 'coffin baths' make for a 'comfortable' cold plunge.

saunair.co.uk
Coffin bath 50.9132, -3.2800

38 Duddlestone Farm

TAUNTON ✽ SOMERSET

The barrel sauna at Duddlestone Farm is run by farmer Ian Lewis. There is a lovely view across open farmland to the Blackdown Hills, and two whisky barrel cold plunges to cool down in. Lambs View, a holiday cottage on the farm, is available for those who want to make a weekend of it.

duddlestonefarm.co.uk
Barrel 50.9840, -3.0922

39 Drift:WOOD Sauna

CLEVEDON ✽ SOMERSET

Paul Kelly has long been involved with the sauna community, but the pandemic made him firm up his plans for Drift:WOOD. After a successful crowdfunding campaign, he converted a horsebox into his sauna and put it on Clevedon Marine Lake. Paul's ethos is very similiar to that of the lake, which is 'run by the community for the community'.

instagram.com/driftwood_mobile_sauna_uk
Marine Lake 51.4349, -2.8694

40 Suvi Sauna

CLEVEDON ✽ SOMERSET

A double-sided barrel sauna at Clevedon Marine Lake caters to the large groups of swimmers who enjoy the tidal pool, fed by the Bristol Channel, in all seasons. Suvi offers 60 and 30 minute slots and the Salthouse Bar & Restaurant provides the snacks.

suvisauna.as.me
Sea 51.4348, -2.8696

41 SiVo Wellness

BRISTOL ✽ SOMERSET

Harry Thacker is an English rugby union player who has long been into contrast therapy for post-exercise recovery. He runs a 'wellness garden' in Leigh Woods in Bristol, which features two saunas that can seat 20 at a time, along with cold plunges and a coffee shop. A separate horsebox sauna and chillers can be taken on the road for events.

sivowellness.com Tubs/ice bath/shower
51.4692, -2.6596

42 Ash Farm

STOURPAINE ✽ DORSET

For Ali Russell, camping has to be luxurious, so when she and her husband Adam decided to open some shepherd's hut accommodation, hot tubs and a sauna on their 120-acre deer farm in Dorset, no details were overlooked. The sauna is located in a shepherd's hut, along with a changing room, fridge and a snazzy cold shower that gives a 50-second blast of ice-cold water from the farm's borehole.

The sauna takes around 40 minutes to heat up – the same time as it takes to do the Antler Walk loop. The Farm's nature-soaked atmosphere and remote location a few miles up a gravel track appeals to people who like it simple, clean and stylish.

ashfarm.org/sauna-hut
Shower/hot tubs 50.8917, -2.1906

43 Swanage Bay Sauna

SWANAGE ✽ DORSET

On the promenade next to the sheltered, sandy beach and cool coffee spot Carve, sits Swanage Bay Sauna. It has a 10-seater sauna for private bookings and a communal sauna that holds six. Its owner, Tracey also runs Studland Sauna Hut and has a loyal following.

swanagebaysauna.co.uk
Sea 50.61113, -1.95765

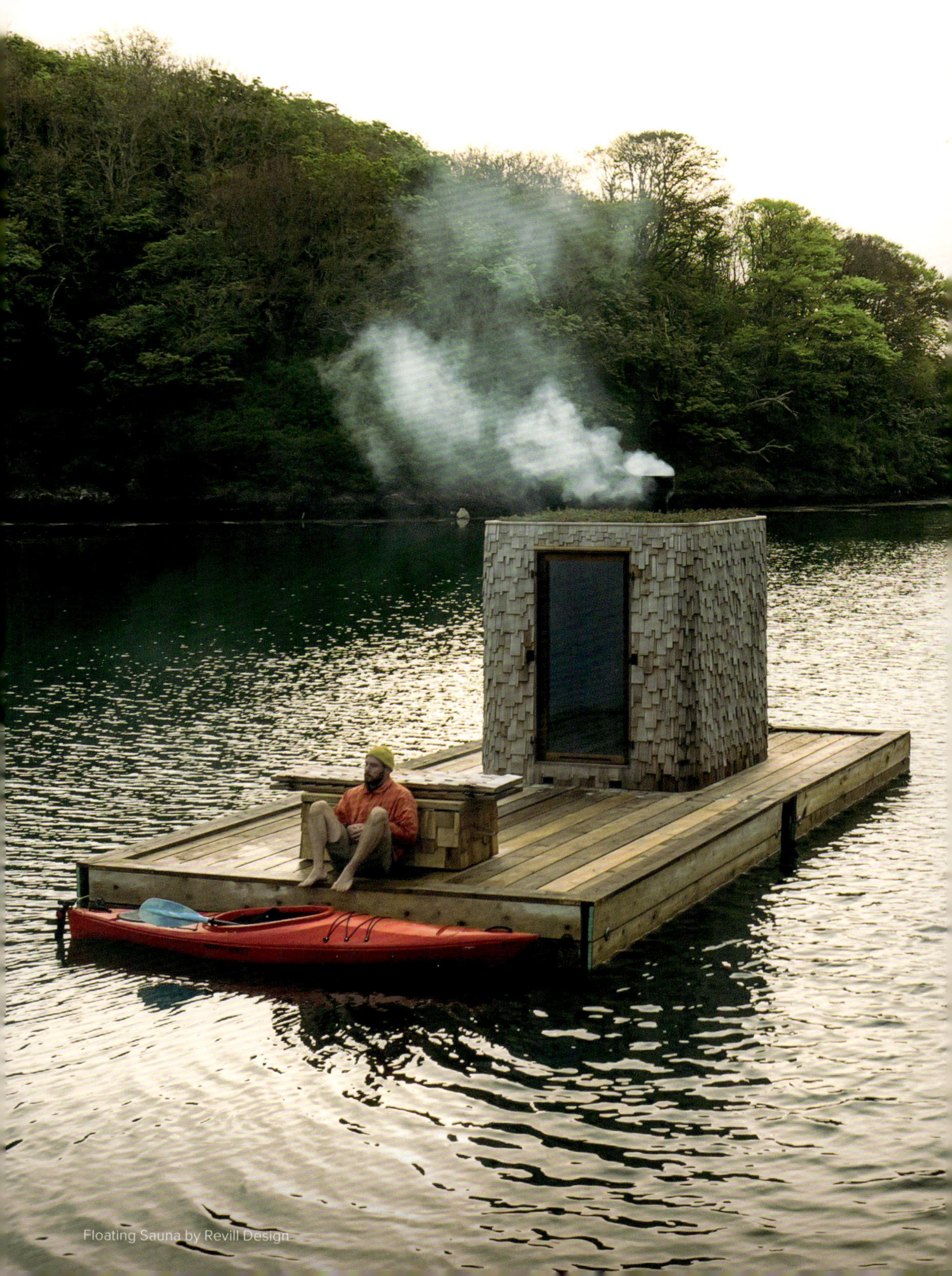

Floating Sauna by Revill Design

44 42 Acres

FROME ❀ SOMERSET

The Wild Weekends at eco-retreat 42 Acres include activities ranging from yoga and meditation to guided walks exploring wildlife, foraging and plant medicine, and swimming in a seven-acre lake. There's also a woodfired sauna and occasional sweatlodge ceremonies (see page 48). When it's not in use for group events for guests the woodland sauna can be booked for others.

42acres.com · Lake · 51.1424, -2.3577

45 Rambling Hearth Sauna

WARLEIGH WEIR ❀ SOMERSET

Oliver and Henry Hall make beautiful saunas at their company Sauna Craft. And they now have their own large mobile sauna, Rambling Hearth, which is available for private hire at events and festivals, and for community sessions at Warleigh Weir. There is a copper shower attached to the sauna, but they always try to pull up next to open water for dipping.

ramblinghearthsaunas.co.uk
Shower/river · 51.3770, -2.3006

46 Wiltshire Wild Sauna

SWINDON ❀ WILTSHIRE

Located at the off-grid Park Farm Campsite, Wiltshire Wild Sauna offers showers and compost toilets. The sauna is constructed from recycled and upcycled materials and features solar lighting.

It was created by sisters-in-law Zoë and Laura Rawlings. Laura's parents own Park Farm, a 300-acre organic dairy farm certified by the Soil Association. Both women understand the mental health challenges in farming and are collaborating with community groups and charities, including local farmers, to provide them with time off and foster a resilient community.

wiltshirewildsauna.co.uk
Shower/bath · 51.5787, -1.9443

47 Rockbox Sauna

VAZON ❀ GUERNSEY

After discovering wild sauna on Seatown Beach in Dorset, Sandy Lawson returned to his native Guernsey and opened a horsebox sauna for six. Horseshoe-shaped Vazon Bay on the west coast is one of the island's best swim spots.

rockboxsauna.com
Sea · 49.4638, -2.6128

48 Sandytoes Sauna

WESTPARK ❀ JERSEY

Blair Talibard, a local surfer, operates and rotates Sandytoes monthly between different beach locations on Jersey. He organises the sauna sessions around high tides so the bathers can jump straight into the sea.

sandytoessauna.com
Sea · 49.2520, -2.1210 & many more

49 Adrift Sauna

ST ANNE'S ❀ ALDERNEY

When Treina Hartell and family moved to Alderney from Scotland, they brought the Adrift Sauna with them and soon became known as the 'Sauna People'. Access to Alderney beaches is limited, so they tend to operate on either of the beautiful Corblets or Braye beaches. Both have good parking facilities and an easy route to get into the sea. There's a very relaxed booking system through phone, social media, or even just popping into Treina's craft studio in St. Anne's.

instagram.com/adriftalderney
Sea · 49.7286, -2.1722

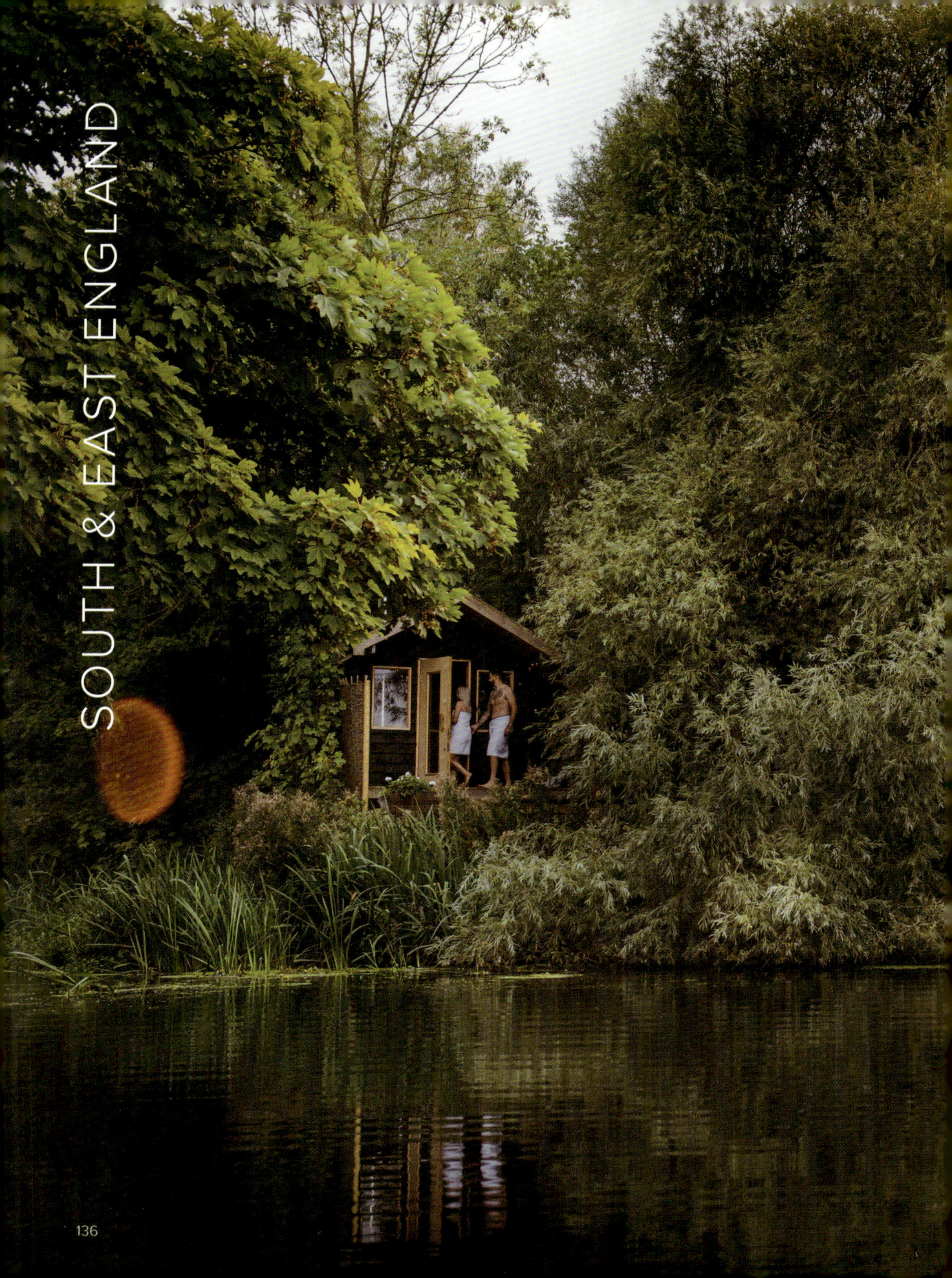

SOUTH & EAST ENGLAND

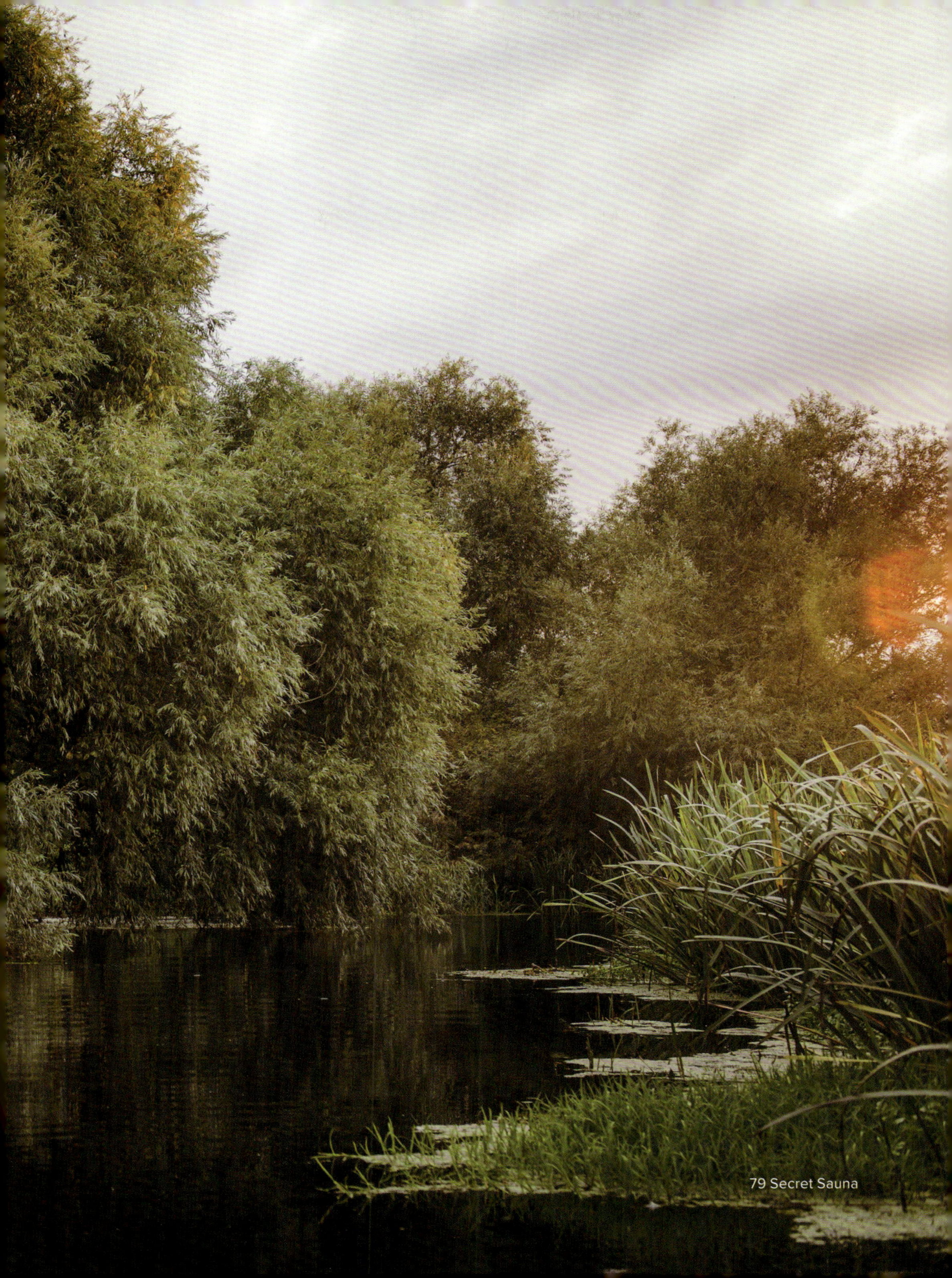

79 Secret Sauna

50

Slomo Sauna

TAPNELL FARM ❦ ISLE OF WIGHT

Slomo Sauna is the latest wellness concept from Rob and Josie da Bank, the husband-and-wife founders of family-friendly festival, Camp Bestival. Such is their passion for yoga, meditation, sauna and open-water swimming that the pair are on a mission to turn the Isle of Wight, where they live, into 'sauna island'.

Slomo saunas pop up all over the island at different times, but a floating sauna, handcrafted by Ben Revill of Rooftop Saunas in Hackney sits on a lake at holiday retreat, Tapnell Farm, along with two Nordic saunas and an ice tank. On the mainland, a Slomo wild spa lives mainly at Elkins Boatyard in Christchurch, but its pack-up-and-go design means it's totally mobile. Wood-fired saunas, ice baths and cold plunges, parasol-shaded seating and beach hut-style changing rooms offer contrast therapy on the move.

For the past two winters, Slomo has been a hot ticket at the Mind Your Brain wellness festival in London's King's Cross, and it will be on the road again this summer at the Slomo Wellbeing Festival at Camp Bestival.

slomo.me · Sea/lake/bath/cold plunge
50.6796, -1.4709 Tapnell Farm
50.7308, -1.7714 Christchurch

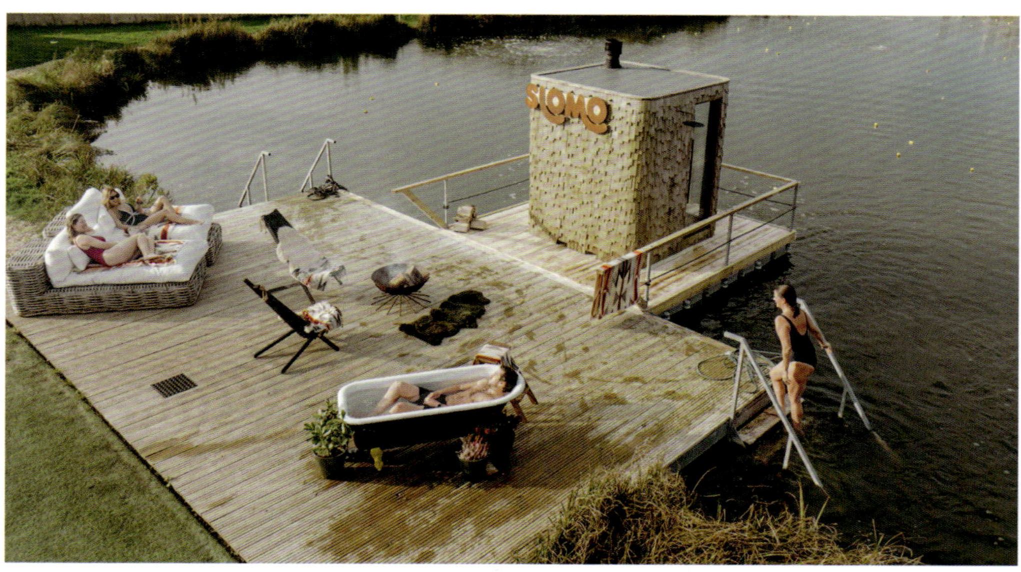

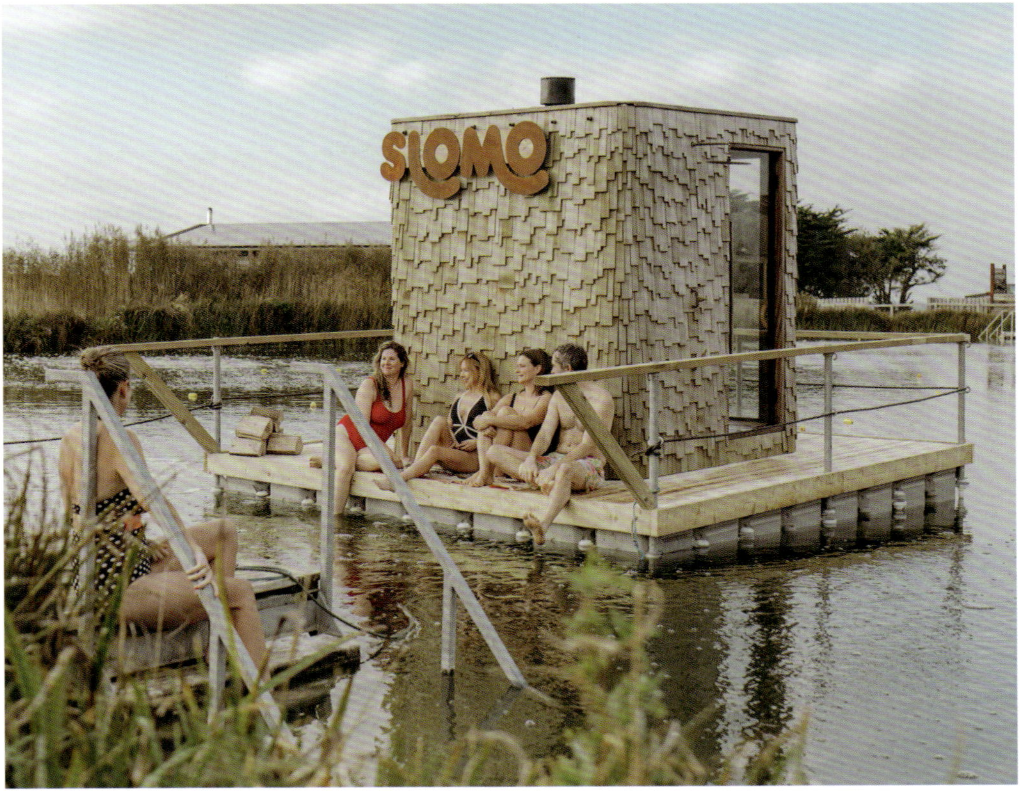

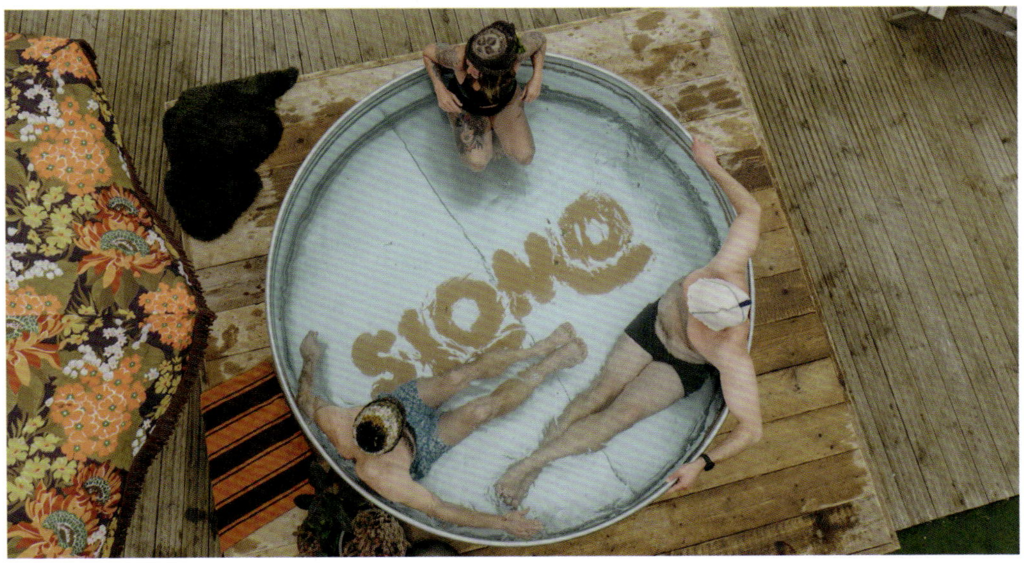
SLOMO

51

Tuhka Talo

ANDOVER ❦ HAMPSHIRE

Tuhka Talo (Finnish for 'ash house') has two saunas in Hampshire: The Fallen Willow Sauna and The Woodland Sauna. Before they founded their own sauna, Jo Caley and her partner, Jonathan Grobler, would privately hire the Saltwater Sauna in Sandbanks and take groups to the coast. They would do yoga on the beach, followed by sauna and sea swimming, breakfast and kayaking. They were the best days ever, and the couple can now host similar activities closer to home in Hampshire.

A sublime setting, a well-run space, an attentive host and a devil-in-the-details design are winning ingredients for a wild sauna, and Fallen Willow has them all. This is why, in 2024, it scooped the Best New Sauna award from the British Sauna Society. It sits amid willow trees next to Mistletoe Lake, a spring-fed swimming lake on private land near Stockbridge. Tucked deep in the forest, two miles from Fallen Willow, is The Woodland Sauna, which comes with ice plunge pools and showers.

Both saunas have built a community around them. 'There's nothing like being in a hot box semi-naked to break down social barriers,' says Jo. 'And I've made great connections and great friends.'

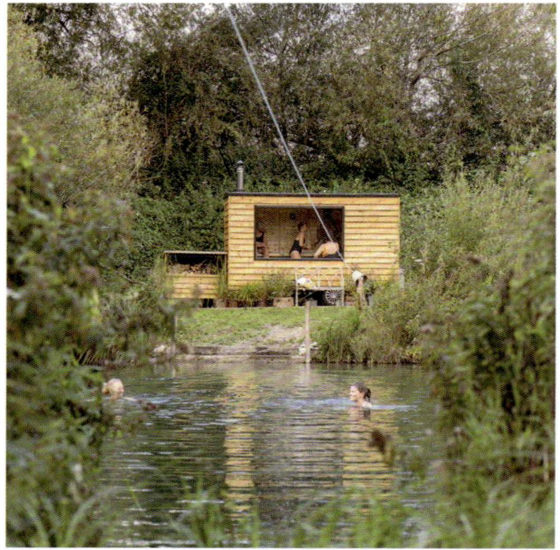

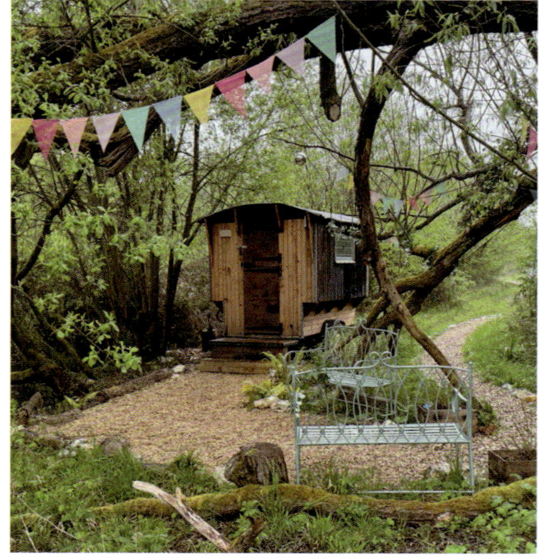

- tuhkatalo.com
- Lake/cold plunge/shower
- 51.1571, -1.4564 Fallen Willow
- 51.1534, -1.4888 Woodland Sauna (approx. locations, exact site explained on booking)

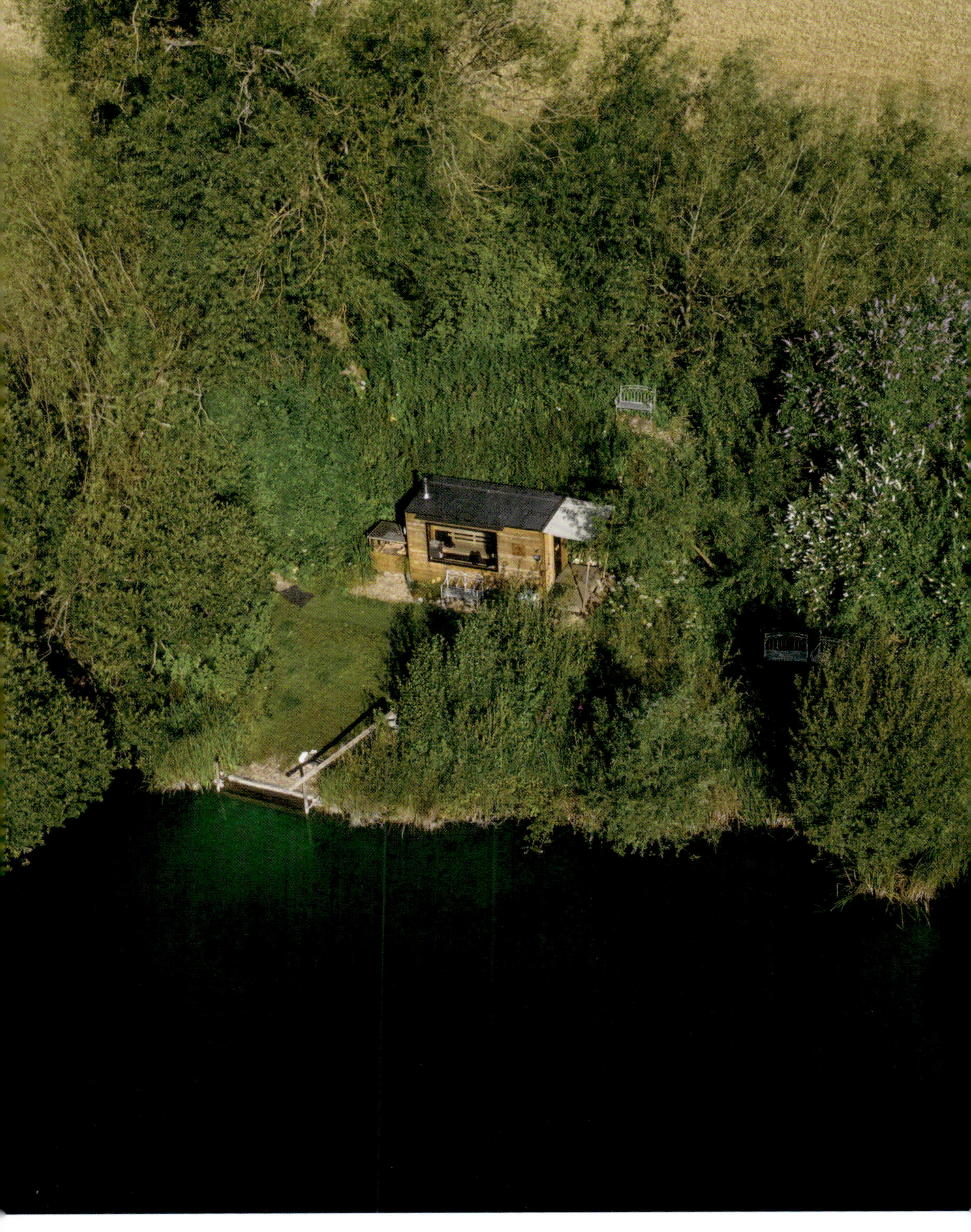

52

Wasing Wellbeing

ALDERMASTON ❦ BERKSHIRE

Trekking down a dirt track through bike pines to a swim and sauna event at the Wasing estate, the forest saunas of Finland come to mind. Not least because on the day of my visit, it was the middle of July, 11°C and raining. Bathers in Scandinavia like to point out that even when the summer disappoints, the sauna never does, and when I spotted a curl of smoke drifting across a glassy pond, I knew today would not either.

Every month, Wasing hosts a Saturday Swim & Sauna, where up to 12 guests can enjoy a two-and-a-half-hour session of wood-fired sauna and lake dips, plus lunch and tea around a campfire. The whole experience is off-grid and back-to-nature (a toilet, shower and bucket shower are nestled in the trees). On this glowering summer's day, the smell of rain-drenched woodland hangs in the air. It's the perfect place for forest bathing too, and a path behind the sauna leads deeper into the woodland past an ancient yew tree.

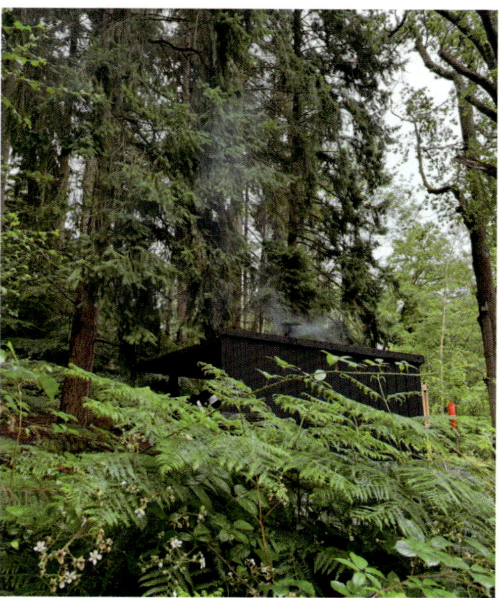

A sauna host is on hand to guide the group, many of whom have never swum in water this cold before. It's 18°C, mostly shallow and has two jetties opposite each other. In winter, these form a perfect crossing point for members of the wild swimming club. Our host gives us a health and safety briefing and advises breathing out on the way into the water, warning that the coccyx and sacrum are particularly sensitive to cold. There's a brown, sludgy biofilm in the water at this time of year that sticks to the skin, and when we come out, we look like prehistoric swamp-people.

Joshua Dugdale and his wife Diana own the 400-acre Wasing Estate and built the sauna in lockdown for themselves and friends. It proved so popular they opened it to the public; anyone can join as a member, or you can hire the whole space privately. It's one of the many wellness offerings at Wasing, along with retreats, meditation, Wim Hof workshops, and the annual Medicine Festival. The estate hosts numerous weddings and concerts too, though when you're in the sauna you feel a million miles from anywhere.

wasing.co.uk
Lake/shower 51.3738, -1.1763

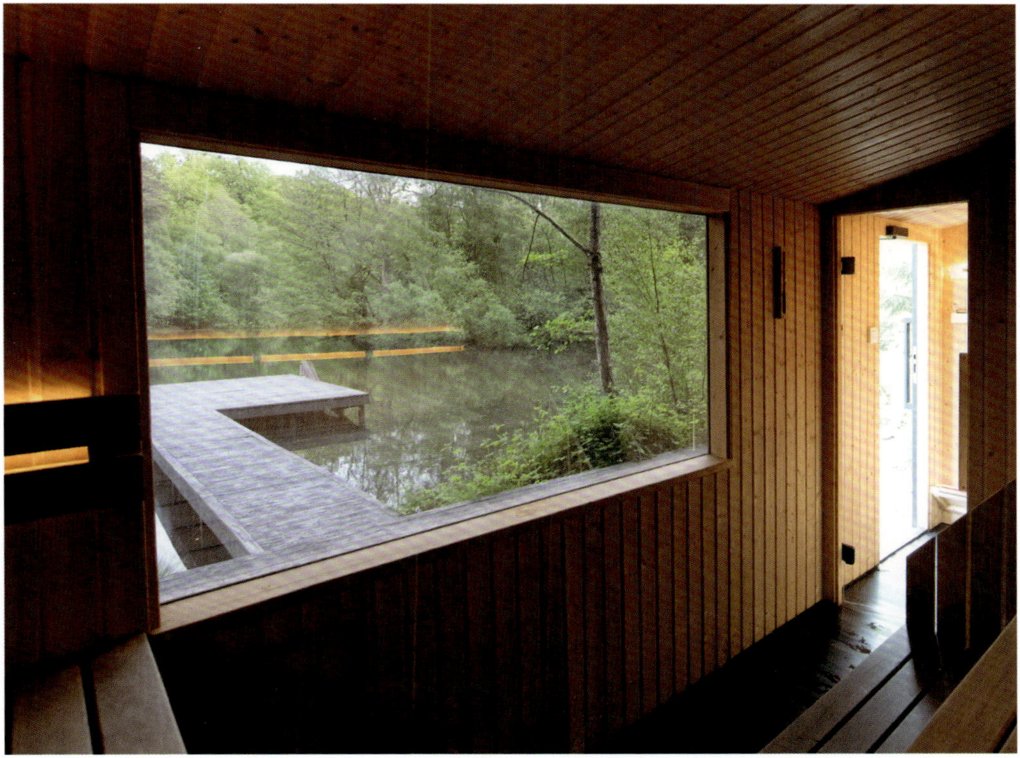

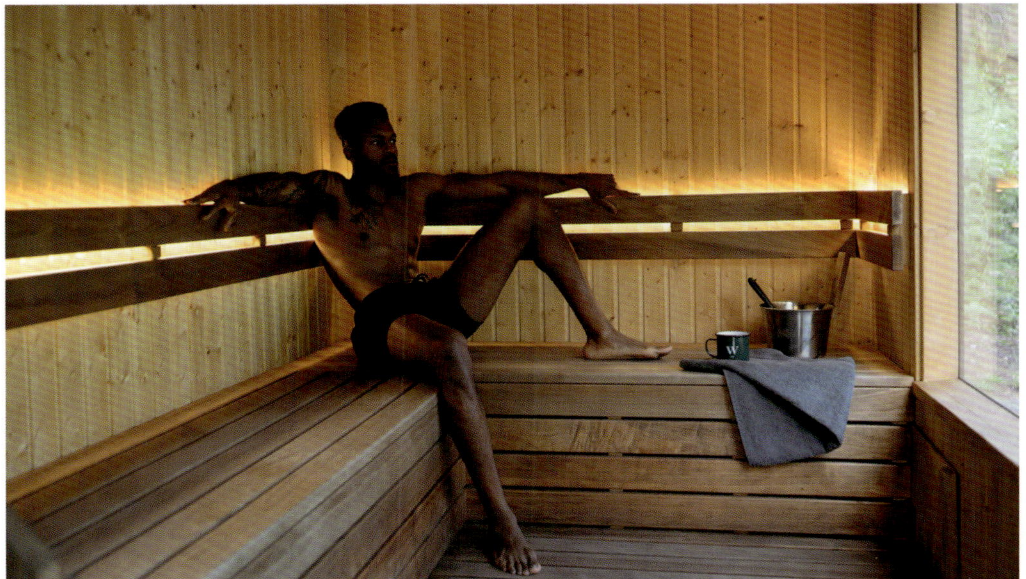

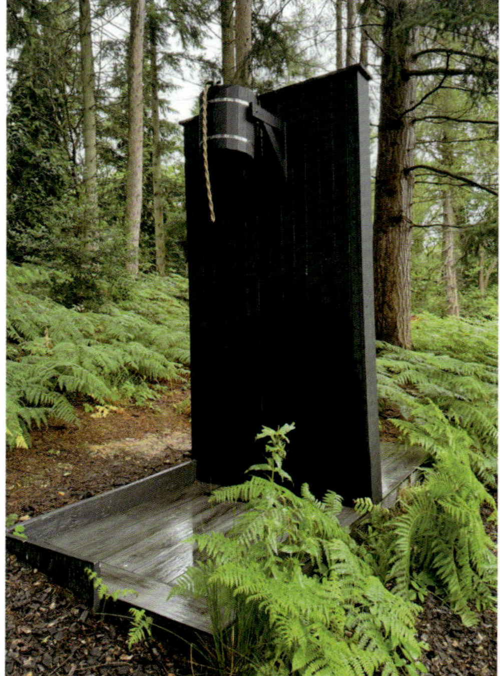

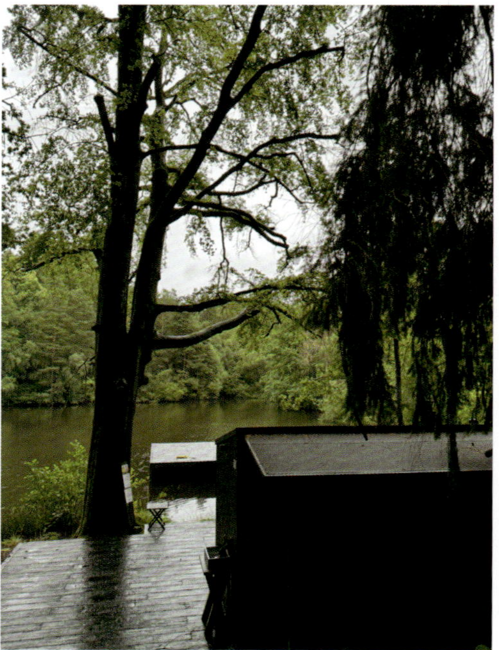

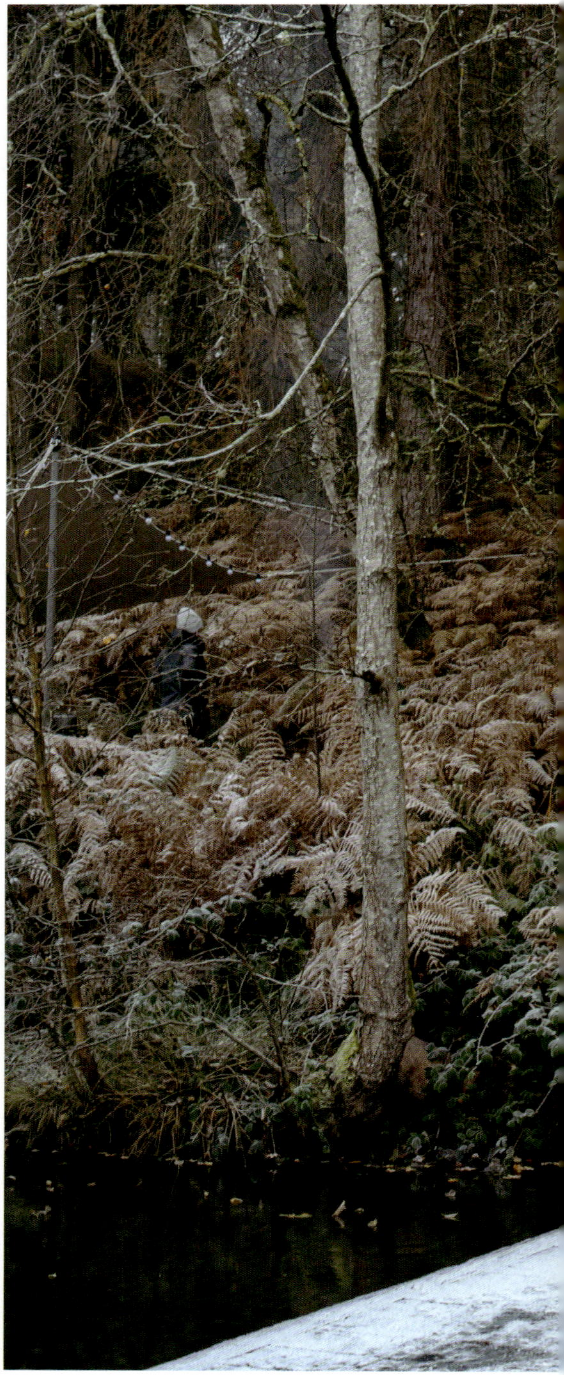

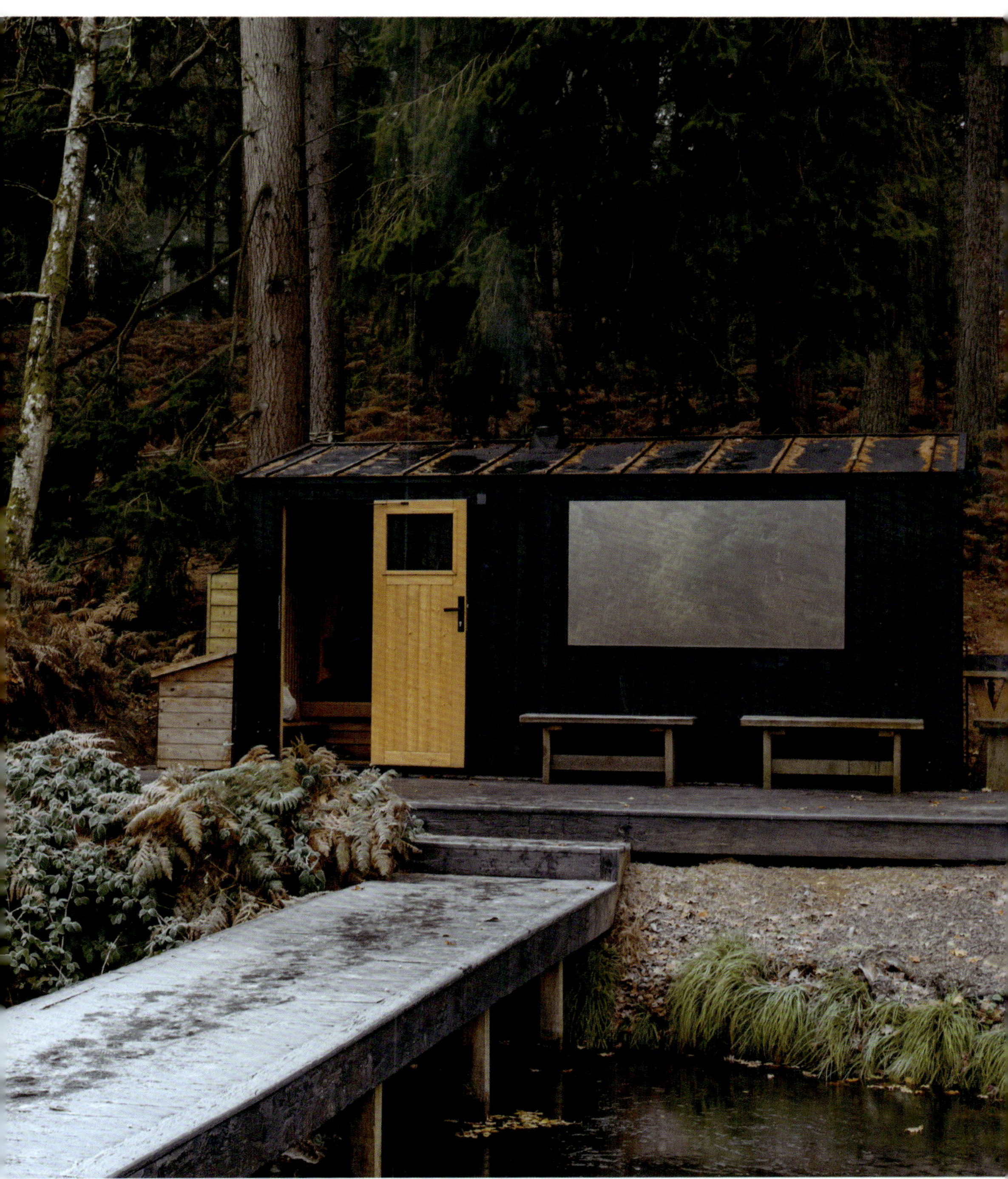

Wasing Wellbeing

53

Fitness at the Farm

FRILFORD ❦ OXFORDSHIRE

This 'outdoor gym' in the Cotswolds does what it says on the tin: what was once an unused field is now a place to exercise in nature. People come to run the mile-long circuit round the farm and work out with ropes, rowers, hammers and tyre weights, all under the guidance of the farm's founder Leah Maclean. It's set up in the round, with a hot tub, a cold plunge and a barrel sauna for post-exercise recovery. Hot showers, cold showers, a changing hut, a bar, BBQ and pizza oven complete the mix. And instead of gym mirrors, wildflowers and trees form the backdrop.

➔ farm-fit.co.uk
Bath/shower 51.6731, -1.3672

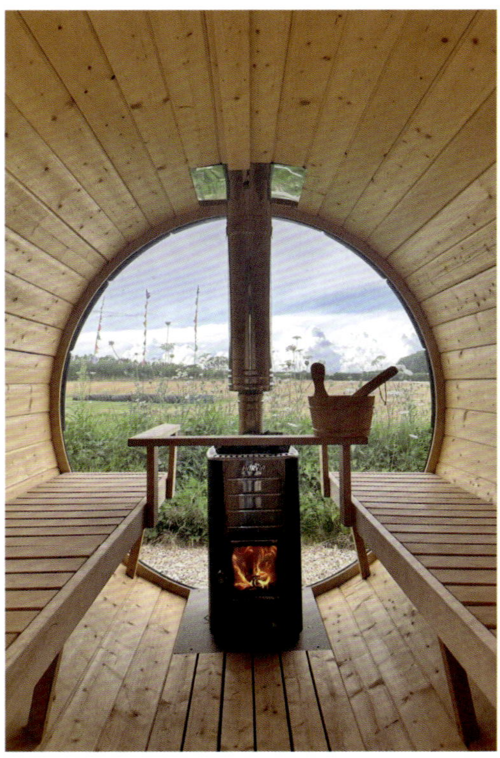

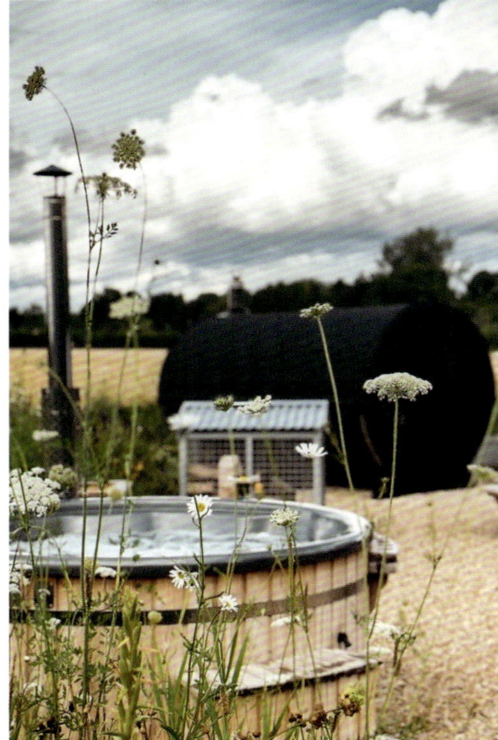

54

Fire, Salt & Sea

WORTHING ❦ SUSSEX

So loved is Fire, Salt & Sea on Worthing Beach that one of its regulars even moved down from London to live right next door. Emma, a therapist from London, met her partner Rebecca in a sauna at a festival in Wales. The steam always carried the reminder of love for them both, and Emma bought a seafront flat so they could sauna and swim together most days. On this pebbly stretch of beach, away from the main town of Worthing, sauna bathers tend to be swimmers too. Despite sell-out community sessions and family-friendly sessions where kids from age five can join, the council hasn't granted Fire, Salt & Sea a permit to stay on the shore overnight, so owner Dave tows the converted horsebox on and off the beach every day and sleeps in his van. There's quite a community of van dwellers on the seafront – and quite a community of sauna bathers too, who know that the best time to visit is at high tide.

firesaltsea.co.uk
Sea/watering cans 50.8077, -0.3822

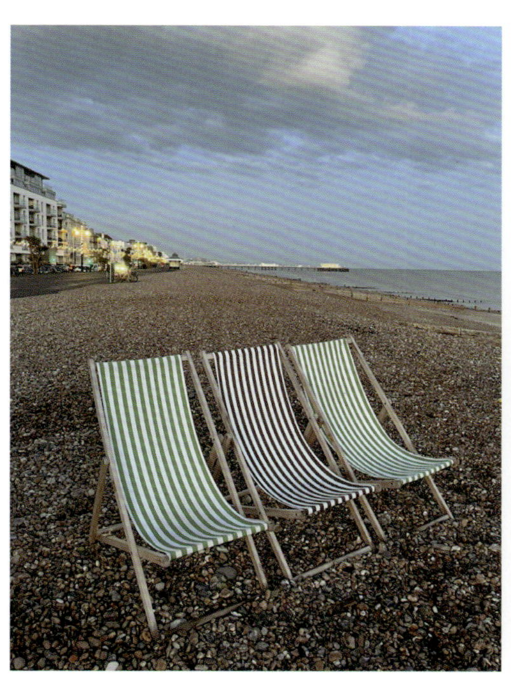

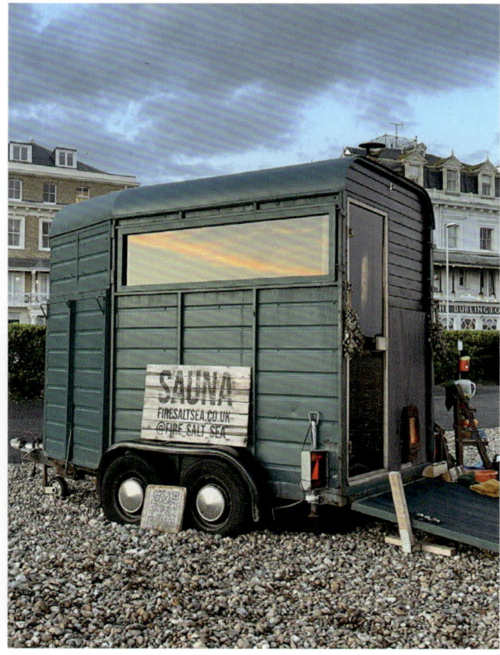

55

The Wild Sauna

WHICHFORD MILL ❦ WARWICKSHIRE

A mill house that featured in the Domesday Book, a stream to swim in, a space for yoga and breathwork, a pond and a beautifully converted horsebox sauna, all make The Wild Sauna at Whichford Mill a destination worth travelling for. Tucked away down a sleepy lane in the Warwickshire countryside, The Wild Sauna started life on a Sussex beach before its creators, Lucy and Tom, bought Whichford Mill and set up their rural B&B. Lucy makes her own shea butter, body scrubs and face masks, while a changing room, a bath filled with spring water and a hot outdoor shower add a touch of luxury. Tom's sister runs The Straw Kitchen, a straw bale café nearby that serves local, ethically sourced food.

Their father, Jim Keeling, is a Master Craftsman who founded Whichford Pottery in the 1970s. A team of 30 craftspeople make Whichford's world-famous terracotta flowerpots, and Jim fires everything in an anagama 'cave' kiln, which is heated for three weeks. In true Korean style, Tom and Lucy crawl in and use the kiln as a sauna once the firings are finished.

➔ whichfordmill.co.uk
River/bath 52.0256, -1.5404

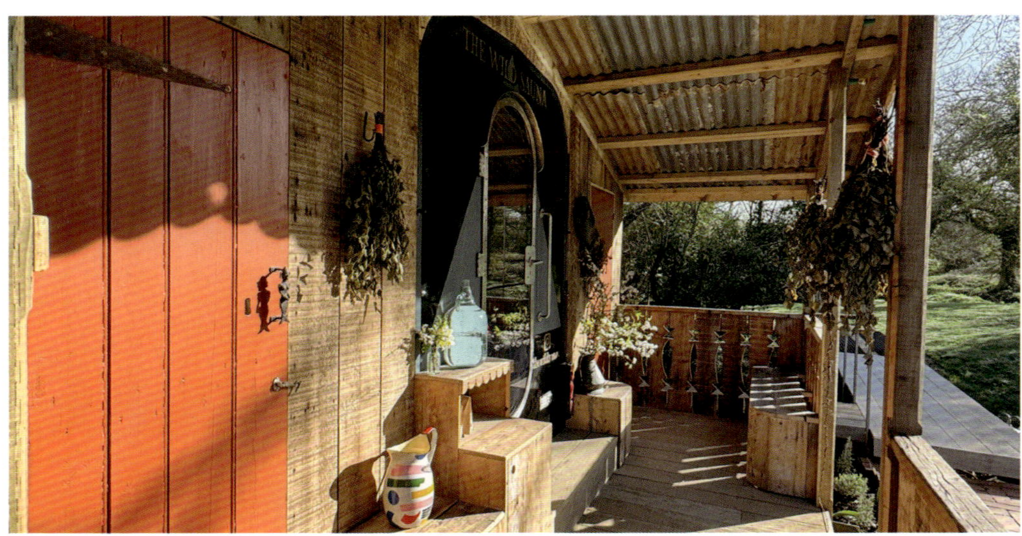

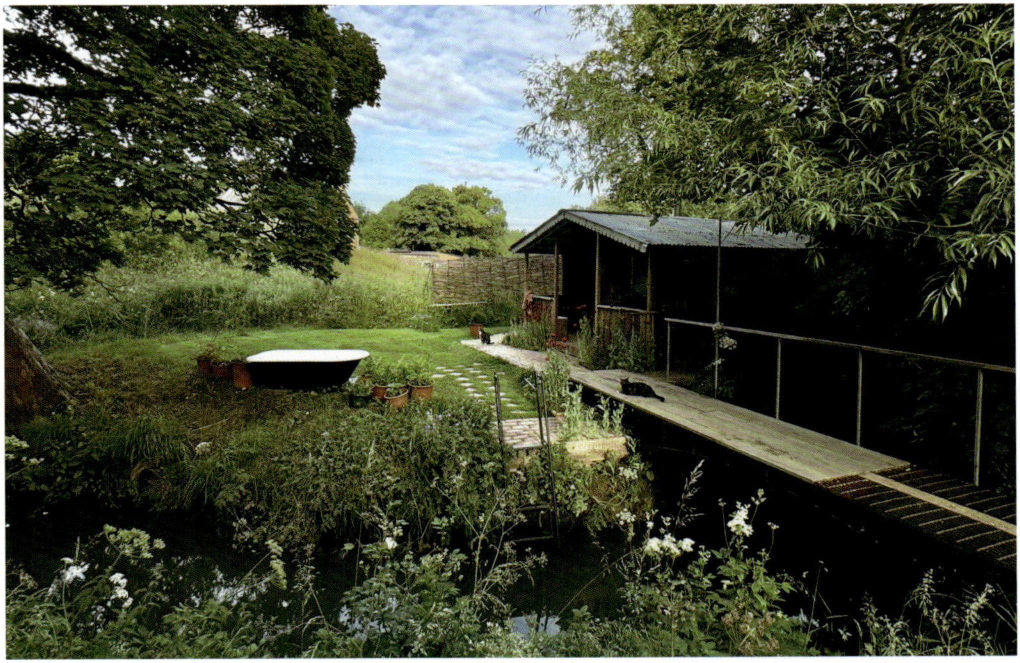

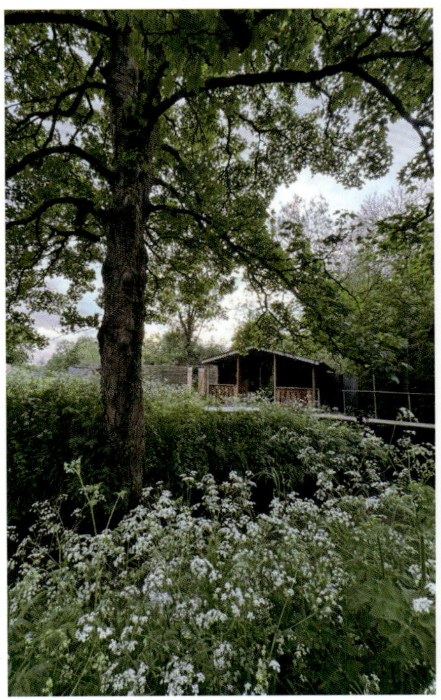

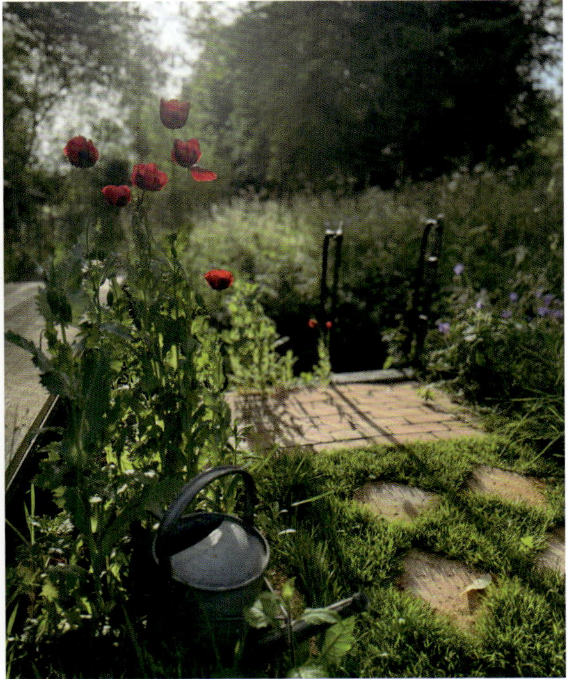

56

The Quays

MYTCHETT ❦ SURREY

The sauna complex at The Quays brings heat therapy to the hundreds of cold swimmers at this well-loved swim spot in Surrey. It consists of two Lithuanian wood-fired saunas that hold 30 bathers in total. Picture windows offer views across the swimming lake, and a walkway leads sauna bathers to a segregated dipping area. Changing rooms, a water fountain, café, external showers and fire pits make it a social spot. A 40-minute sauna and dip costs £10, with reduced rates for those who have paid for a swim; and the saunas can be hired for private bookings.

➔ quayswim.co.uk
Lake 51.2949, -0.7372

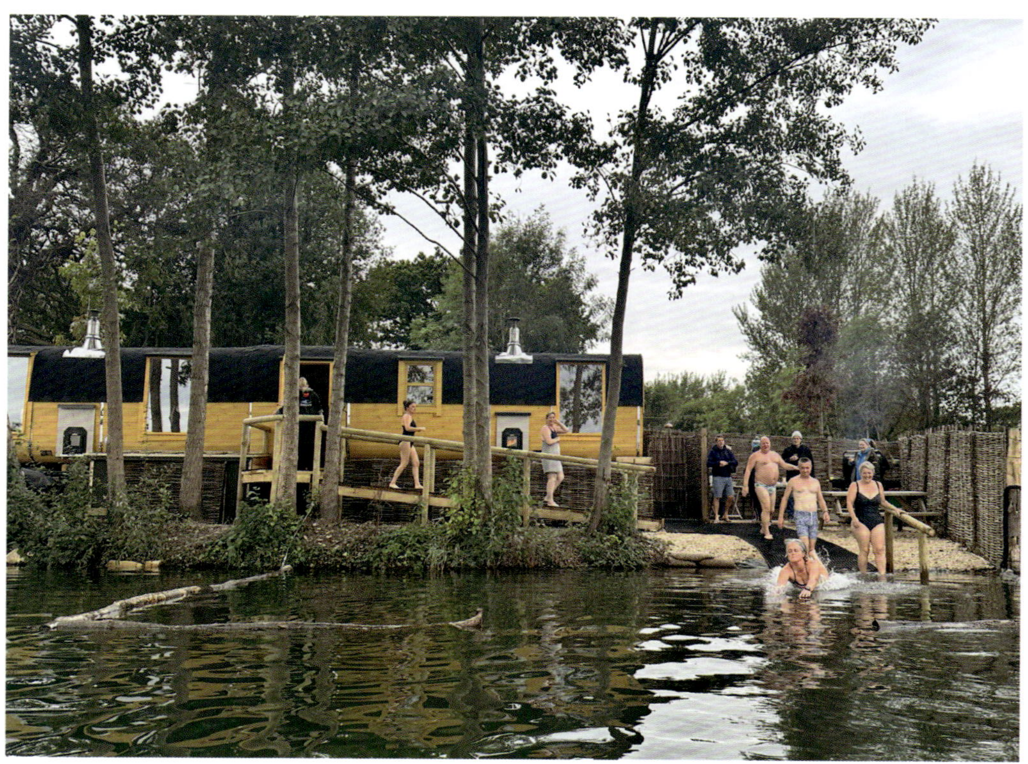

57

The Nomadic Sauna

SHOREHAM-BY-SEA ❦ SUSSEX

'The Nomads' are friends and sauna operators with three sites on the south coast. Dan is a member of the GB 24hr Ultra Running Team, and finds sauna helps muscle recovery; he has been having a sauna every day for about seven years. So hooked on the heat did he become, that he and his partner Charlotte, along with friends Tess and Karn, decided to build their own. 'We thought, let's do something ourselves. The worst that can happen is we have a sauna on the beach and we get into it every day.'

Karn, a carpenter, took care of the builds, and Nomadic was born on the beach, first at Kingston Beach, near Shoreham-by-Sea, then Seaford, and then for the summer at Pells Pool in Lewes. (Opened in 1861, Pells is the oldest freshwater outdoor public swimming pool in the UK, and is fed by a spring.) Neither of the Nomadic beach sites has planning permission, so every day the owners drive the saunas on and off the shore. They also run a permanent spot on a private lake at Swanborough near Lewes.

Dan is an *aufguss* master and competes in international show *aufguss* (see page 38). His Boris Johnson routine (and blonde wig) has cult status, and his 'secret sauna rave', where bathers were given white gloves and whistles, sold out in seconds. Like all *aufguss* masters, Dan knows his aromatherapy oils too. He mixes his own and puts them to use at Nomadic's sell-out *aufguss* shows.

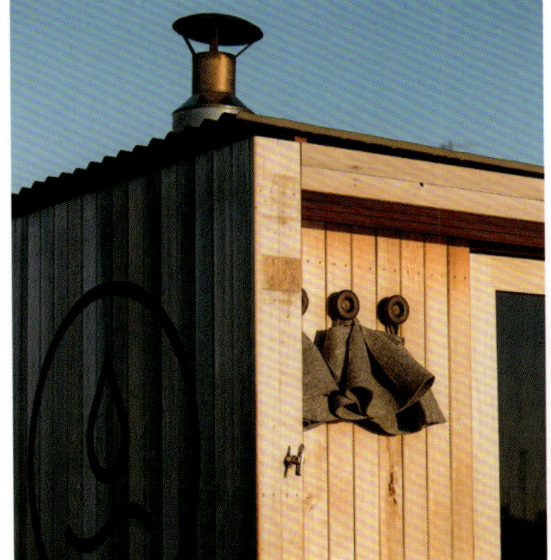

- thenomadicsauna.co.uk
- Sea/bath/dip tank (winter)
- 50.8307, -0.2480 Kingston Beach
- 50.8554, 0.0004 Swanborough
- 50.830, -0.2480 Seaford Beach

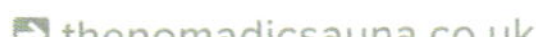

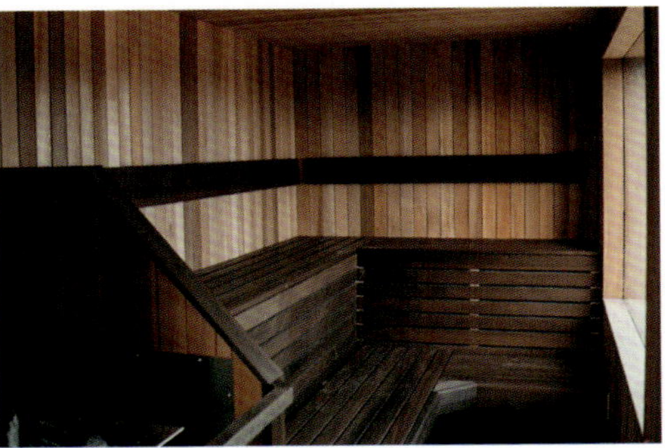

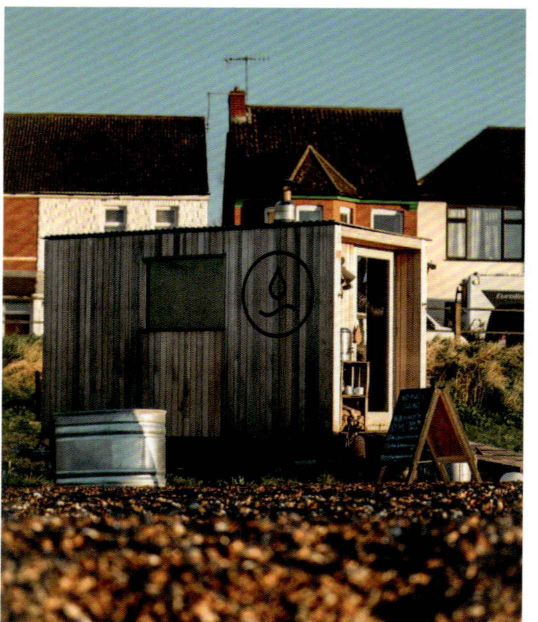

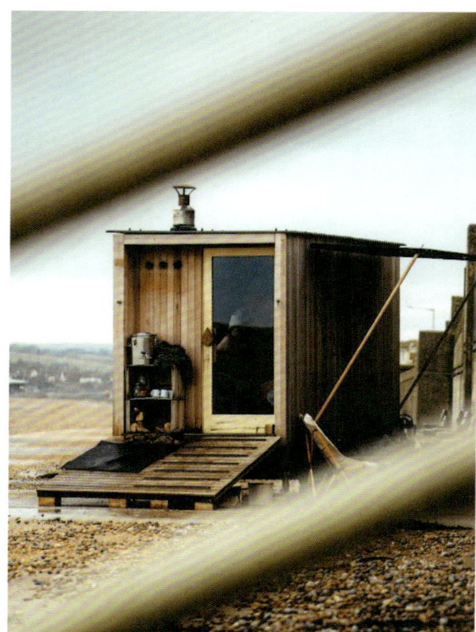

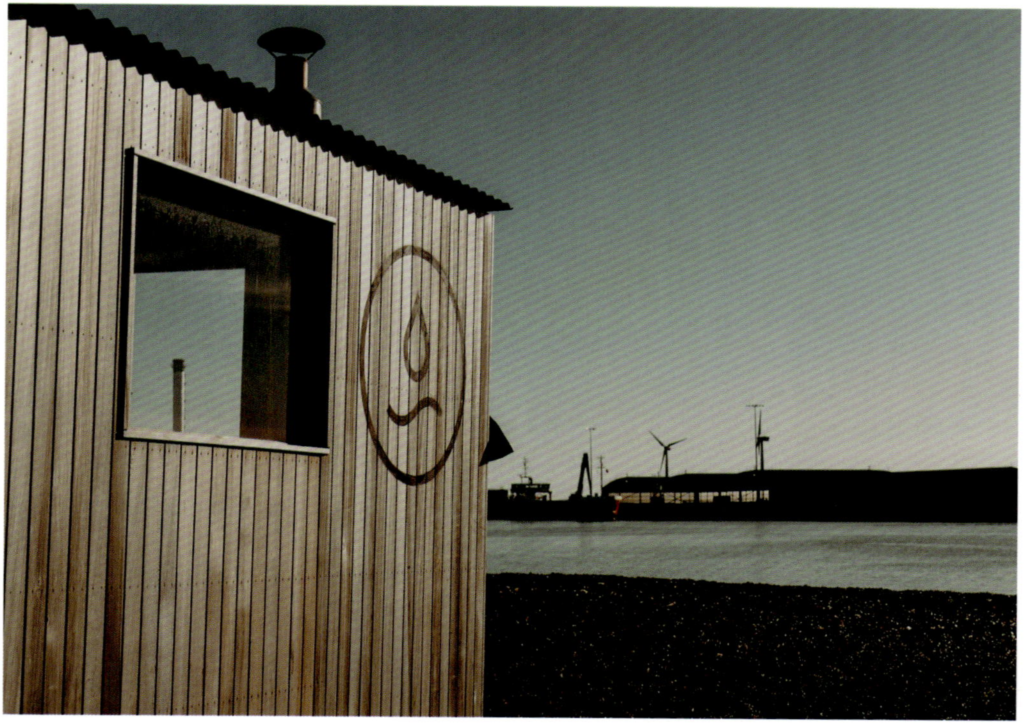

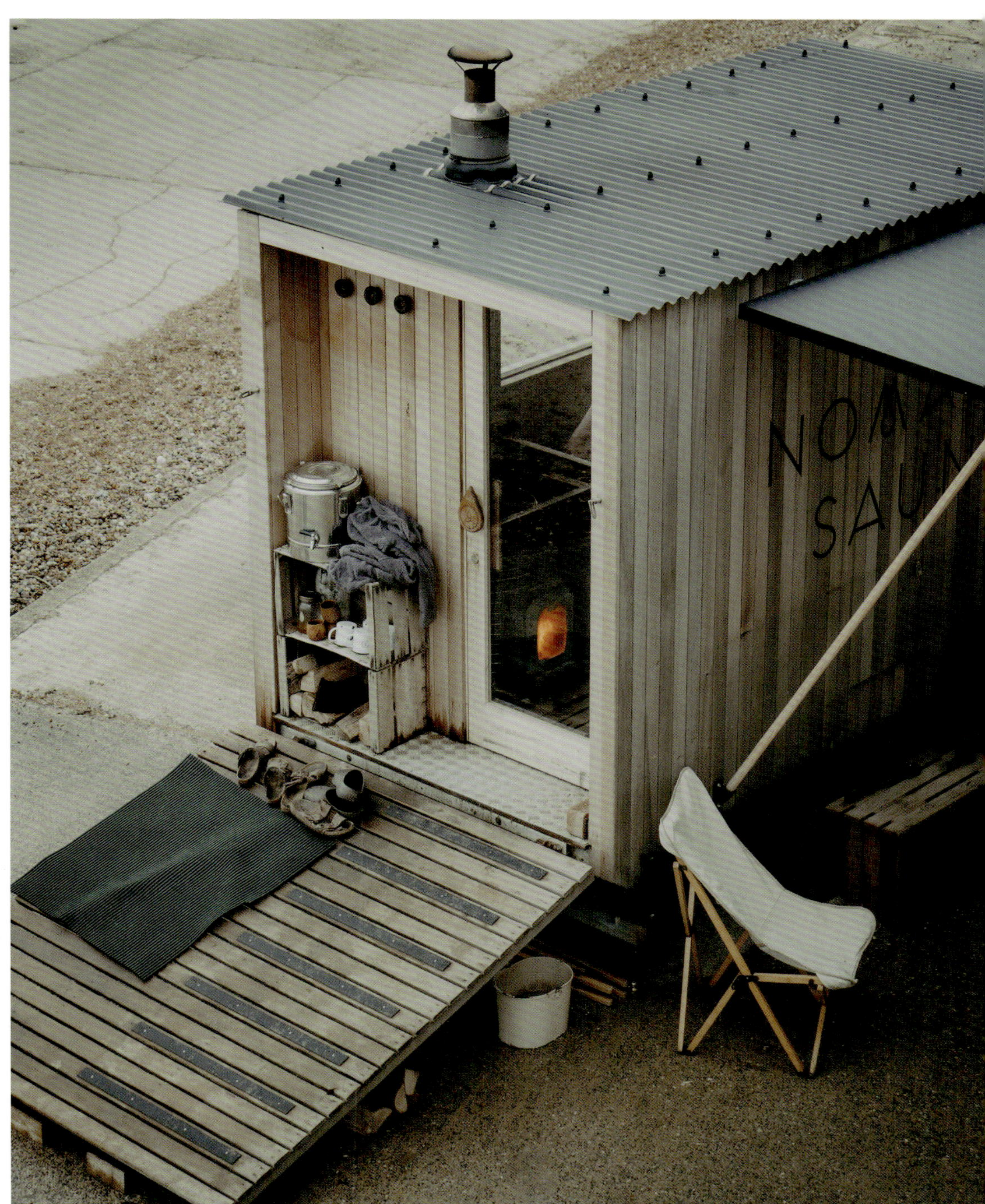

The Nomadic Sauna

58

Kindred Sauna

HORSHAM ❦ SUSSEX

Knepp in Sussex has always been ahead of the curve. This 3,500-acre estate started animal-led rewilding 20 years ago, and endangered species such as nightingales, turtle doves and purple emperor butterflies, along with English longhorn cattle, Tamworth pigs, Exmoor ponies and deer now occupy the landscape in abundance. No surprise then, that it would be quick to welcome a sauna to its grounds.

Kindred Sauna is owned by Marianne Drake who works part-time in the NHS and part-time in the sauna. She knew she didn't want to be on the crowded Sussex beachfront, and she's not a fan of the 'dressing gown and prosecco' spa day. She wanted trees and nature, and Knepp is steeped in both. A stylish horsebox conversion, Kindred sits on the 60-person campsite at Knepp on the edge of an ancient wood, next to a wild swimming pond and a wildflower meadow. Food is available at Knepp Wilding Kitchen.

kindredsauna.com

Shower/pond 50.9708, -0.3632

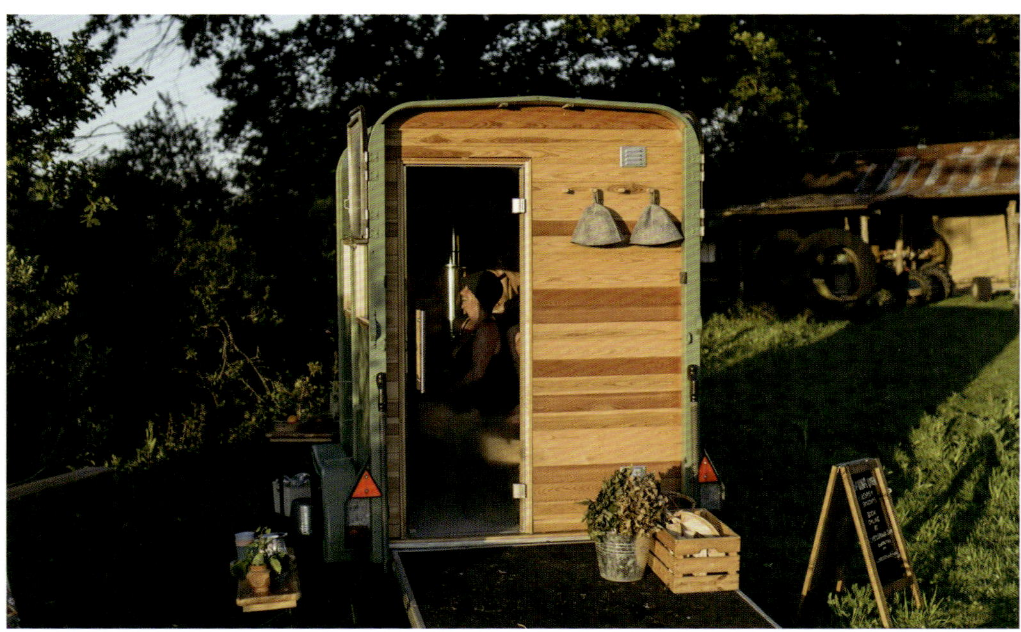

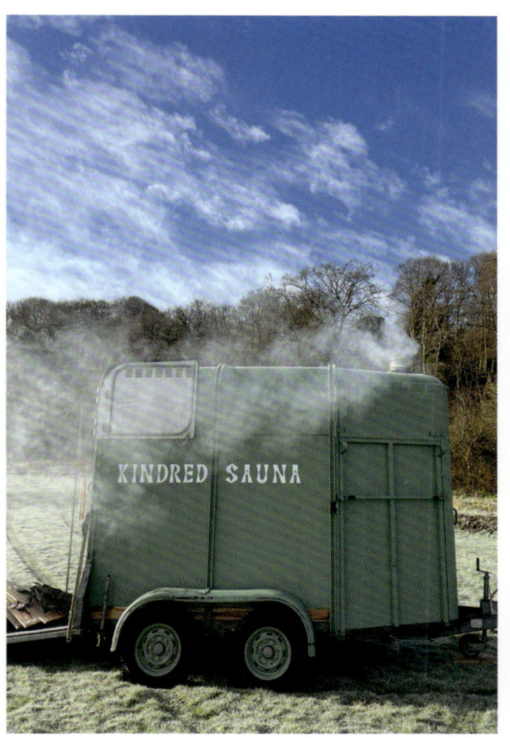
KINDRED SAUNA

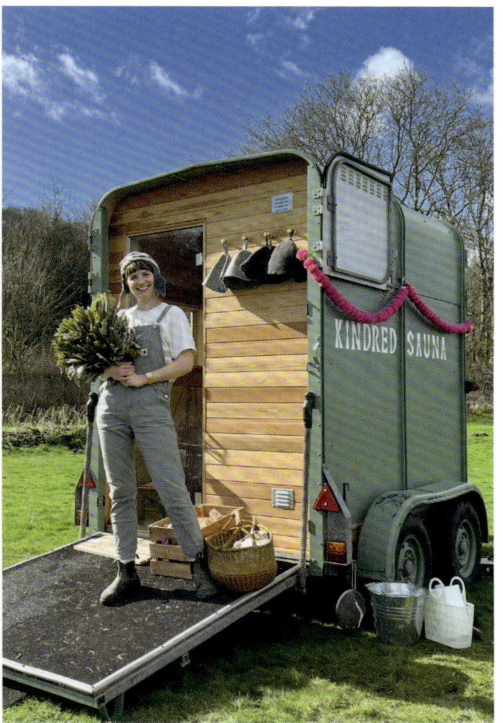
KINDRED SAUNA

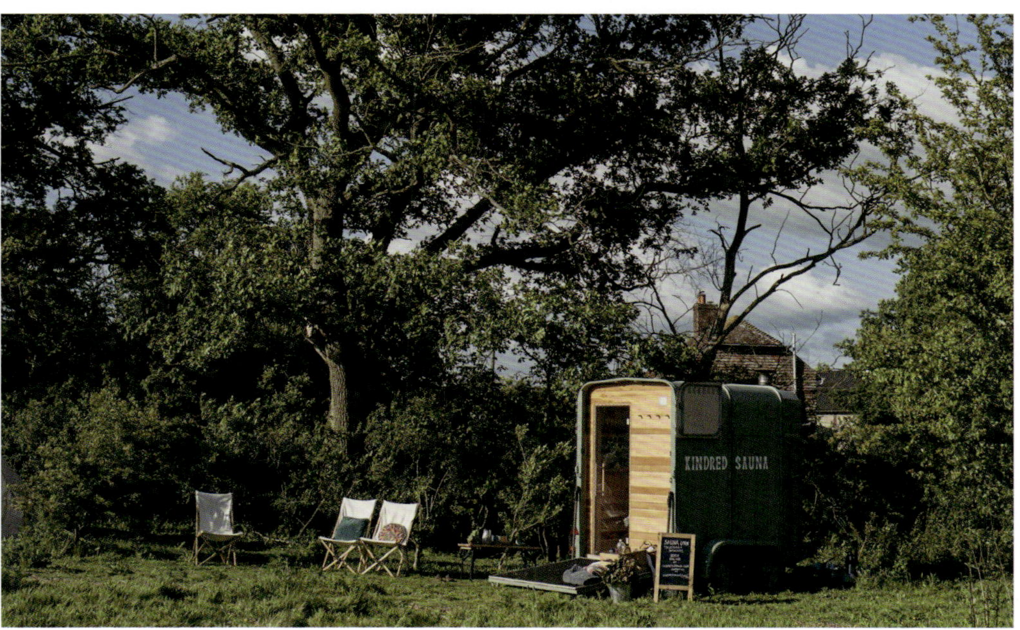
KINDRED SAUNA

59

Saunadelic

HOVE ❦ SUSSEX

Hove Lagoon is a hive of activity, even on moody days when red warning flags blow horizontally all along the Sussex shoreline. Normally, bathers at Saunadelic jump in the waves, but when the weather sets in, they rinse under cold showers, or dip into the lagoon, which is waist-high and fed with seawater. There's a strong sense of community around the lagoon: it is home to a water sports centre, fitness classes take place on the promenade, and the Big Beach Café is legendary.

Saunadelic is at the centre of it all. Its founders trained at Beach Box (61) and host a range of rituals and ceremonies, even teaming up with local chefs to run a Sauna Supper Club where flavours echo sauna fragrances. They equate the sauna to the coffee shop, where there are many to choose from, but they are all different.

saunadelic.uk

Sea/lagoon/cold plunge 50.8267, -0.1987

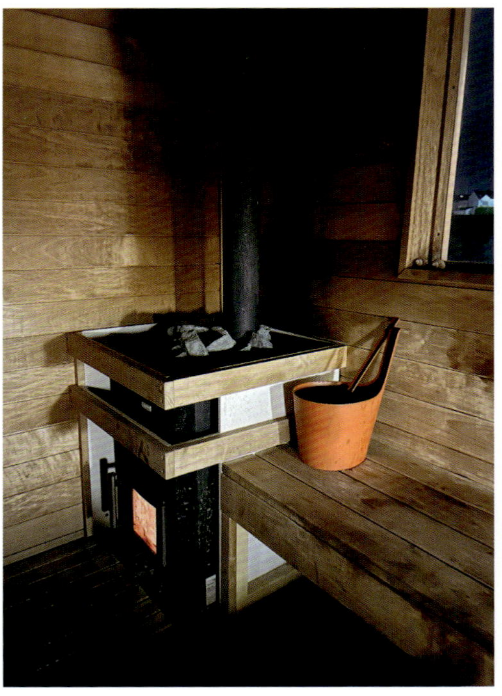

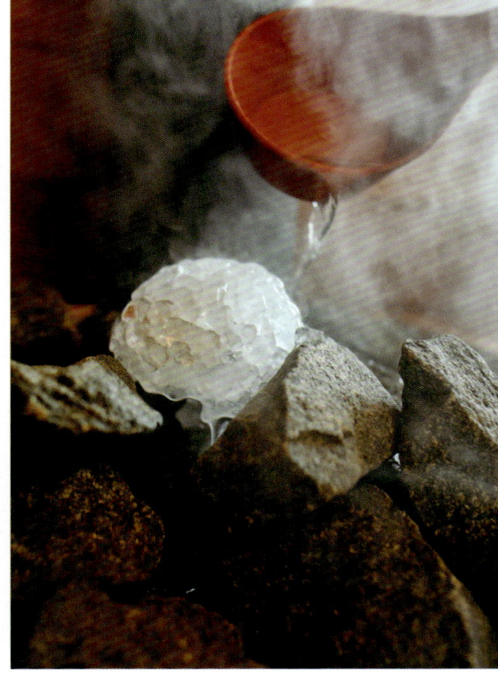

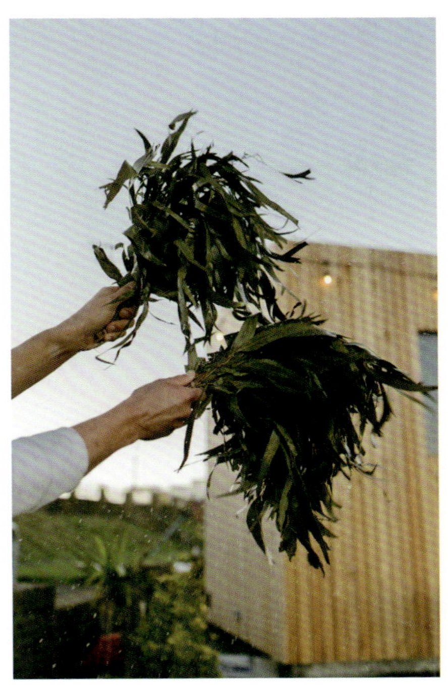

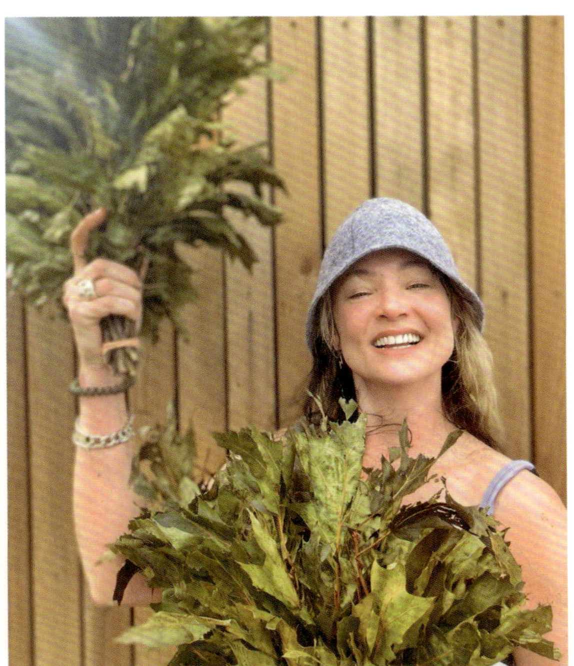

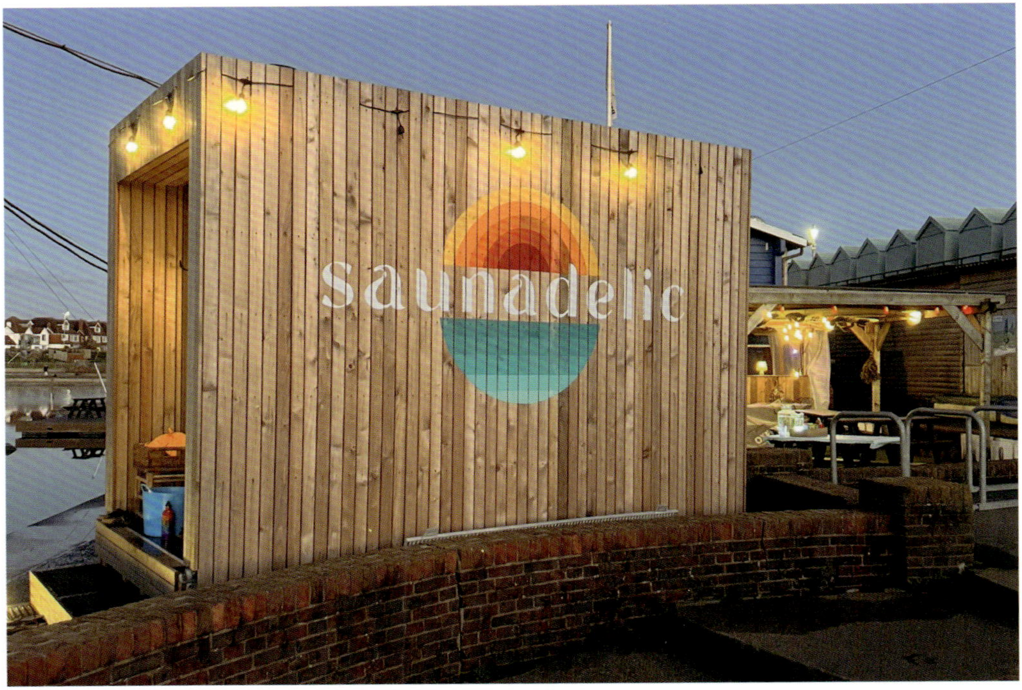

60

Luna Hut

BRIGHTON, EASTBOURNE & WORTHING ❦ SUSSEX

Everybody has their sauna epiphany, and for Laura Brown and Mike Lord, it happened in a large, sea-view sauna in Cork, Ireland. Having previously run a rural spa in the Sussex countryside with his partner, Laura Brown, the couple were used to making things from scratch. And so they built Luna Hut, which has a large picture window, space for sixteen bathers, and a covered porch. Every winter, from November to March, they park up next to Sea Lanes, a cool complex of bars and offices, an open-air lido, and Luna Wave Yoga Studio, which Mike and Laura also run. Together, yoga and sauna seal the connection between mental and physical health; similarly, Sea Lanes' physiotherapists use Luna Hut to offer combined massage and sauna sessions. Matting running down to the sea makes the sauna wheelchair accessible and compatible with Sea Lanes' commitment to disabled access for pool and sea swimmers alike. Other Luna locations include the seafront at Eastbourne and the Splashpoint Leisure Centre in Worthing, and a new Luna complex with multiple saunas, cold plunges, food and events is opening in Brighton.

➔ lunahutsauna.co.uk
❄ Sea/shower 📍 50.8170, -0.1233 Brighton
📍 50.7652, 0.2899 Eastbourne
📍 50.8120, -0.3615 Worthing

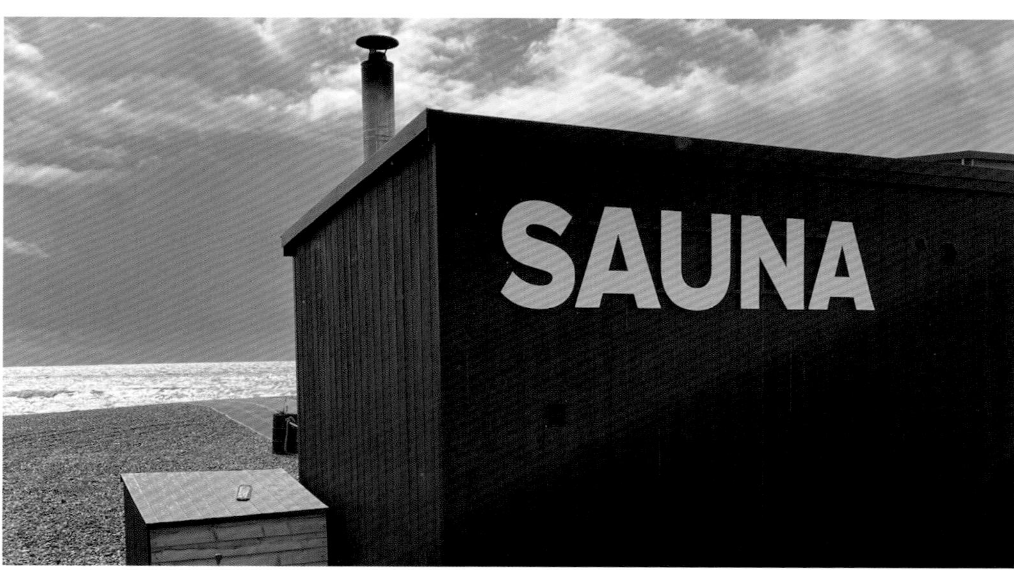

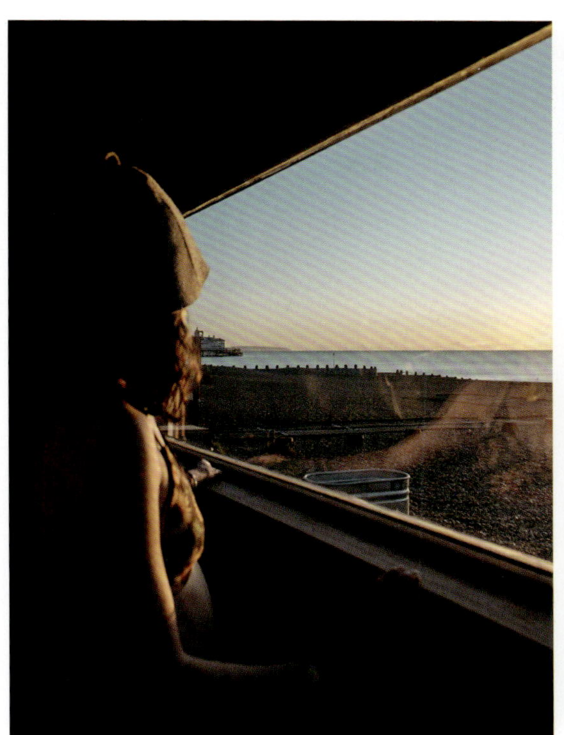

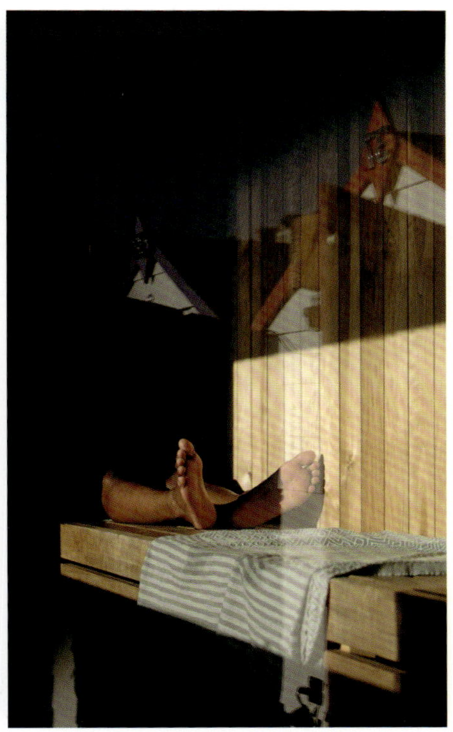

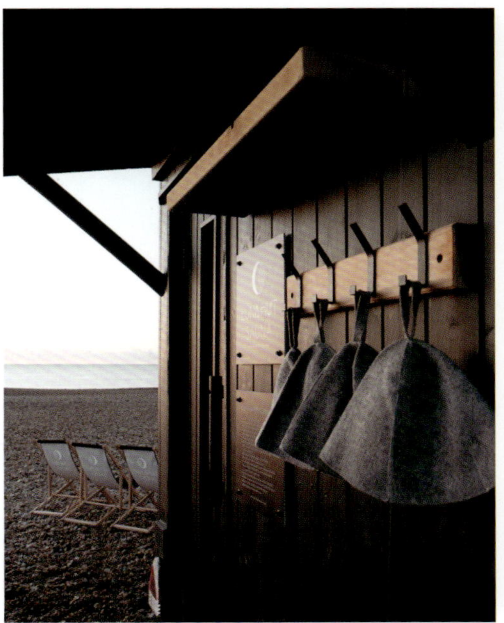

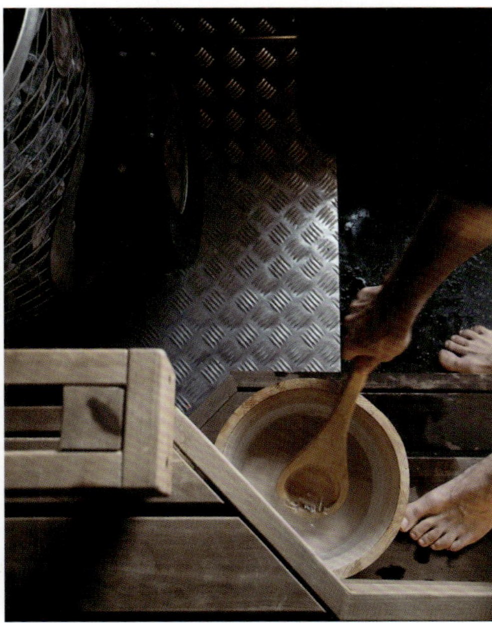

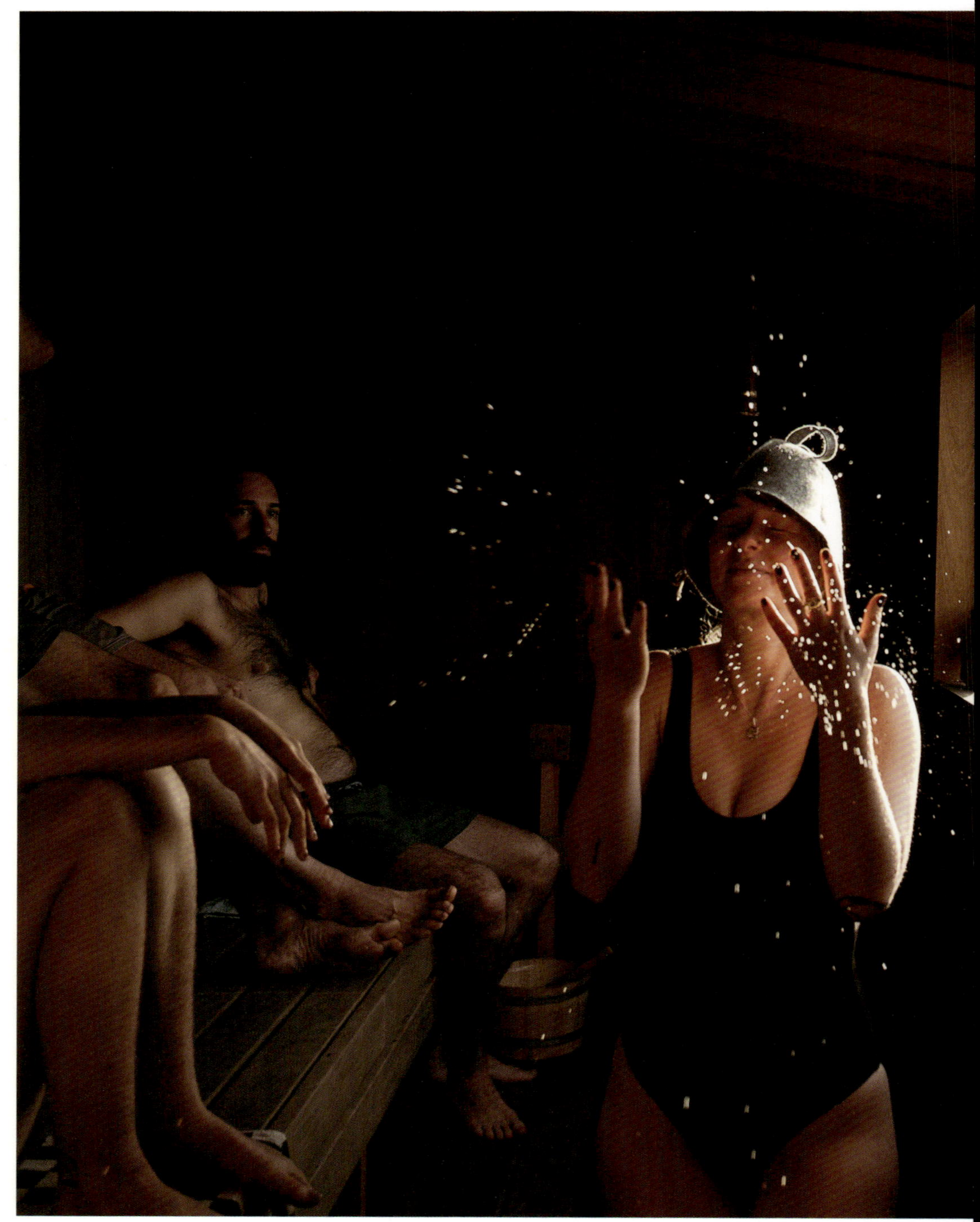

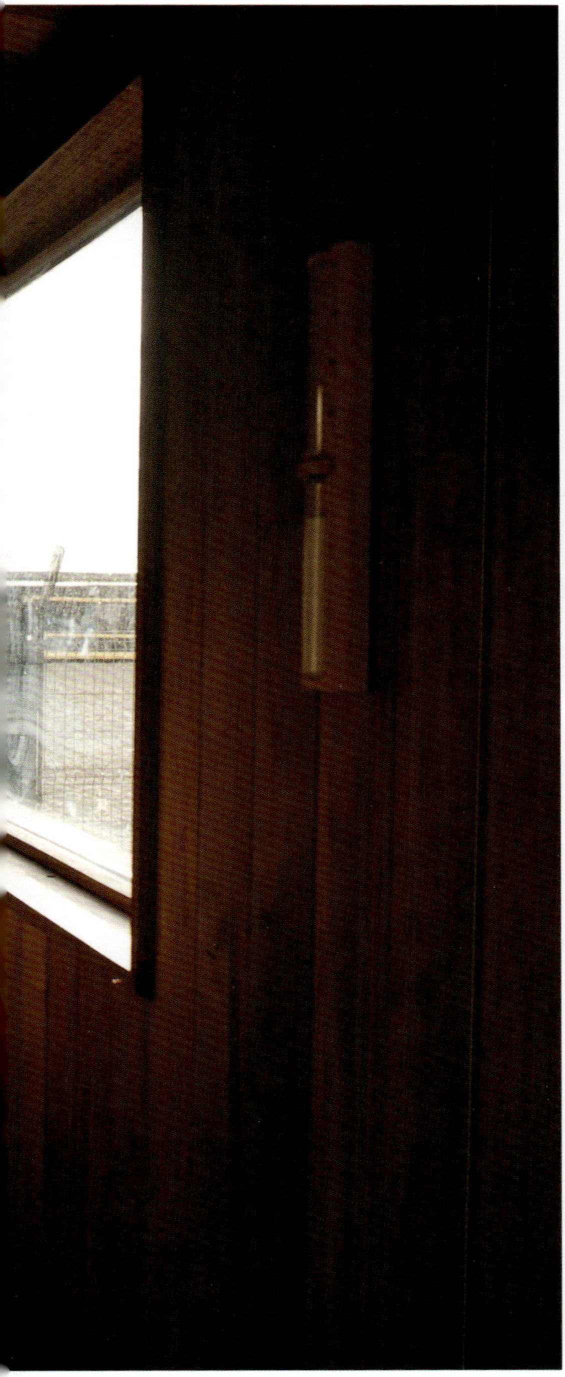

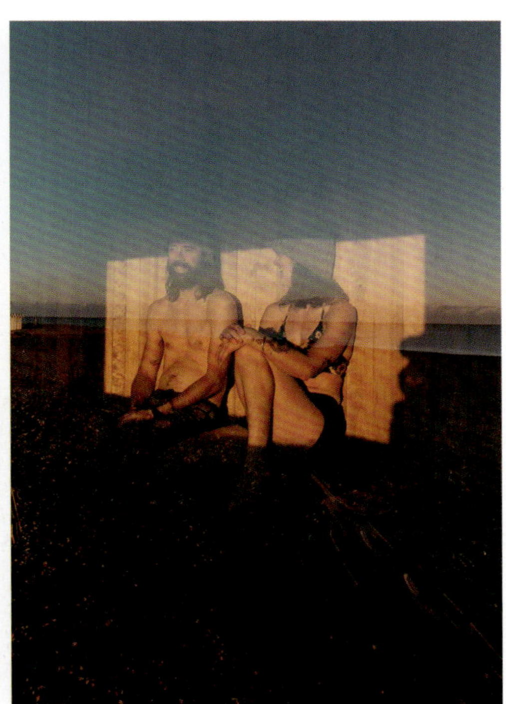

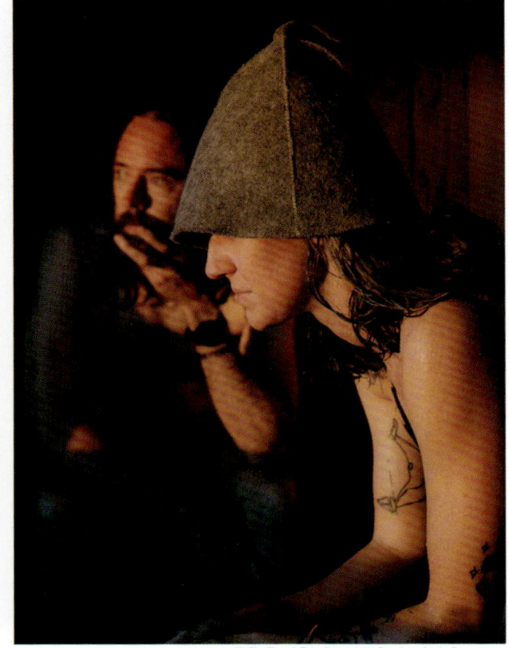

61

Beach Box Sauna Spa

BRIGHTON ❦ SUSSEX

The arrival of Beach Box Spa in Brighton in 2019 marked the moment when hot and cold found each other in the UK. What started as a horsebox sauna temporarily wheeled into action for the Brighton Fringe Festival the year before, became so popular that it never left. One horsebox was joined by another, and another: now three wood-fired saunas huddle around a fire pit and stone seating circle, offering sun-soaked views of the pier and easy access to the sea. (For tree lovers, they have recently introduced a weekend-only woodland sauna in nearby Battle.)

When it comes to wild saunas, Beach Box is the trailblazer; and there's not much that its founder Liz Watson doesn't know about what makes a good sweat. She is a driving force on the UK scene, training staff in proper know-how, and bringing experiences from other sauna cultures into the mix. Think *aufguss*, leaf whisking, salt scrubs, sound baths and more. Talk to almost any sauna operator and they will have settled on a bench at Beach Box at some point. It's a place of sauna epiphanies, an incubator of ideas, and a training ground for a new generation. Above all, it's a very fine place to work up a sweat and stare at the sea.

beachboxspa.co.uk
Shower/sea/baths/cold plunge
50.8161, -0.1203

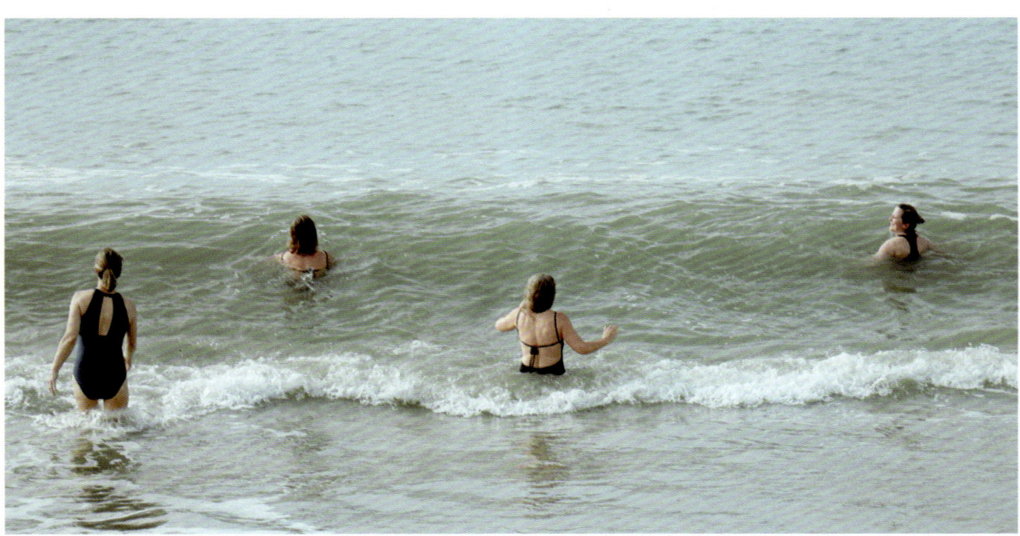

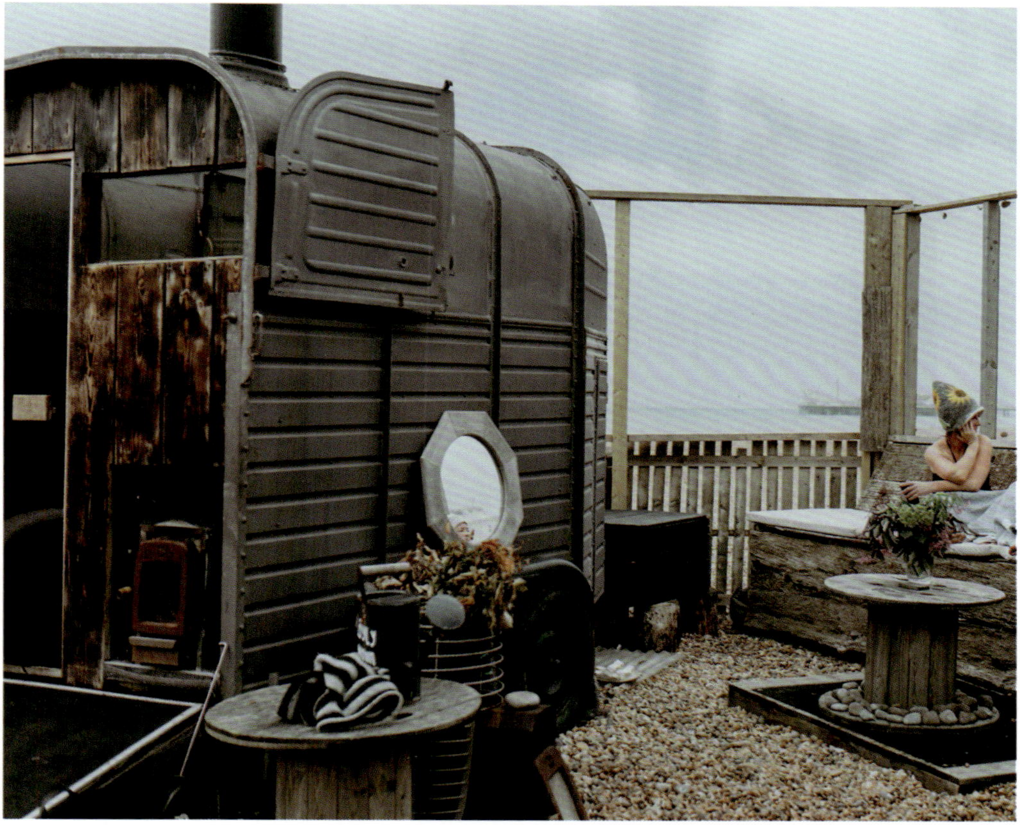

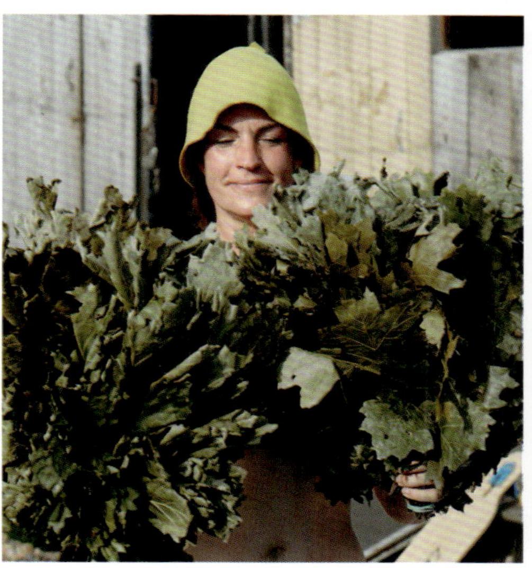

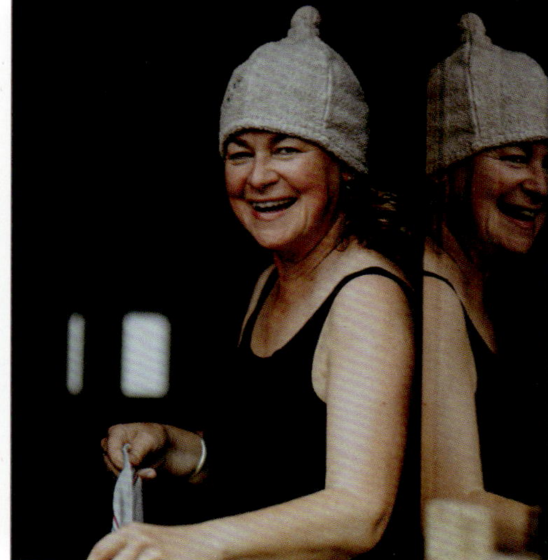

62

Stanmer Sauna Garden

STANMER ❦ SUSSEX

A group of women in changing robes gather round a fire, and Bella pops her head out of the sauna with a jar full of raw honey and frankincense that she has been using as a scrub. She had been foraging that morning for goose grass, a lymphatic tonic that comes into its own in early spring, and she is also armed with rosemary, bay, birch whisks from Lithuania and flowers. People gather round Bella when she explains their health giving properties and how she will use them in the sauna. She runs the first non-profit sauna seeded by the Community Sauna Network, which sits on council-owned land on the Stanmer Estate outside Brighton. The land is open to anyone on low incomes to develop community projects, and there are more than 20 to date. Neighbours include herbalists, musicians, potters, eco-therapists. Add these to the Victorian walled gardens, farm shop, cafés and packed programme of events, and Stanmer Estate is unsurprisingly a popular destination in the Sussex countryside.

➔ instagram.com/stanmersaunagarden
❄ Cold plunge ⌖ 50.8720, -0.1099

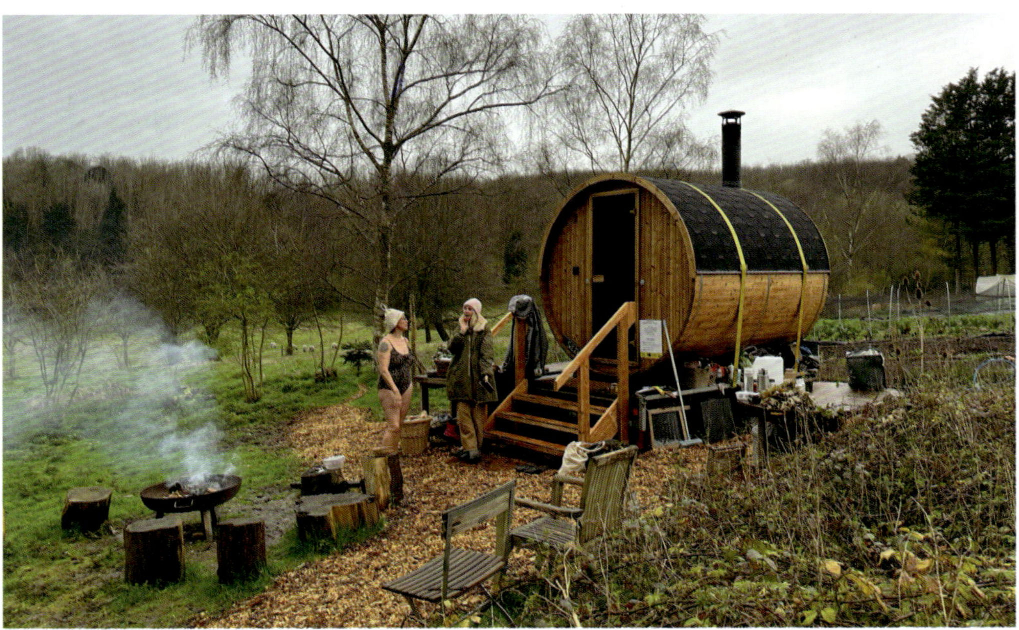

63

Sonder Sauna

THAME ❦ OXFORDSHIRE

While a plastic sauna may not sound plausible, these low-cost, polycarbonate sweatboxes are a popular option with handy types who like to experiment. They are also easier to transport, weighing around 400kg rather than the 2,000kg of a horsebox.

Kathy Thomas runs Sonder Sauna in the wellness area at Lopemede Farm. She inherited the see-through sweat box from the previous owner Aspen saunas. It's open seven days and there are donations-only sessions for people who might not be able to afford the regular fee. This 200-acre property farms wagyu beef and sheep and supports local businesses that offer connections to nature – think 'rogue' yoga, a 'feral' choir, tree planting and more.

➔ sonderexperience.co.uk

❄ Cold plunge/ shower 📍 51.7623, -0.9921

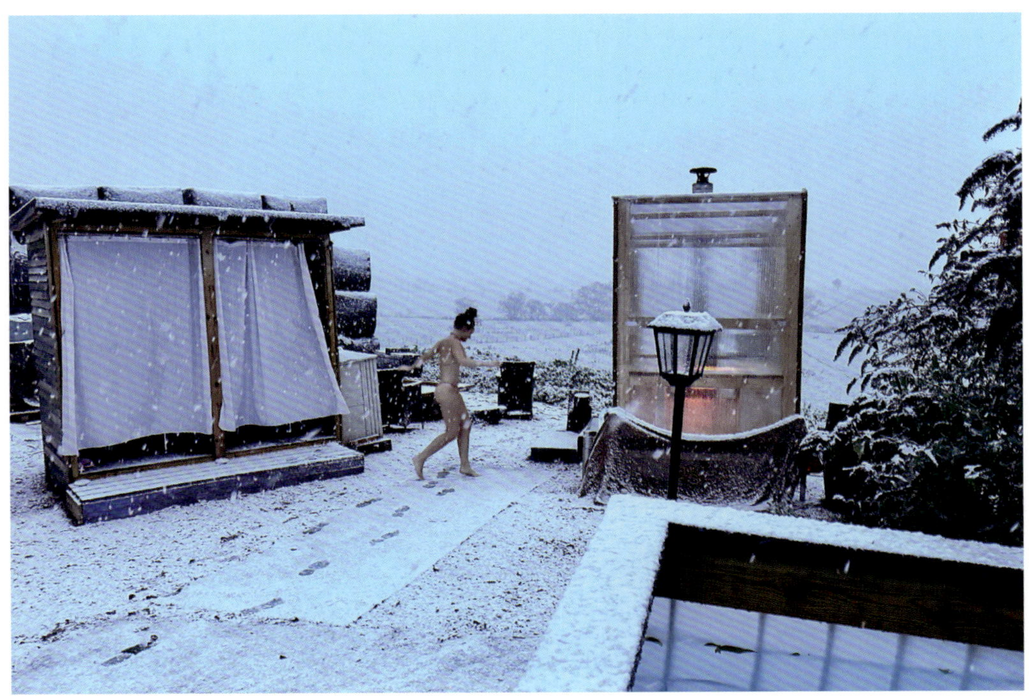

64

Wild Spa Wowo

UCKFIELD ❦ SUSSEX

With its three saunas, Wild Spa Wowo is a landmark address for sauna cognoscenti. Its founder, Katie Bracher, has been at the forefront of the sauna scene for more than a decade, co-founding the British Sauna Society and Beach Box Sauna Spa in Brighton, and advising many sauna start-ups in Sussex and beyond.

In 2021, Katie set up her summer spa in the woods at Wowo campsite and launched sauna master training sessions. To date, around a hundred UK sauna masters have trained with her.

But Wowo is a place you can enjoy if you're a sauna newcomer, too. Tucked away in the trees, its entrance is marked by an archway of stag oak branches. 'It's a cathedral of nature,' says Katie, who operates off-grid and builds her saunas predominantly in upcycled materials. 'It's about the nature connection, and we offer steam rituals and treatments that reflect that, incorporating leaf whisking, freshly foraged summer plants, clay masks and salt scrubs.'

The Forest Room is a steamy 40°C greenhouse where group training sessions take place, and the heat is gentle. A hotter sauna is found in the ten-seater trailer, and there's also a clay-lined *pirtis* sauna. *Pirtis* is the Latvian and Lithuanian word for sauna, and Katie runs training sessions with Birutė Masiliauskienė of the International Bath Academy in Lithuania. They specialise in leaf whisking and forage for birch and other seasonal plants to make their own whisks and scrubs. Lithuania was the last country in Europe to adopt Christianity (in the late 14th century), and its pagan roots are celebrated in *pirtis*. 'Before we started building churches, spiritual places would have been in nature, in groves of trees and so on,' Katie explains. 'For me, the origin of sanctuary and sanctum comes from nature.'

Special events range from full moon and solstice sessions to women-only and family sessions, massage in the forest glade and outdoor yoga. Cooling down slowly and chilling out is an essential part of the sauna experience (and one that is sometimes overlooked on a freezing windswept beach). A session lasts three hours at Wowo, and a large cold plunge, a cold bathtub, rainfall and waterfall showers, hammocks and chill-out areas guarantee a digital and real-world detox.

The camping fields around the Wild Spa are dotted with yurts, shepherd's huts, bell tents and geodomes; the whole site has a laid-back, festival vibe. 'It is said that every hour in the sauna is like a day's holiday,' says Katie, 'so you really do come for a mini break.'

➔ wildspawowo.co.uk

❄ Cold plunge/shower 📍 50.9926, -0.0068

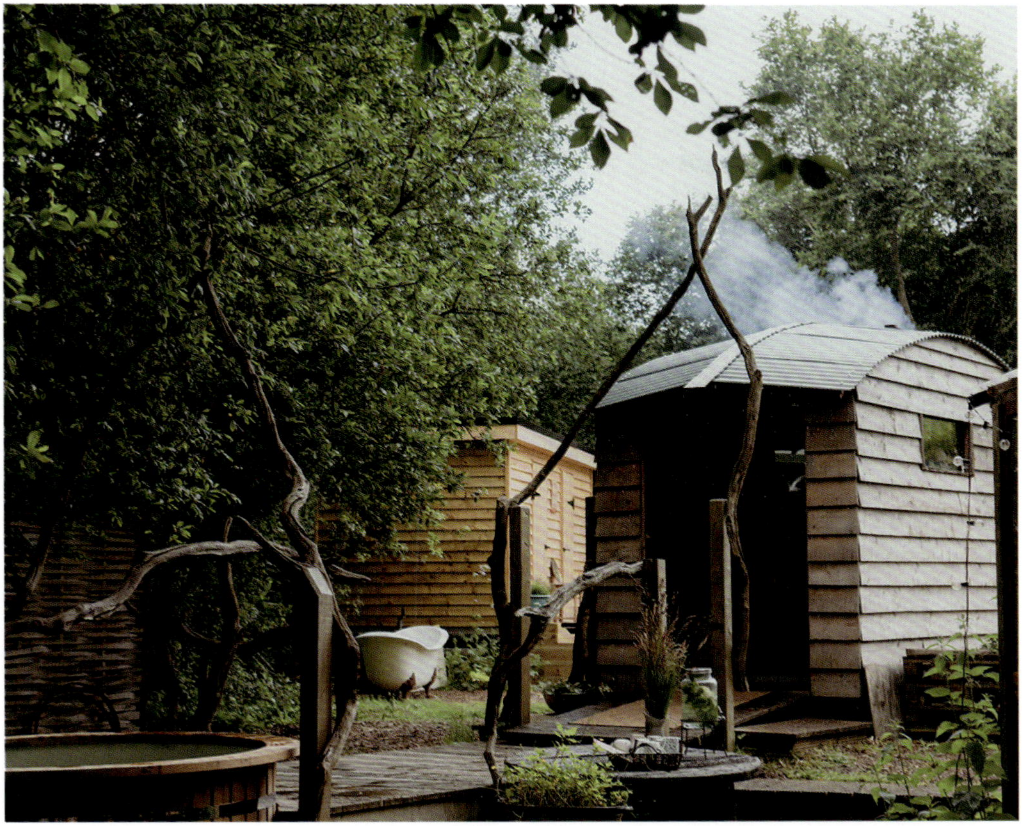

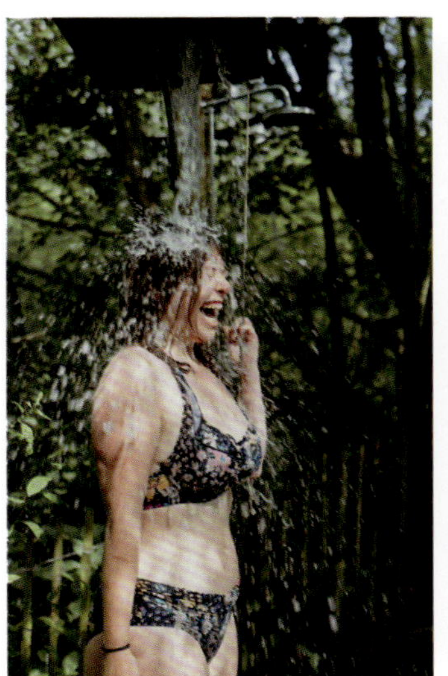

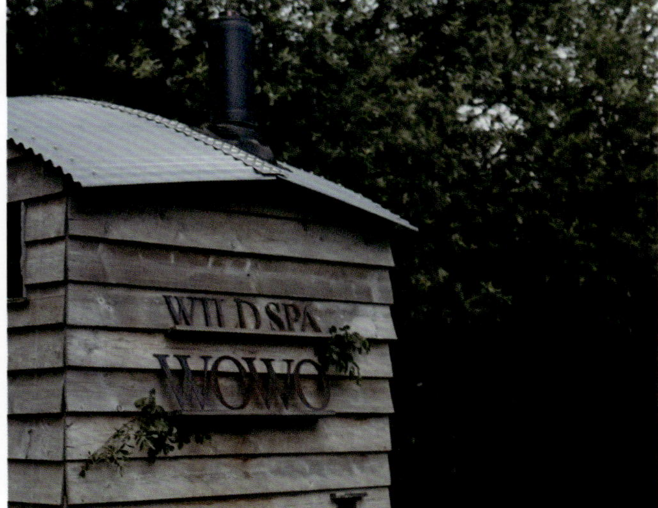
WILD SPA
WOWO

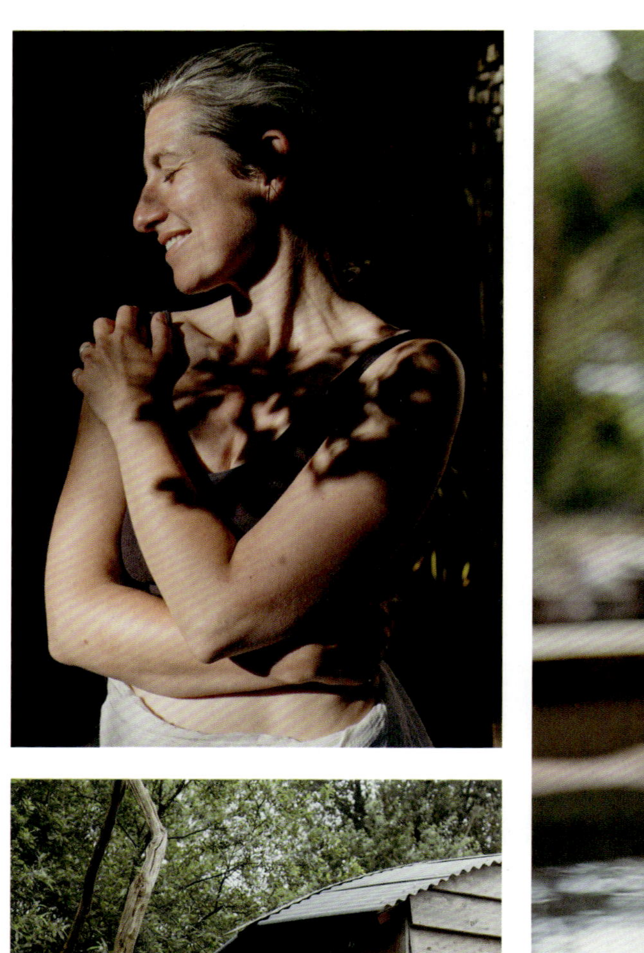

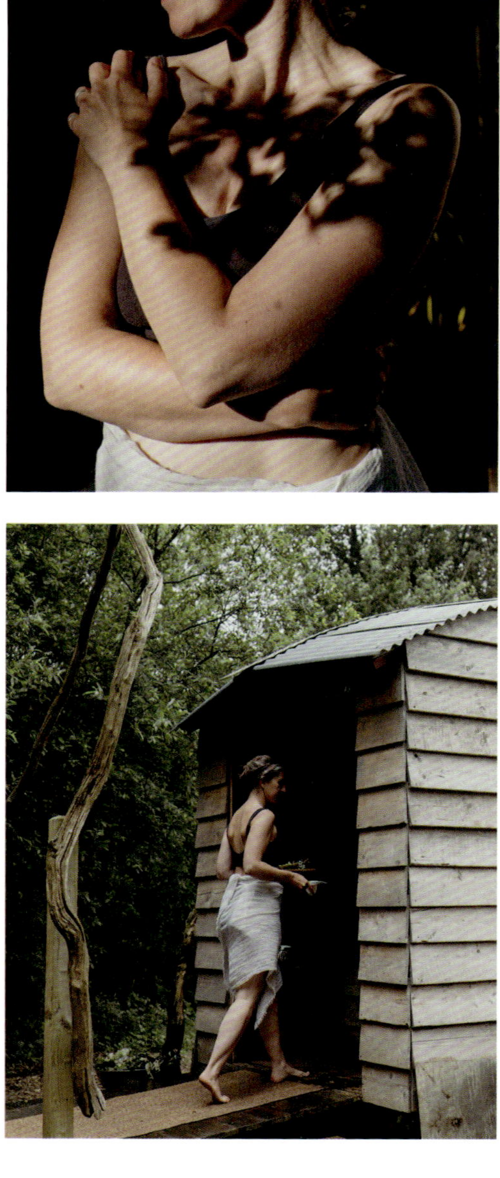

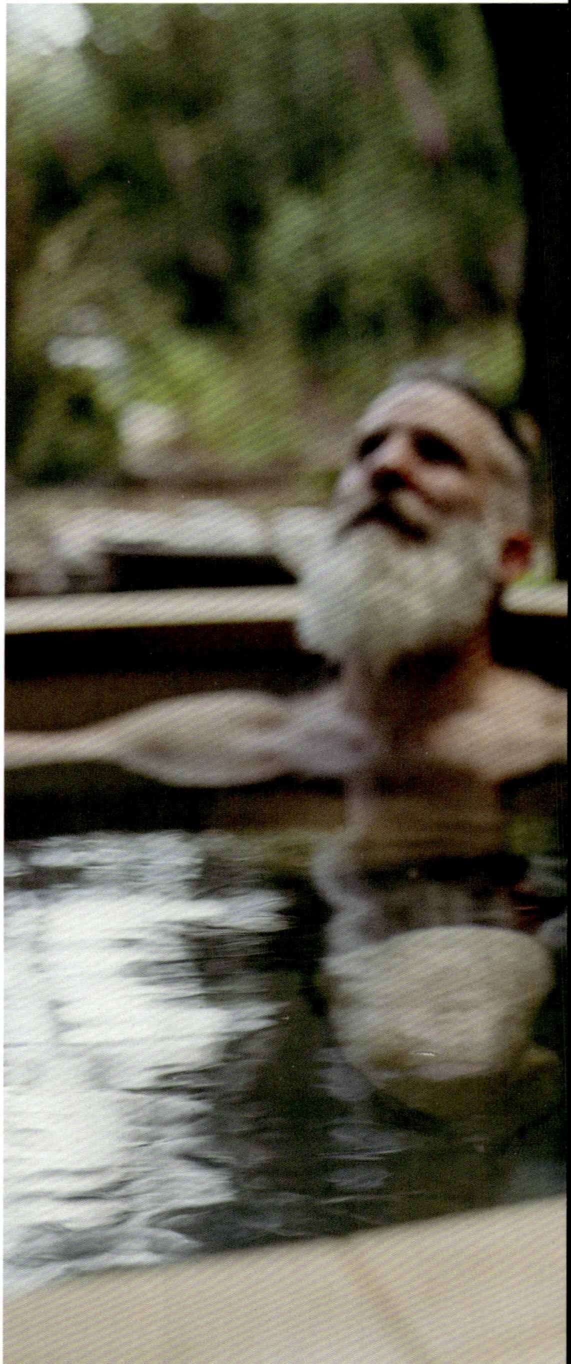

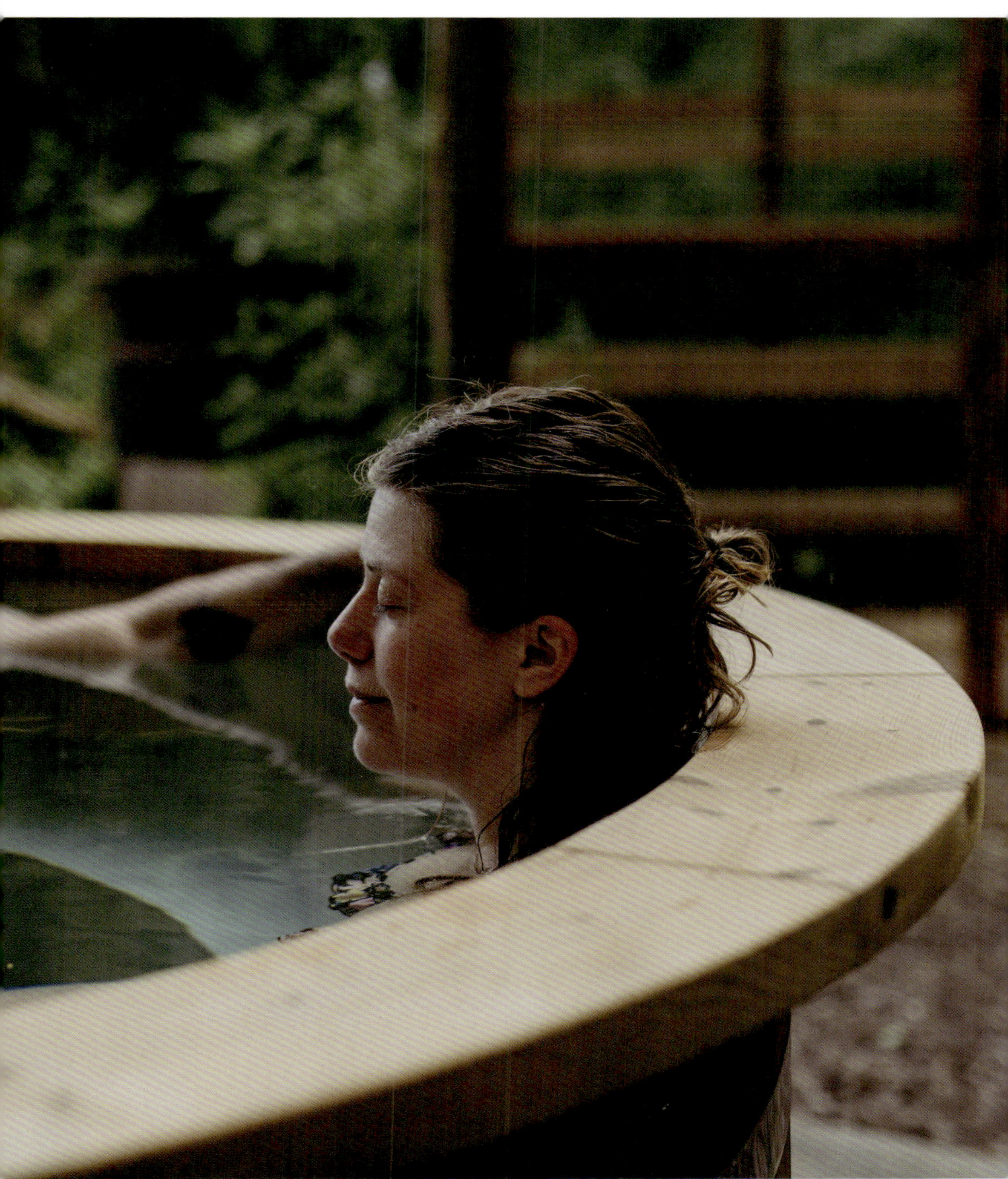

Wild Spa Wowo

65

Sauna Yoku

CUCKFIELD ❧ SUSSEX

Sauna Yoku takes its name from *shinrin yoku*, the Japanese concept of forest bathing, and Japan and Scandinavia feature heavily in the design of this converted horsebox. Owner Charlotte Monkhouse is a trained yoga, meditation and breathwork teacher, and she hosts moon events, guided wellbeing sessions, mini yoga retreats and other groups in both the sauna and the stretch tent next to it. Bathers can cool off in an idyllic swimming lake, which in summer is open to paddleboarders and campers at the Holmstead Himalayas campsite. The sauna has use of the campsite's toilets, changing rooms and showers, and in summer Charlotte installs a cold shower. Views across the South Downs are stunning, and the setup feels rustic and wild despite being a stone's throw from Haywards Heath.

➔ saunayoku.com
❄ Cold shower/lake ⚲ 51.0228, -0.1723

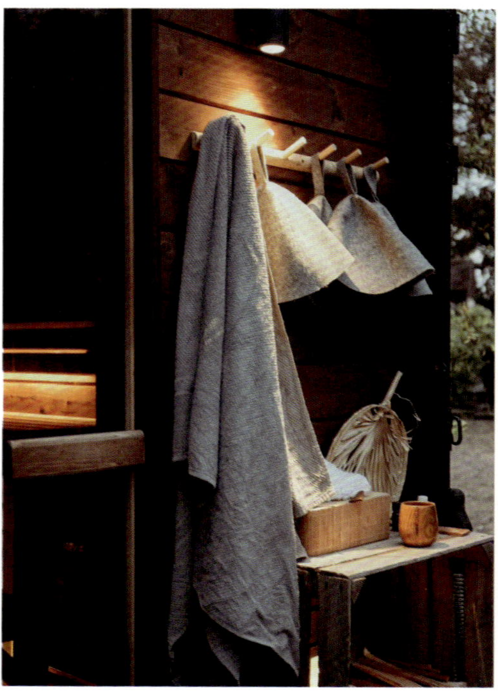

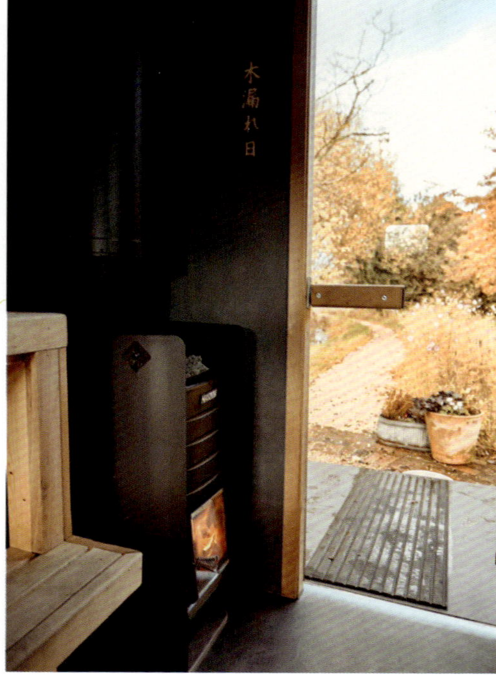

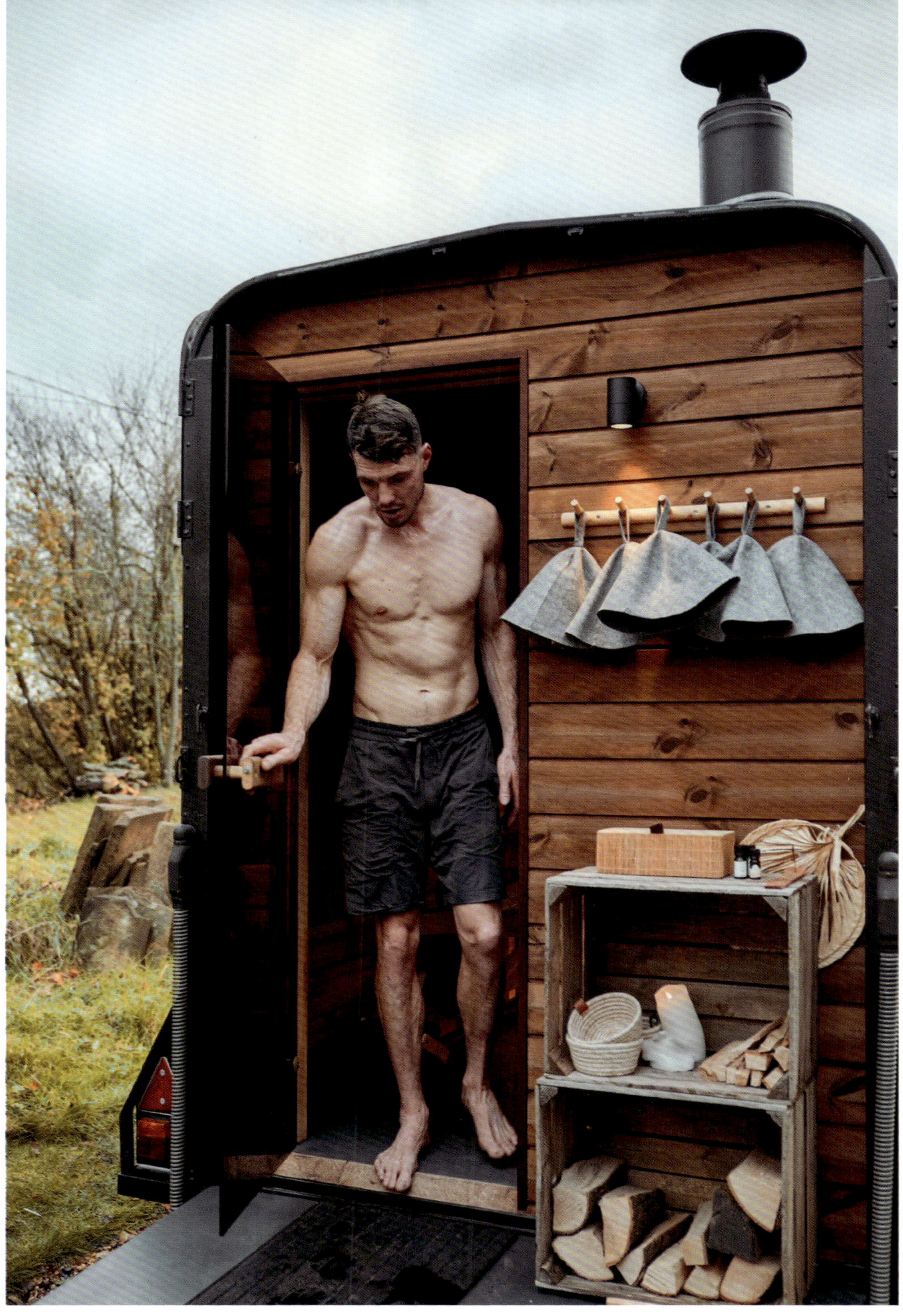

66

The Drying Shed Sauna

CATSFIELD • SUSSEX

The Drying Shed Sauna sits nestled in secluded woodland next to a stream, a pond and cold plunge at Architect's Holiday, a countryside escape in East Sussex. Architect, Will Gowling created it as an experimental project alongside three holiday cabins on his family's 24-acre farm. The sauna is made from red-stained larch shingles and takes its name from the shingle designs found on rural grain stores around the UK. It seats four, who perch on a bench made from a fallen silver birch and is lined with alder to match the surrounding woodland. Will got into sauna bathing through a Norwegian friend, and when he designed the first of the three cabins at the retreat, he liked the idea of a sauna so he could use it too. The Drying Shed Sauna is available to both cabin guests and non-guests.

architects.holiday/sauna

Shower/cold plunge /river 50.9003, 0.4507

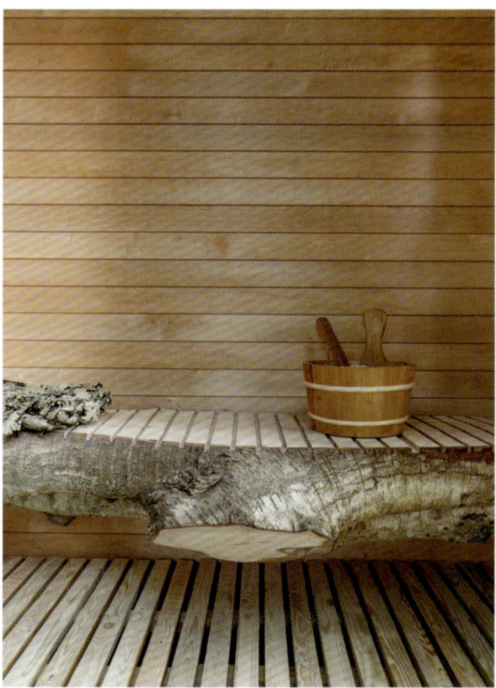

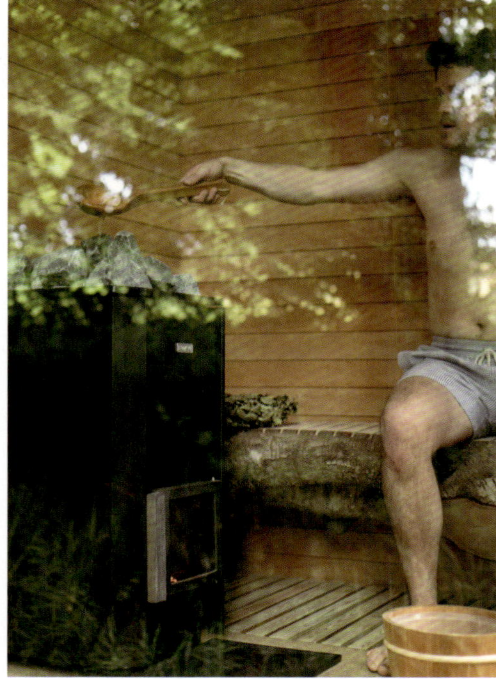

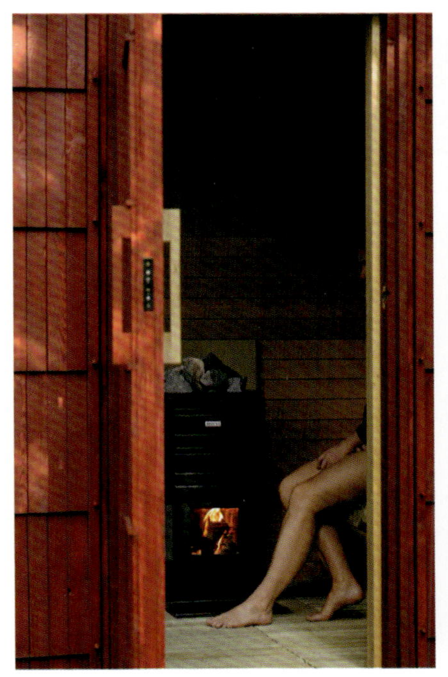

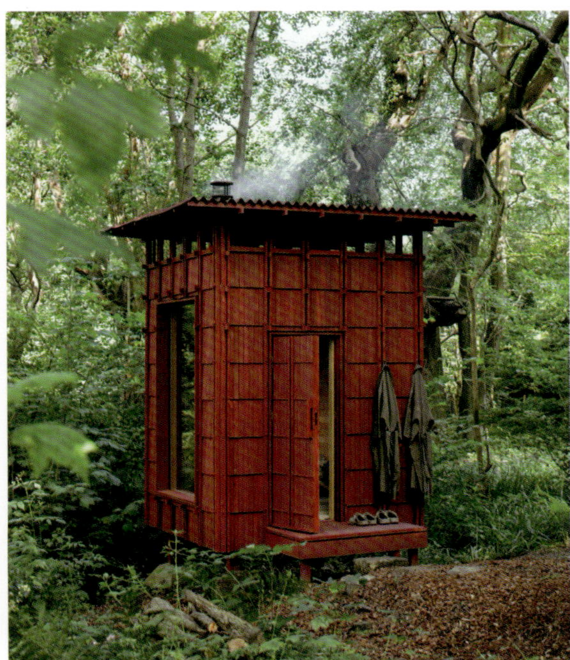

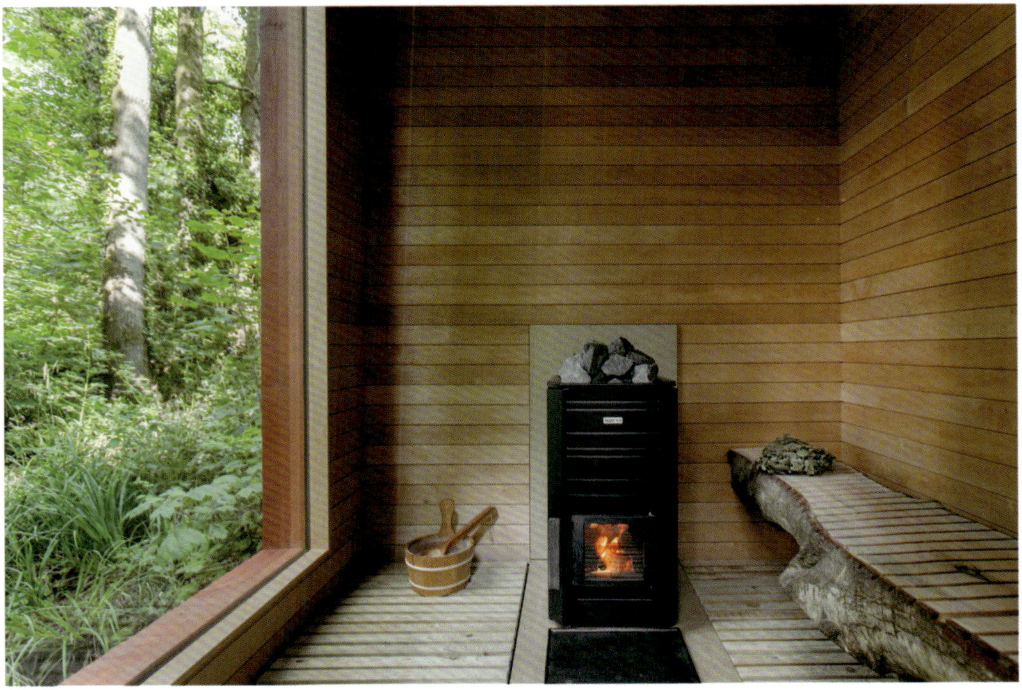

67

Samphire Sauna

HASTINGS ❦ SUSSEX

The first sauna to get a permanent home on a seaside pier anywhere in the UK (congratulations, Zoya and Nell).Samphire also offers an unexpected oasis of calm, especially at 8am, when the rest of the pier is still closed, and the town has yet to wake up fully. The beaches are dotted with cold swimmers who come from all along this stretch of coast, from Hastings to West St Leonards, to plunge into its more sheltered waters. They then head up to one of the two four-person saunas to bag a bench and warm up. As the pier wakes up, so does the sauna. And when the swimmers and pre-work crew leave, Samphire fills up with birthday gatherings, groups of friends, and strangers who come to connect in the steam. It's a sociable spot that has formed the backdrop to many a new friendship. 'We offer a buzz & connection to those that want it and moments of zen to those that need it,' says Zoya.

Like many UK saunas, Samphire was a lockdown project, and two years in the making. Founders Nell and Zoya are part of Hastings' lively creative scene; so too is the pier, which, although originally built in 1872, was rebuilt in 2017 (after damage from a fire in 2010). With its expansive deck that opens onto the sea, using timber reclaimed from the fire-damaged original, its minimalist design won the acclaimed Stirling Prize for Architecture.

Summer evenings at the end of the pier are alive with skaters, concerts, and a string of outdoor events. The saunas, screened off with deck chairs and a sun terrace/yoga space, feel private and cocooned. From here, you can witness the action without being part of it, and when the tide is in, you have the unique sense of being on the prow of a ship, offering uninterrupted views of the sea from the sauna bench. A cold shower unit with a bucket shower caters to those who don't want to cool off in the sea, and there are plenty of places for post-sauna drinks and snacks to find around town afterwards.

Samphire Sauna first popped up in Bodiam, then Eastbourne, then in Bexhill on the famous De la Warr Pavilion in 2022, but the pier is a top spot not just because it's exactly halfway between St Leonards and Hastings Old Town, but also because the Hastings Act prohibits anyone from setting up a new business between Bexhill-on-Sea and Rock-a-Nore beach in Hastings, meaning that Samphire is one of the few saunas to be found anywhere along this stretch of coast.

➔ samphiresauna.co.uk
❄ Sea/cold plunge 📍 50.8521, 0.5726

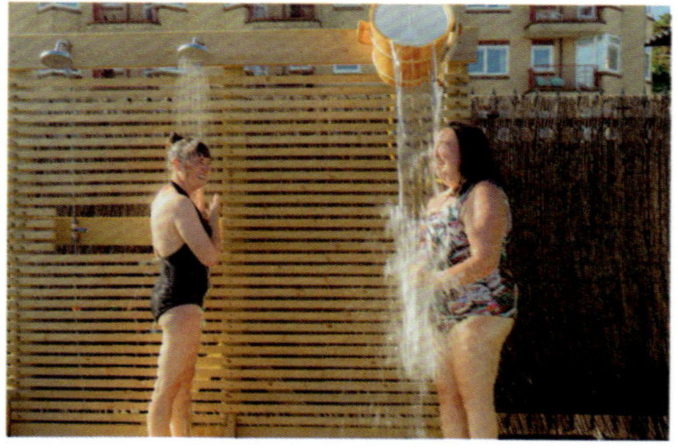

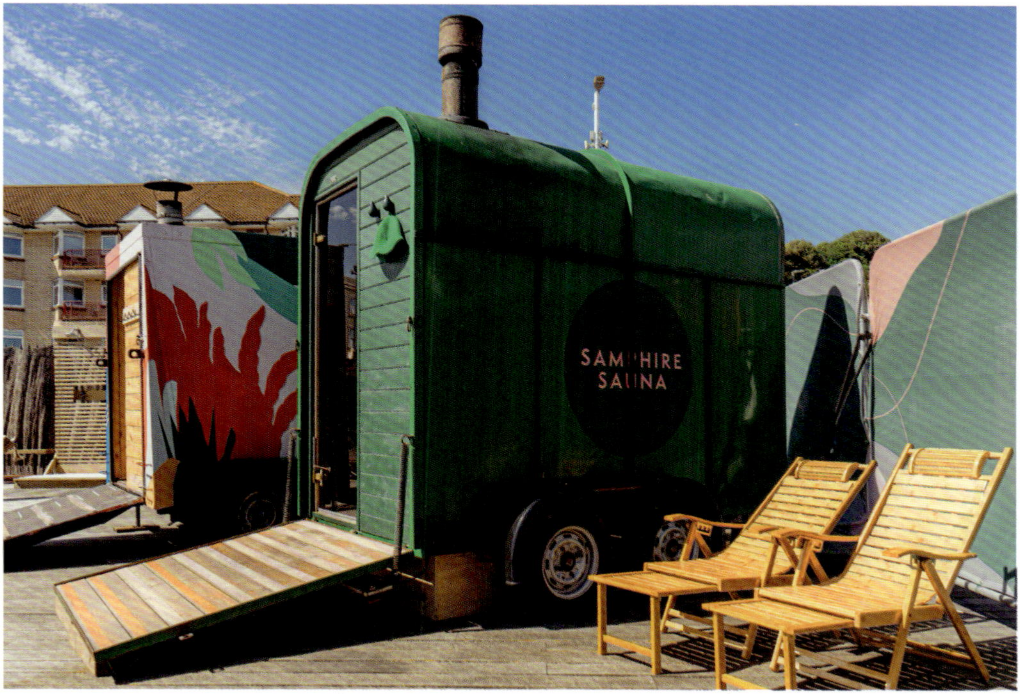

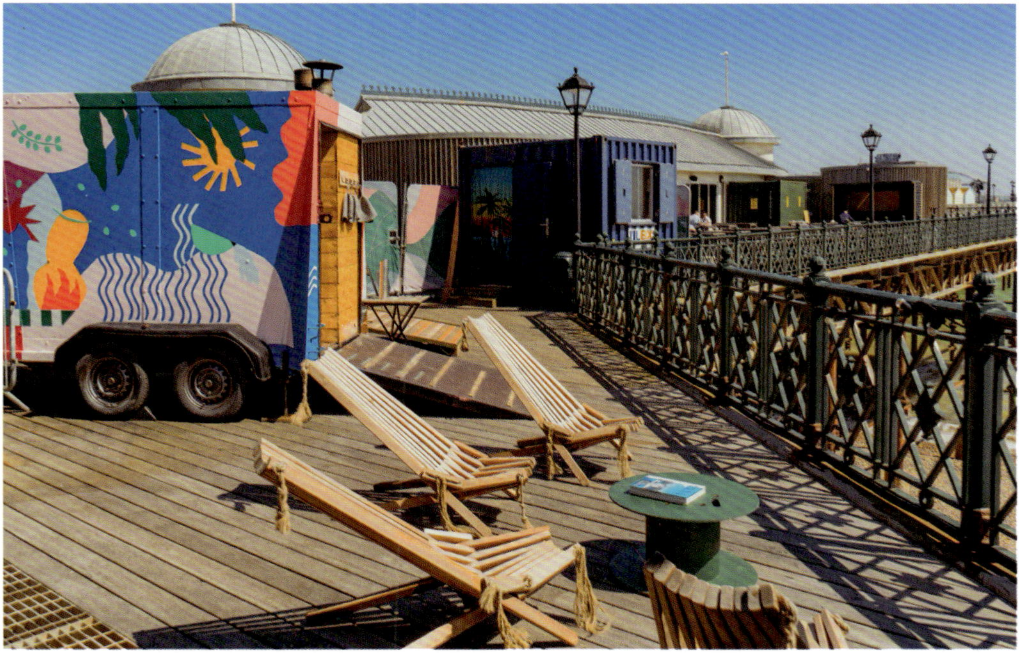

68

Sauna Social Club

PECKHAM ❦ LONDON

The clue's in the name of this sauna space located under a railway arch in south London. It's a place to connect with new people, disconnect from tech, and enjoy music and socialising without alcohol. ('Sober curious' is a growing wellness trend). Founders Benji, an actor, and Nikki, an ambient DJ, were inspired by sauna clubs in Berlin and by the listening bars of Japan, which prioritise sound over conversation. They conjured 'Japanavia style' interiors and built a sauna for 14. As well as offering contrast therapy (the backyard holds two ice baths, hot showers and a bathtub), the couple use the sauna as a creative space to 'play' – think *aufguss*, sound baths, queer yoga, poetry nights and more – all to the backdrop of ambient tunes.

➔ saunasocialclub.co.uk
❄ Ice bath/bath 📍 51.4695, -0.0624

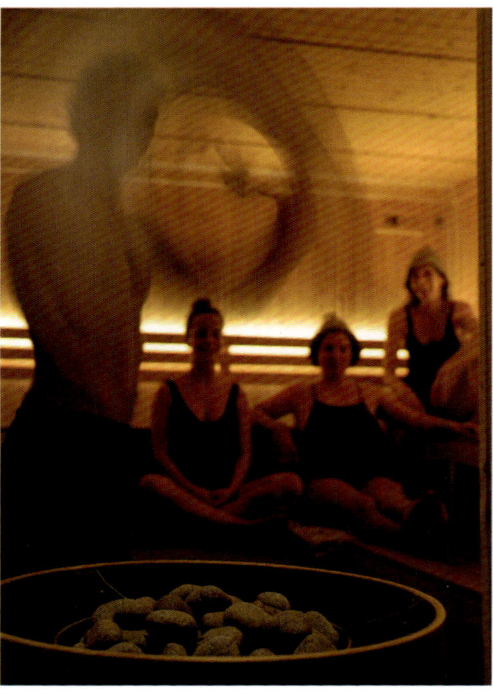

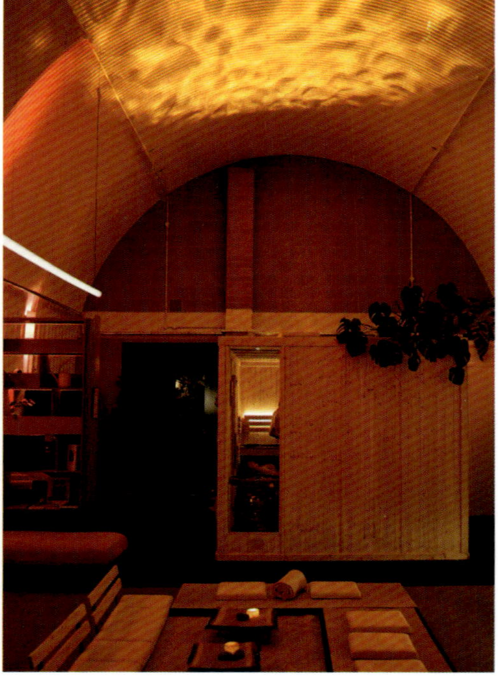

69

Community Sauna Baths

HACKNEY, STRATFORD & MORE ❦ LONDON

It's hard to underestimate the impact and influence the not-for-profit Community Sauna Baths (CSB) has had on the UK sauna scene. Since opening in the backyard of a former public baths in Hackney Wick more than three years ago, CSB has become a world-famous sauna destination, with sister sites in Bermondsey, Stratford, Peckham, Camberwell, and Walthamstow.

More than just a place to sweat, CSB is a welcoming space where people come together to relax, connect, and share experiences. It has become a true community hub, fostering a sense of belonging and wellbeing through the simple act of gathering in the heat. Many ideas are aired in the steam at CSB: think myth-telling saunas, sound bath saunas, pagan ritual saunas, trans saunas, sauna life drawings, and queer poetry nights. CSB works with the NHS and charities to offer free sauna sessions to those who might benefit the most, ensuring that warmth and wellbeing are accessible to all.

CSB has recently founded the Community Sauna Network (CSN), a Community Interest Company dedicated to supporting and empowering community saunas across the UK. CSN aims to create a robust and resilient network by fostering collaboration, resource sharing, and advocacy, as well as funding new community saunas. Thanks to the efforts of CSB and CSN, other places – such as Bristol, Devon and Inverness – are starting their own fires, bringing similar affordable, inclusive and authentic sauna experiences to their local communities.

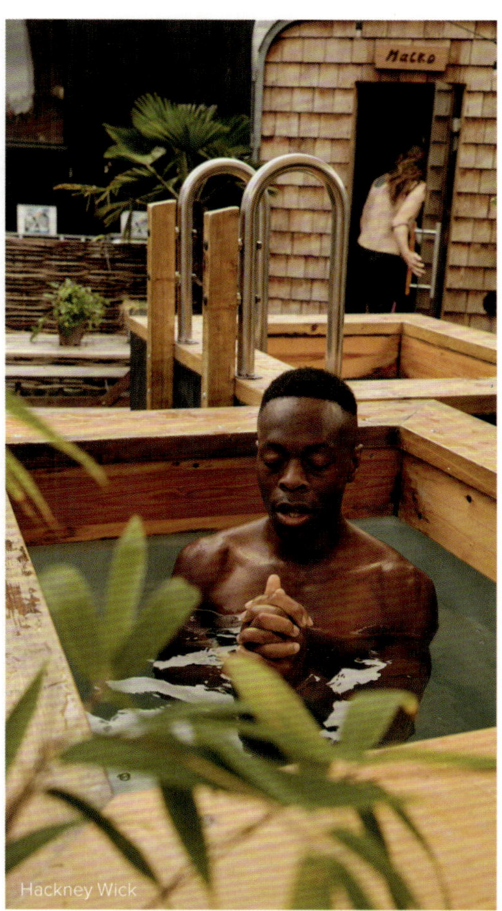
Hackney Wick

- community-sauna.co.uk
- Barrel/ice bath/showers
- 51.5471, -0.0293 Hackney Wick
- 51.5459, -0.0065 Stratford + more

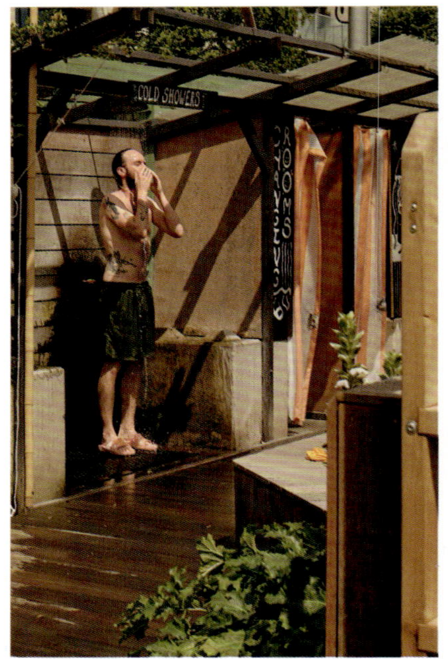

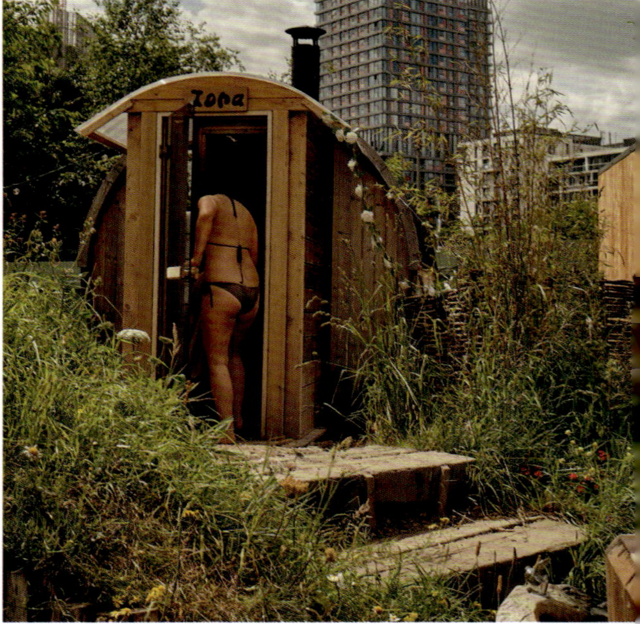

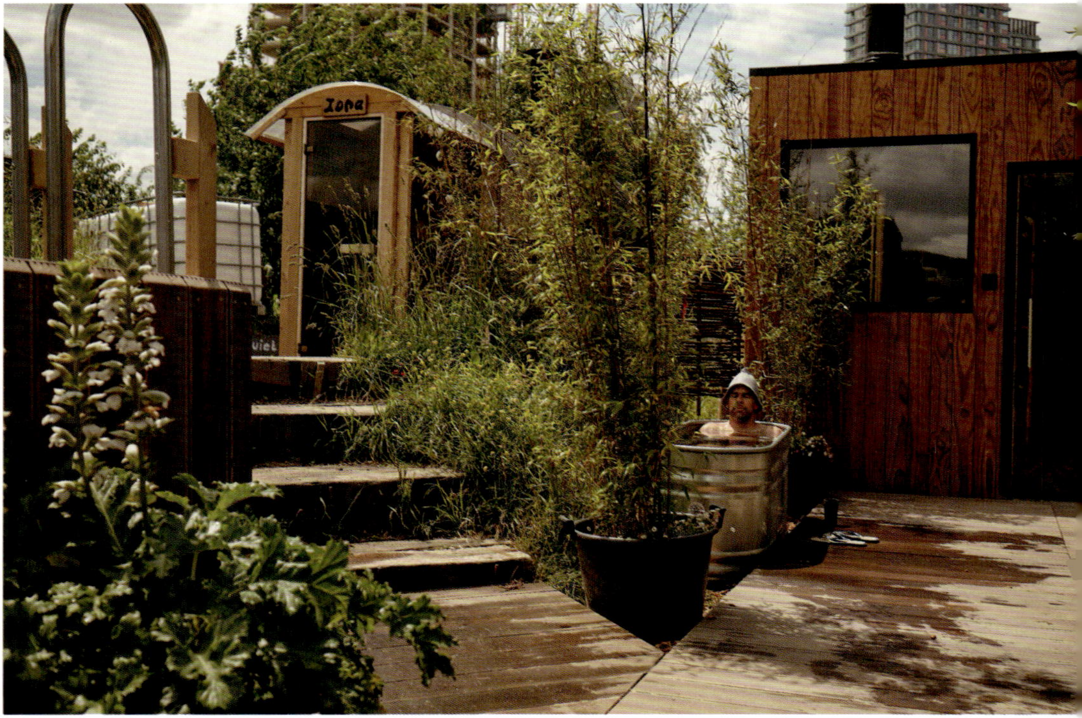

Community Sauna Baths Stratford

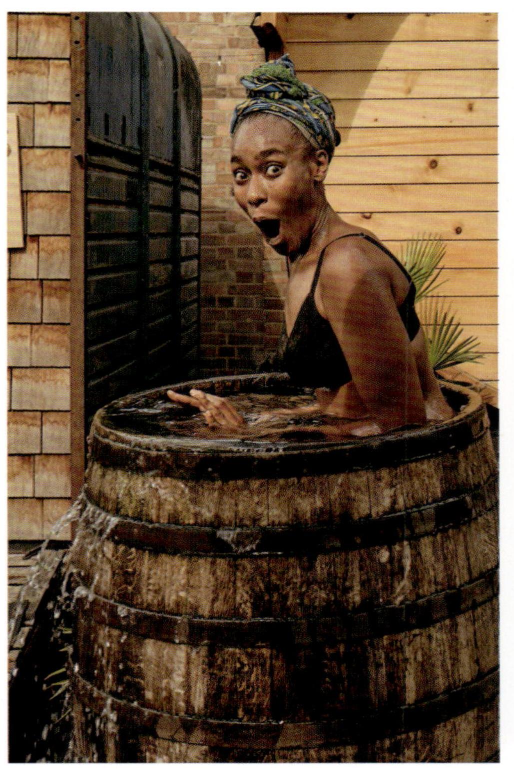

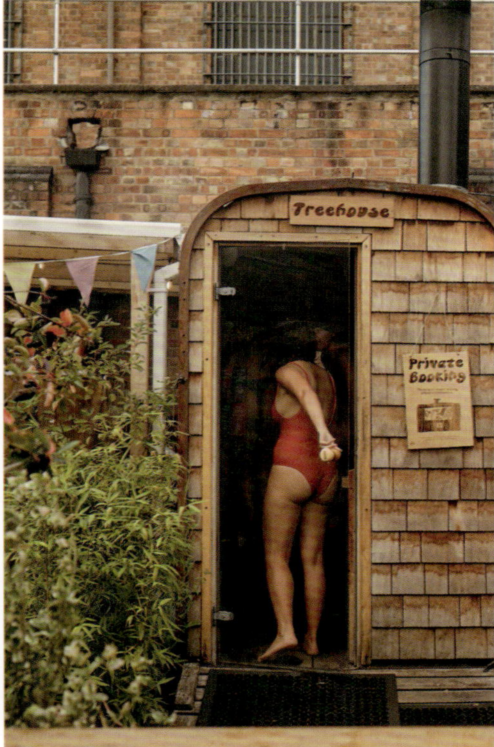

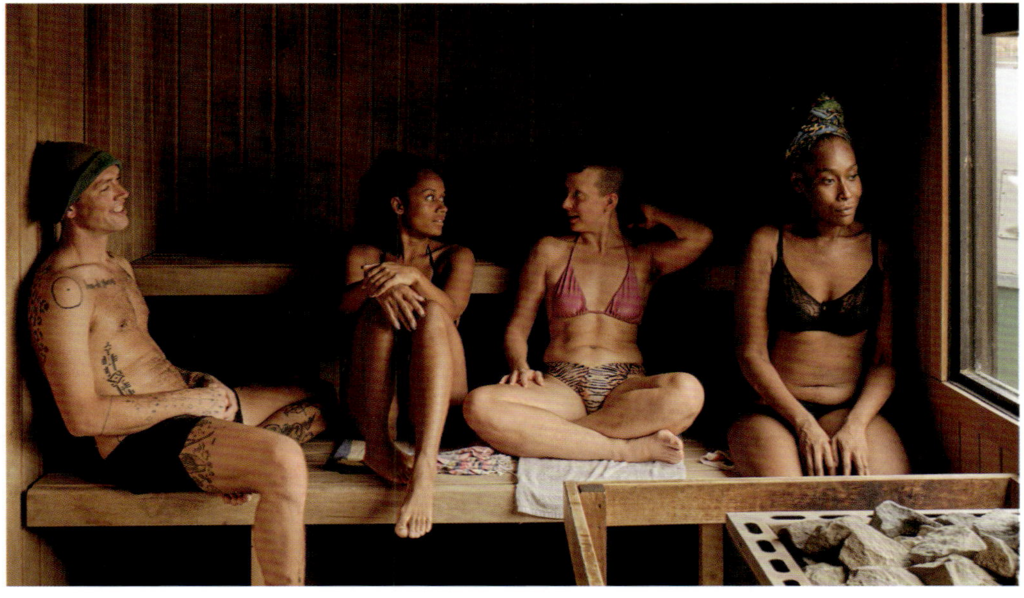

Community Sauna Baths Hackney Wick

70

Rooftop Saunas

HACKNEY & BRIXTON ❦ LONDON

For a city sauna with a view, nowhere beats London's Rooftop Saunas. What started out as four snug hot boxes on a disused Hackney rooftop has grown into a complex of eight saunas, six cold plunges, four drench buckets, warm showers, changing rooms and fridges stocked with drinks. Netil 360 rooftop bar and pizzeria next door provides bathers with many options to refuel, and the views of cranes, gas holders, graffiti and traffic below make for an uninterrupted and intriguing urban landscape. This spring, a sister Rooftop Saunas opened with the same set up on the 11th floor of an office block in Brixton. Both spots appeal to groups of friends who block book for a catch-up and to those who like the raw rooftop buzz. In 2023, Hackney Rooftop hosted the UK's first-ever Sauna Summit, bringing together more than 200 pioneers from the sauna world. Its creator, Ben Revill, is a carpenter who likes to experiment – he also created Slomo's floating sauna (50). For him, the only way is up.

→ rooftopsaunas.com
❄ Barrel/drench bucket/shower
📍 51.5374,-0.0573 Hackney
📍 51.4643,-0.1134 Brixton

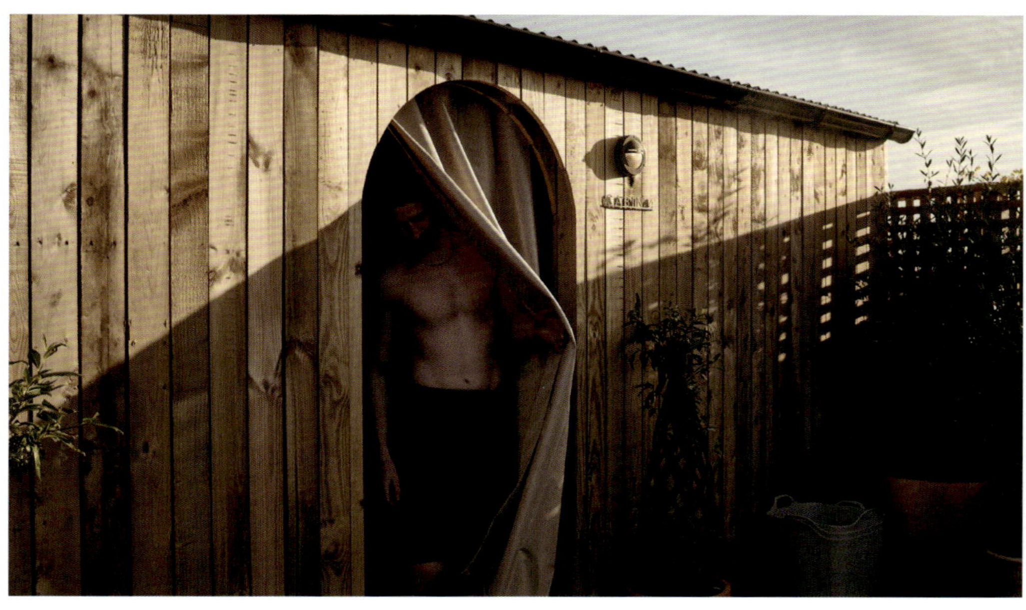

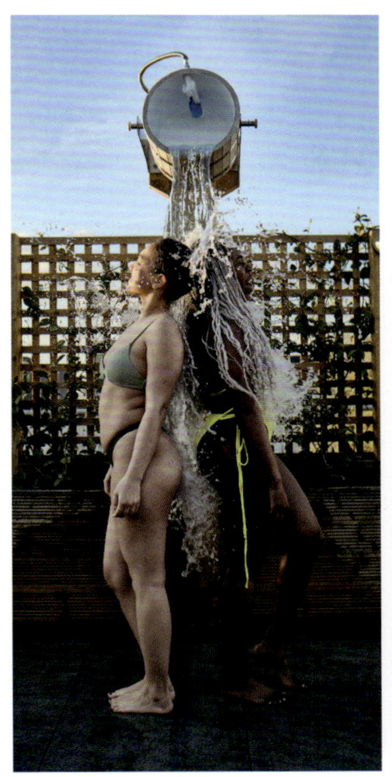
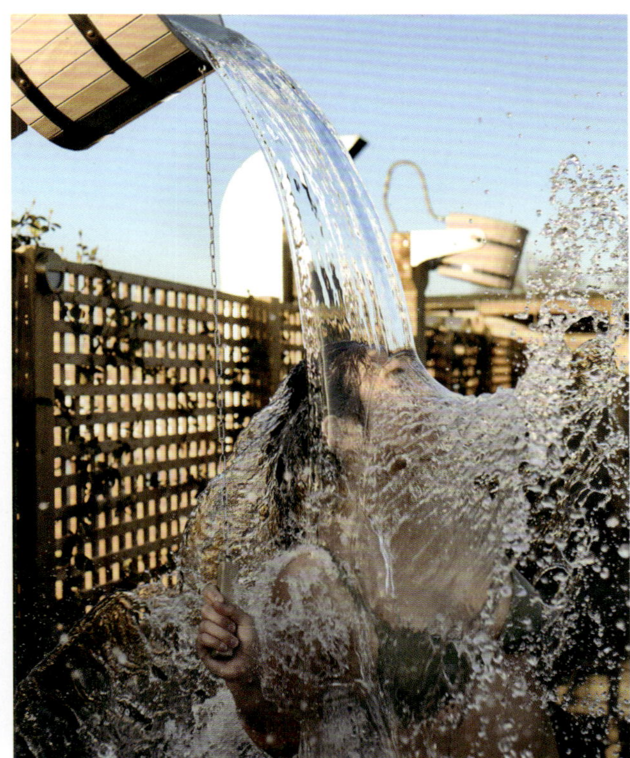
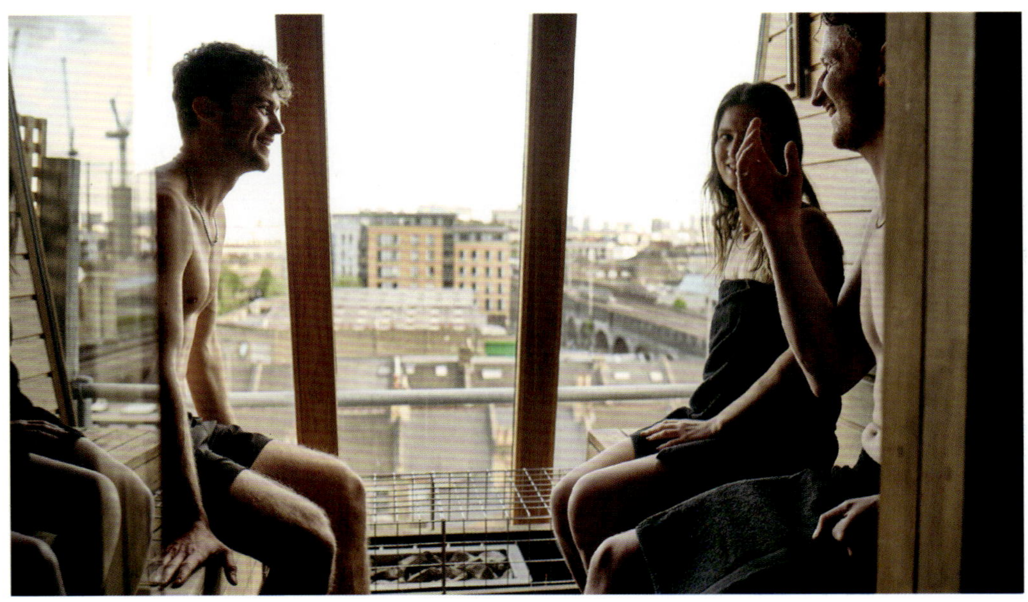

71

Sweheat Sauna

ROYAL VICTORIA DOCK ❦ LONDON

Are you a biohacker who likes to time your hot and cold immersions and exit the sauna when your watch tells you to, or are you a go-with-the-flow bather who exits when your body says enough? Victoria Maddox, the founder of Sweheat in London's Royal Victoria Dock, is firmly the latter. A sauna aficionado who has been on the wild sauna circuit for more than a decade, she discourages timers in Sweheat's two saunas, nudity is not discouraged, and *löyly* is plentiful (all of which please the local Lithuanian community, who are regulars).

Next to the sauna set-up is the Wakeup Docklands wakeboarding park, and together the outfits provide hot, cold, sport and relaxation at Western Beach. There are showers and a large communal cold plunge at Sweheat, but many prefer to dip in the dock, which is regularly tested for cleanliness. Sweheat regular Jon Byrne runs Wakeup Docklands and explains his attitude shift from biohacker to sweat-bathing evangelist: 'I have had spinal surgery, double knee surgery, hip surgery and torn many ligaments. The cold is great for sharpening the mind and bringing down inflammation, but I can soften in the sauna,' he says. 'I try to get customers who sauna after boarding to leave their timers outside, because the sauna feeling doesn't leave you when you stop the clock.' Victoria knows this, which is why at Sweheat, time really does stand still.

➔ sweheatsauna.co.uk
❄ Cold plunge/dock/showers 📍 51.5058, 0.0165

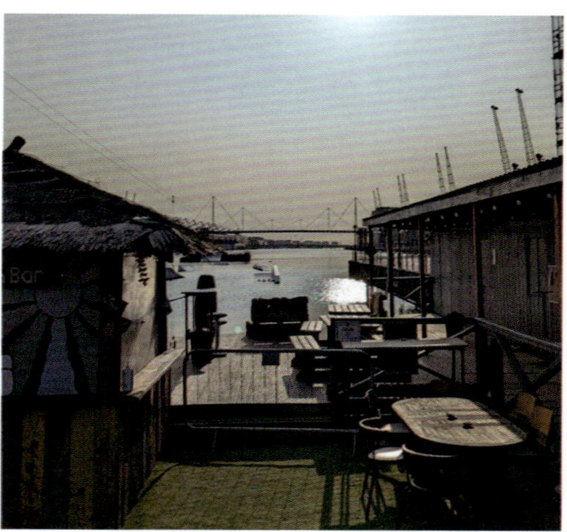

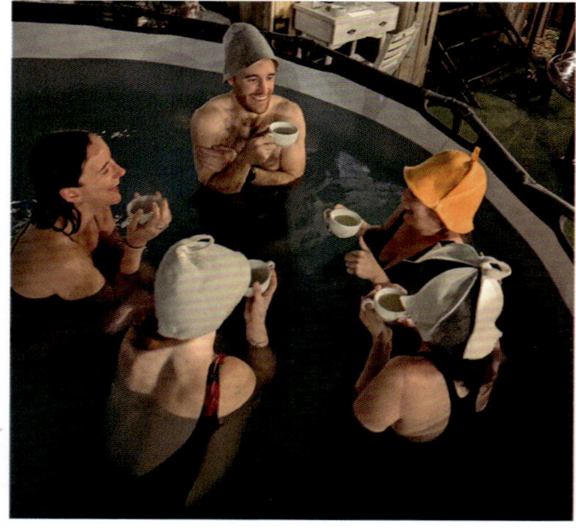

72

Heal Saunas

THETFORD FOREST ❦ SUFFOLK/NORFOLK

Sam and Molly Medley got married at local wild spa PAUS (75), and set off on a sauna odyssey. They travelled the UK, Ireland and Scandinavia in their van, hosting nature-based sauna rituals in the UK before returning home to Cambridgeshire. With his experience in carpentry and construction, Sam then built a ten-person wood-fired sauna and named her Hilde after a Norwegian sauna practitioner they had met on their travels. The couple forage ingredients and make all their own sauna products, and Molly's scrubs made of coffee, honey and brown sugar, and of sea salt and orange peel have become signature treatments.

➔ healsaunas.co.uk
❄ Cold plunge/shower ⊙ 52.4344, 0.6630

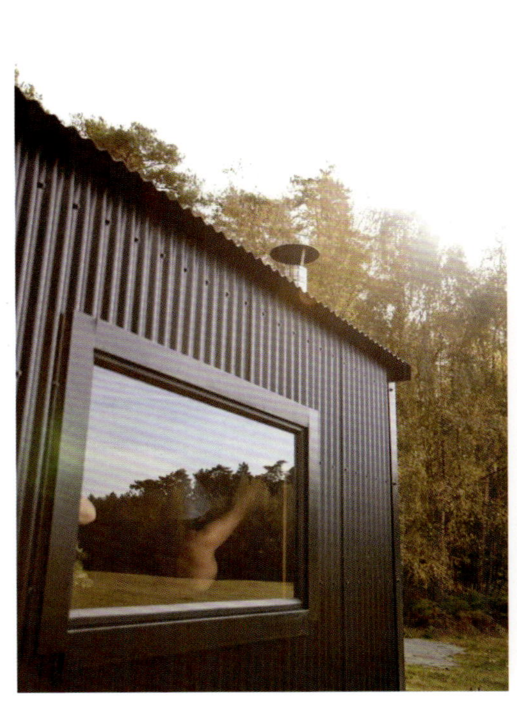

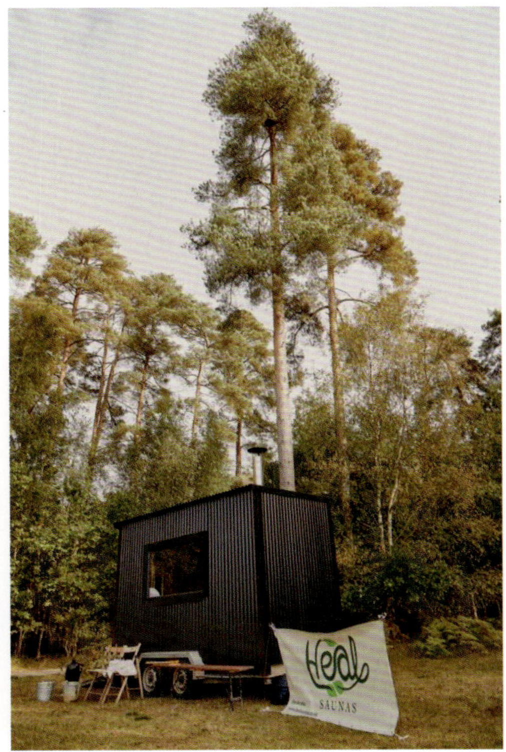

73

Suku Sauna

TOWSTER ❦ NORTHAMPTONSHIRE

Inspired by the unsupervised Kuuma saunas on the canals of Amsterdam, brothers George and Josh Taylor decided to create a similar version on family land near Milton Keynes. They commissioned a carpenter friend to build them a sauna for six to ten people and set it up with two buckets, a cold plunge, and a cold shower next to a lake, where dipping will shortly be an option. Upon booking, bathers receive a text message with the sauna door code, and they are left to their own devices. Throwing water on the rocks and cleaning up when they're done are both encouraged. Does this autonomous approach work with Brits? "We try to avoid too many guidelines, and most people like it," says George, who is planning to develop it into a wellness site with wild swimming and padel courts. There's a security guard on site who checks bookings and helps in an emergency, and cleaners go in once a day. Enabling bathers to enjoy full freedom while taking responsibility is the model of advanced sauna nations, so let's hope the UK follows suit.

sukusaunas.co.uk

Cold plunge/bucket 52.1111, -0.9316

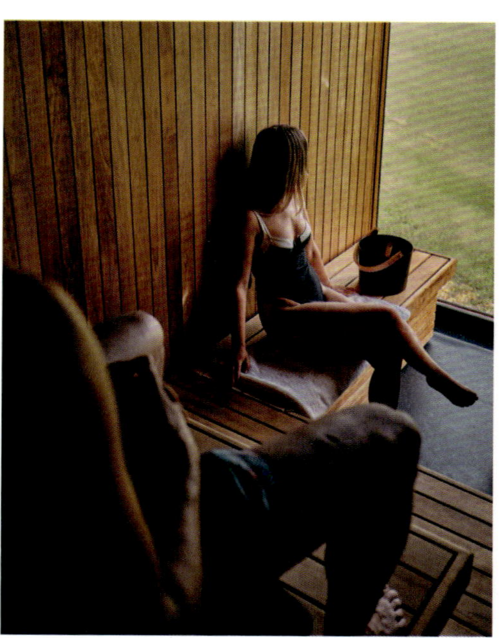

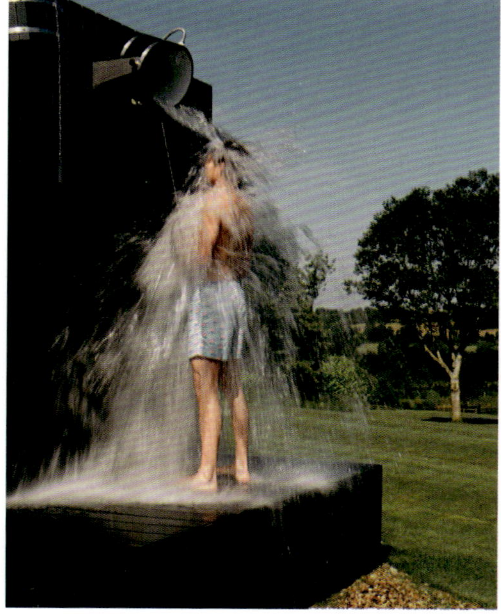

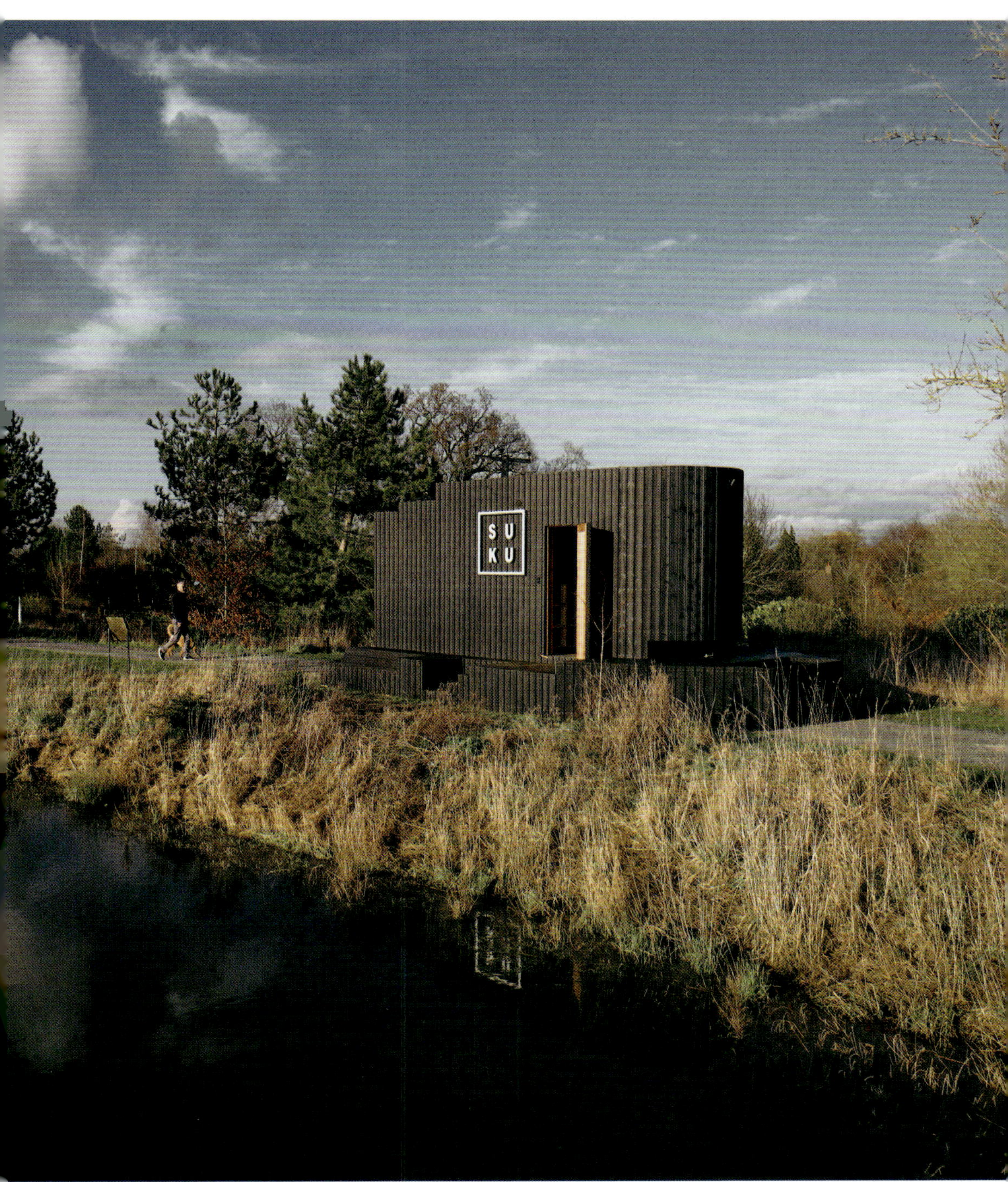
S U
K U

74

PAUS

CAMBRIDGE ❦ CAMBRIDGESHIRE

PAUS (pronounced 'pause') is one of the original wild spas. Just 20 minutes from Cambridge, PAUS sits on a hilltop surrounded by 24 acres of meadows. Founded in 2018, it is the permanent venue of Bathing Under the Sky. Czechoslovakian founders, Alexandra and Bart, have spent 15 years crafting wood-fired hot tubs and saunas and touring their wood-burning pop-up spa to events and festivals across the UK. There's not much they don't know about wild spa experiences.

At PAUS, 12 wood-fired hot tubs and four saunas share the hilltop spot with ice baths, three large plunge pools, and cold showers. There are a host of bathing options, a bistro, and nature walks with panoramic views.

The largest sauna, Tauko Gaia, seats up to 16 people, while two other barrel saunas cater to smaller sessions. A fourth – the Waterside Sauna – is nestled under mature trees and can be hired for private gatherings, special occasions, and woodland events. The meadows have been regenerated from a sterile golf course; they include a 1km barefoot sensory trail and a grass maze. The Hilltop Bistro serves delicious dishes made with seasonal produce grown on-site; where a homemade 'post-sweat' electrolyte drink developed by the in-house nutritionist is popular with sauna bathers.

PAUS makes for an excellent day trip – a perfect combination of clean and luxurious, while feeling unfussy and exposed to the elements. With hot showers with Faith in Nature toiletries, towel and bathrobe hire, deck chairs and sun loungers, and a cold water 'playground' in the planning, it echoes the sort of affordable day spa that, in the UK at least, feels hard to come by.

➔ paus.life

❄ Cold plunge/shower 📍 52.1835, -0.0481

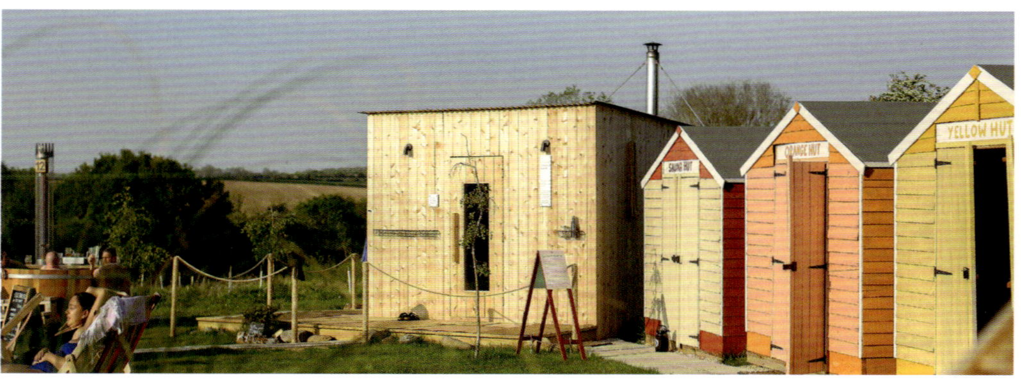

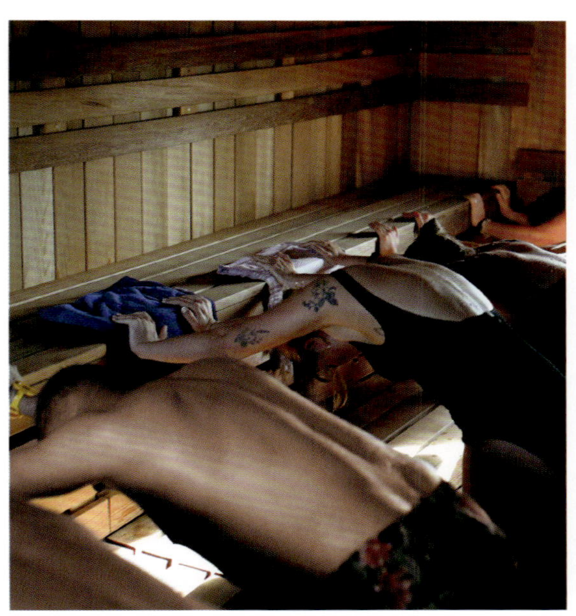

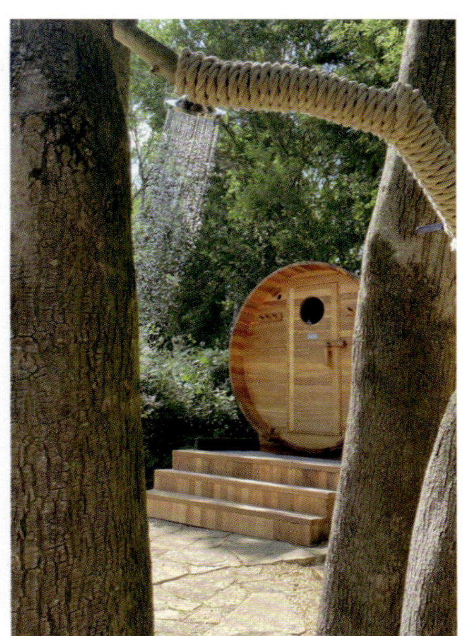

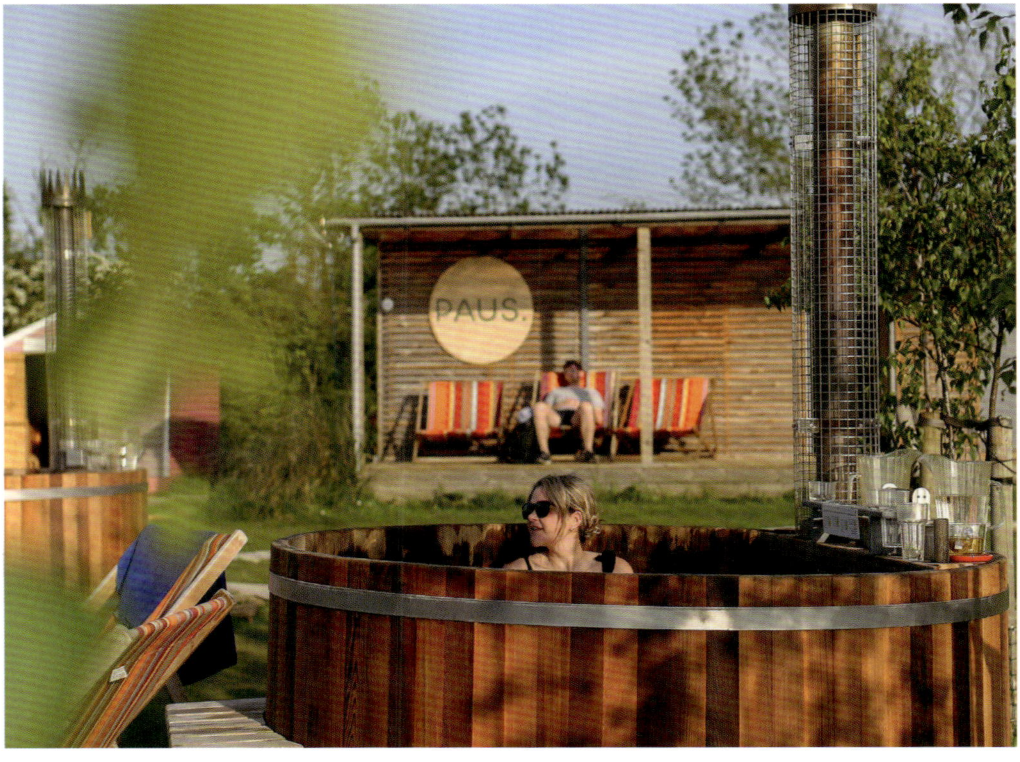

75

The Hot Box Co

PENSHURST ❦ KENT

Jack Botting lived in Japan for four years where he developed a love of *onsen* (hot springs). After returning to the UK and realising that 'winter here is not exactly exciting, like it is in Japan', he bought a barrel sauna and located it at Kingdom, a 13-acre wellness and activity forest in the Kent countryside. A cold plunge, bucket shower, running water, solar panels and a wind turbine complete the off-grid set-up. 'It's a space for the community to come together,' says Jack. 'We're not for the hardcore. It's aimed at as many people as possible: easy access, a simple experience and a gateway for lots of people who haven't tried sauna before.'

The larger Walled Garden sauna can be found at the Walled Garden Wellness Centre in Tonbridge.

thehotboxco.co.uk Cold plunge/shower
51.1618, 0.1625 Penshurst
51.2162 0.2323 Tonbridge

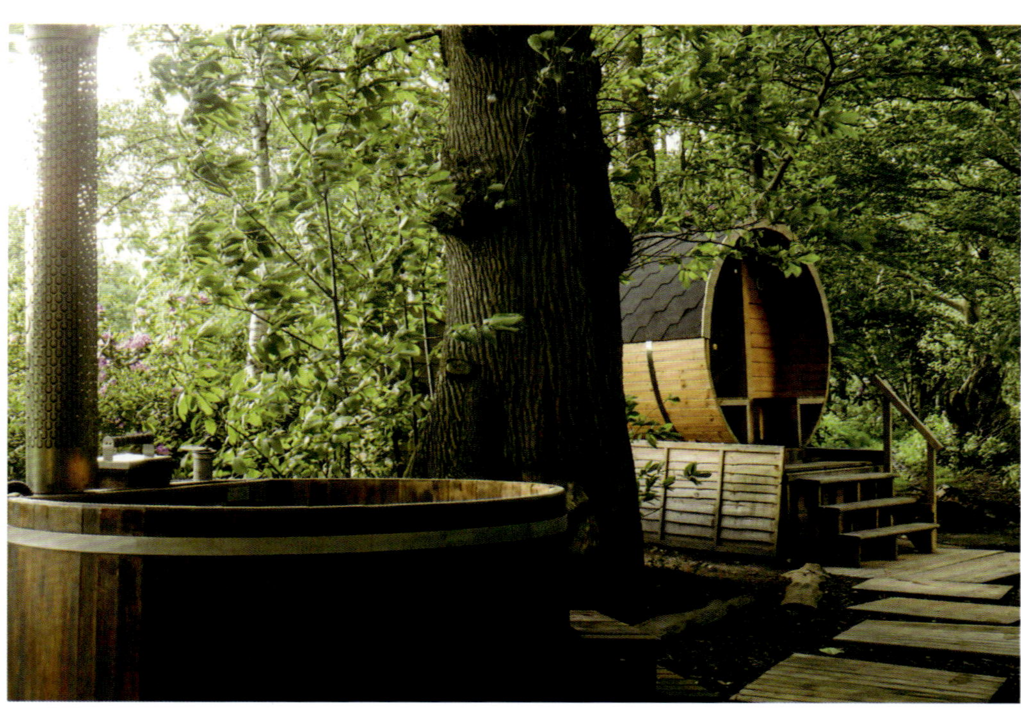

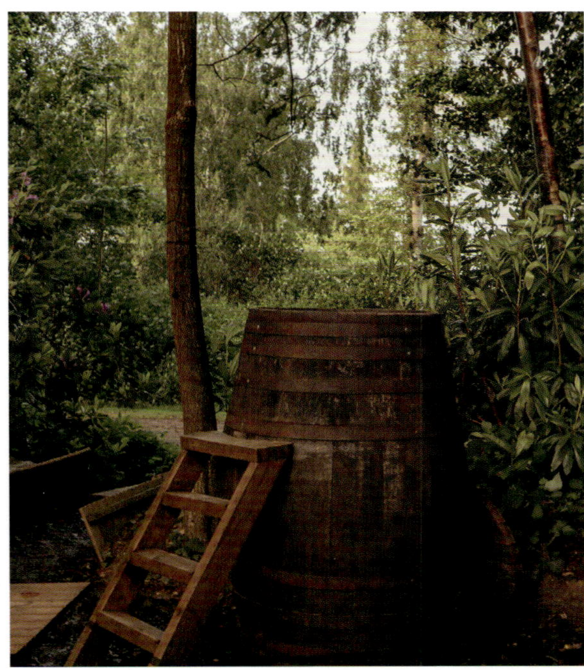
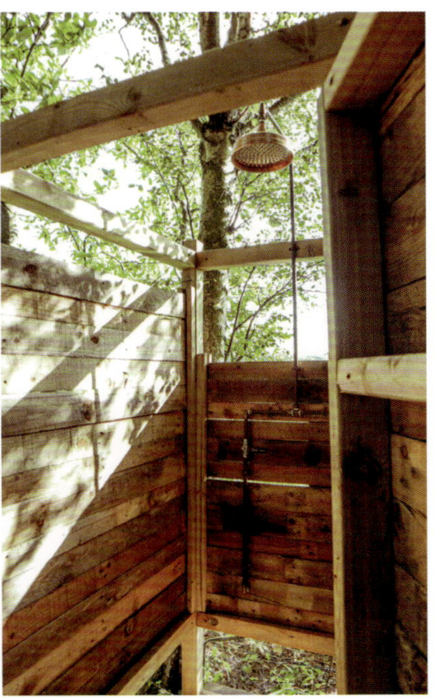
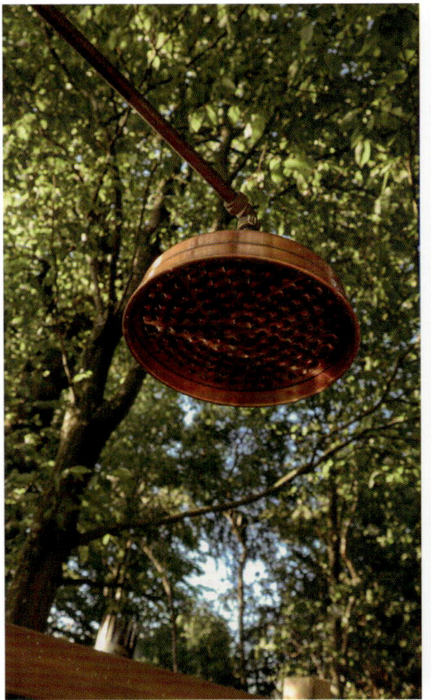
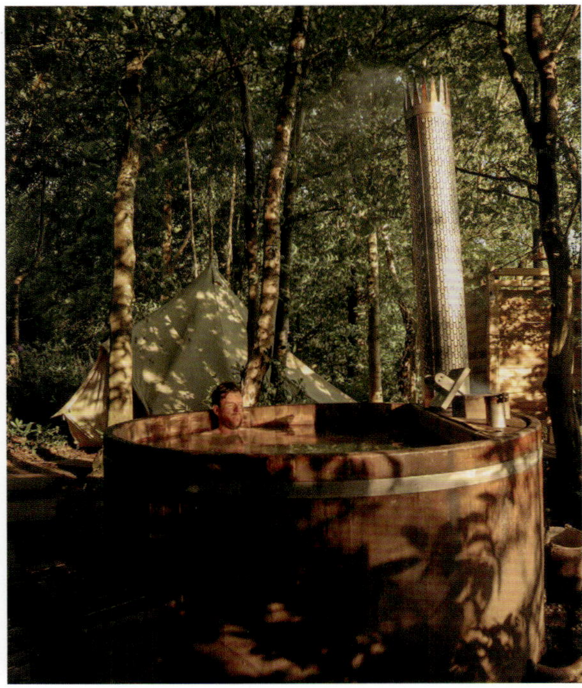

76

Rebels Dover

DOVER ❦ KENT

With its distinctive doodle art graphics and tattooed owner, Rebels Dover is a sauna, coffee shop and creative community hub on the esplanade at Dover. Founder Tim Smithen is an artist, musician and tattooist. He had been running Steampunk Sauna in Folkestone for two years when the Port of Dover and Dover Town Council asked him to take over the disused toilets on the esplanade. It's a busy spot: a starting point for swimmers heading across the English Channel, and for rowers and athletes who train on the beach.

Tim turned the block into a ten-seat sauna and a cool café that serves toasties, beer and good coffee. Events range from art shows to vintage clothing fairs; a 'Sauna Sisterhood' session caters specifically for menopausal women.

Tim's mobile woodfired sauna 'Steam Punk Sauna' is in the process of returning to its original site on the beach in Folkestone.

And on the topic of tattoos, how do they fare in the sauna? 'It's sun exposure, not heat, that causes tattoos to fade,' says Tim – and he should know.

➔ instagram.com/rebels_dover
❄ Sea 📍 51.1250, 1.3222

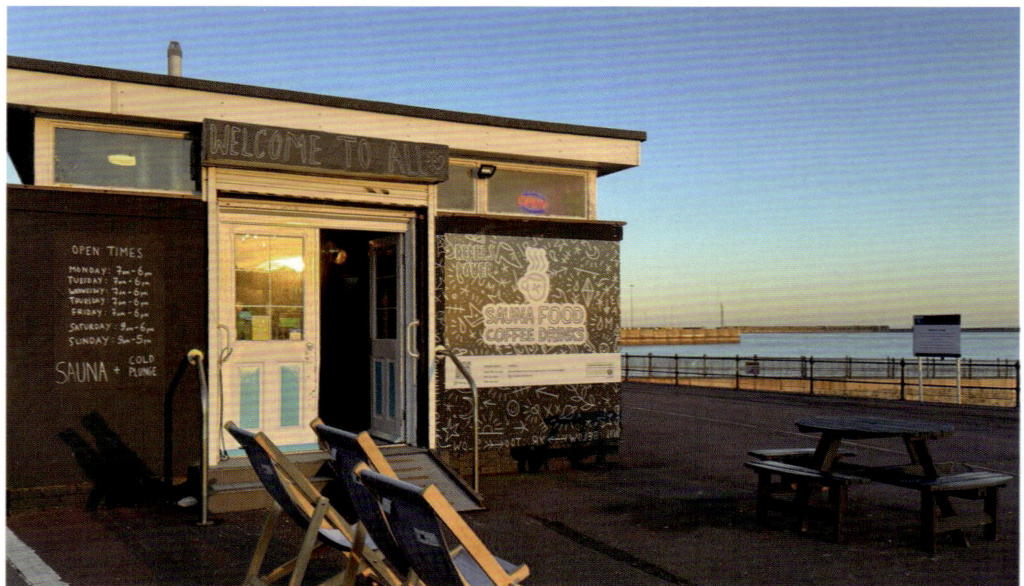

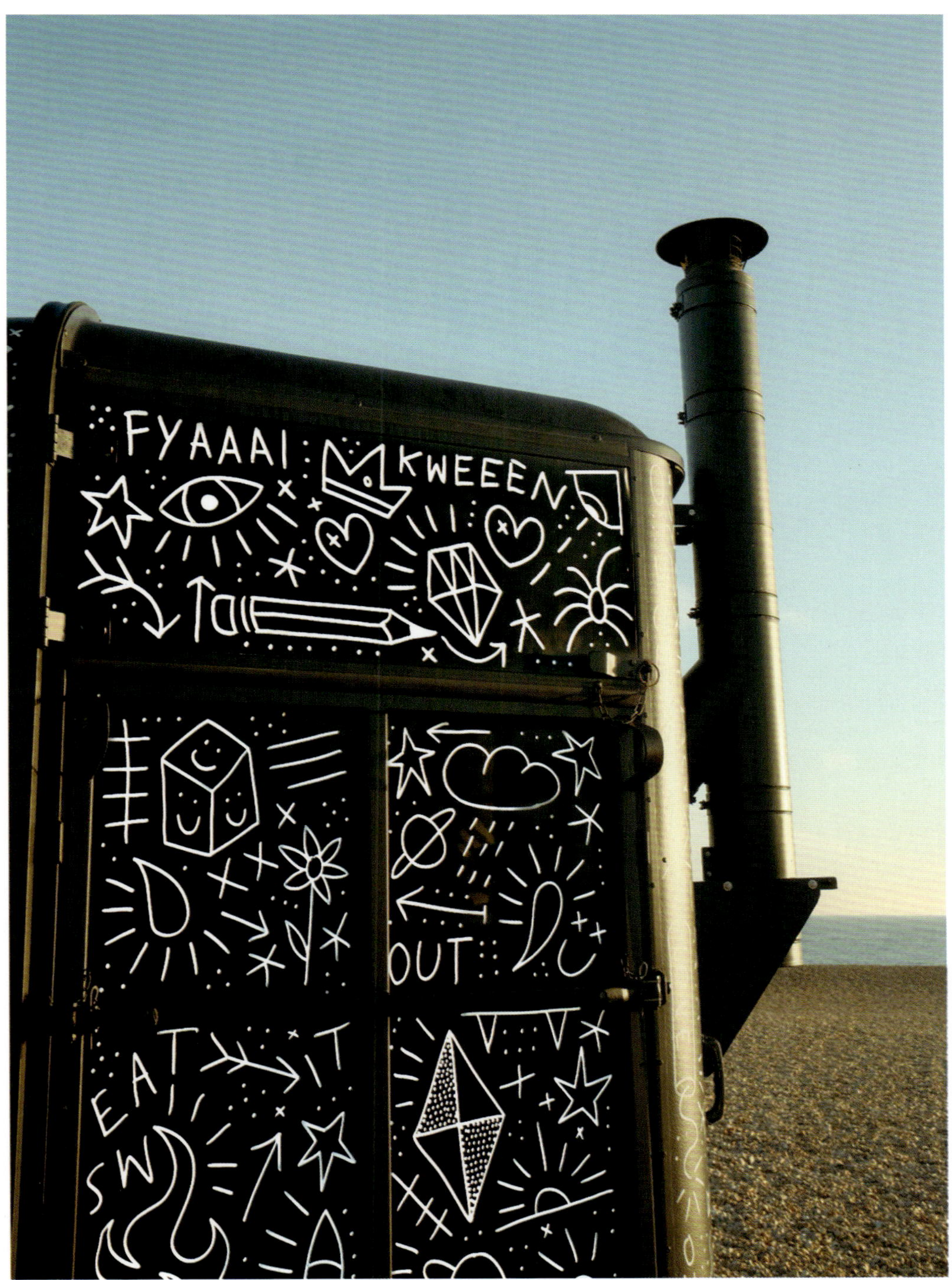
FYAAAI
KWEEEN
OUT
EAT
SW
IT

77

Sea Scrub Sauna

MARGATE & WHITSTABLE ❦ KENT

Sea Scrub was founded by Robin Bartlett and his cousin Luke (who lives in Oslo and has seen the floating sauna boom first-hand). 'Luke recognised that our climates and cultures aren't that different, and in the UK, for nine months of the year, it's not nice outside,' says Robin. So the pair bought a barrel sauna without anywhere to put it, wrangled for 14 months for a plot, and ended up on a packed-out Margate Beach in the height of summer. No one came. They survived by selling lollies and ice creams. Fast forward 18 months, and how times have changed. Now, Sea Scrub has added a swish electric sauna, two cold barrels, changing rooms and running water to the mix, and has even expanded to Whitstable.

Sea Scrub welcomes hen and stag parties, cold swimmers, tourists and celebs. A visit from local artist Tracey Emin early on was a game changer; she showed her support by posting pictures of herself post-sauna, colostomy bag in full view.

'In the winter, when the only souls on the beach were dog walkers wrapped up, hunched over, you now see bathers in swimsuits, walking around, shoulders back, wind and rain in the face and just loving life,' says Robin. 'There's no other way to access that than with the sauna.'

seascrubsauna.co.uk
Sea/barrel/cold plunge
51.3870, 1.3735 Margate
51.3630, 1.0257 Whitstable

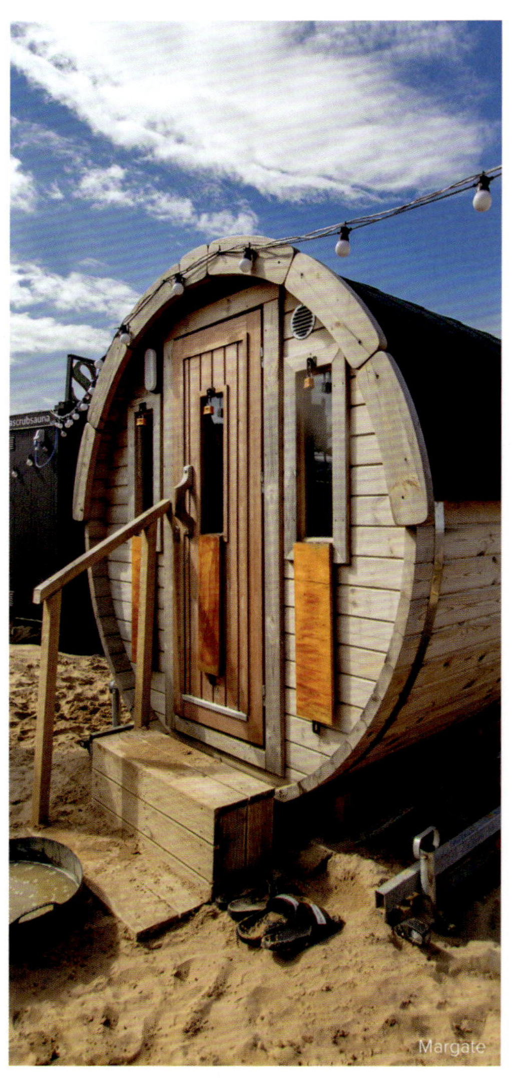
Margate

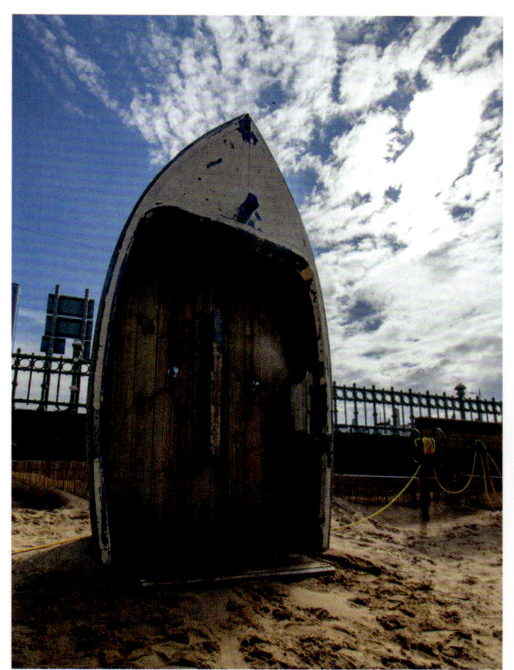

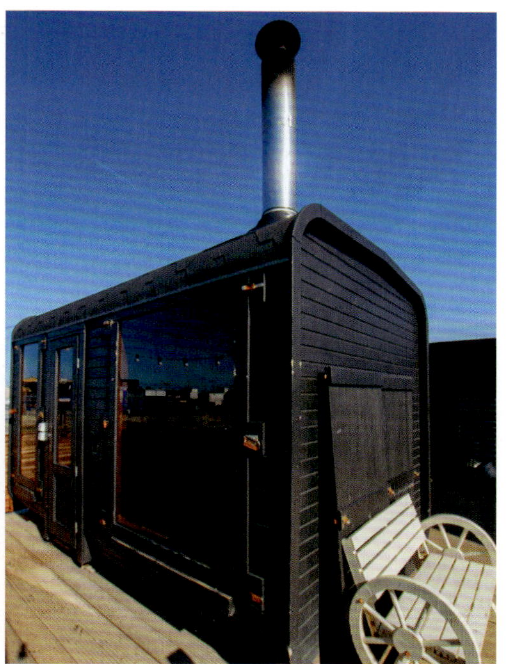

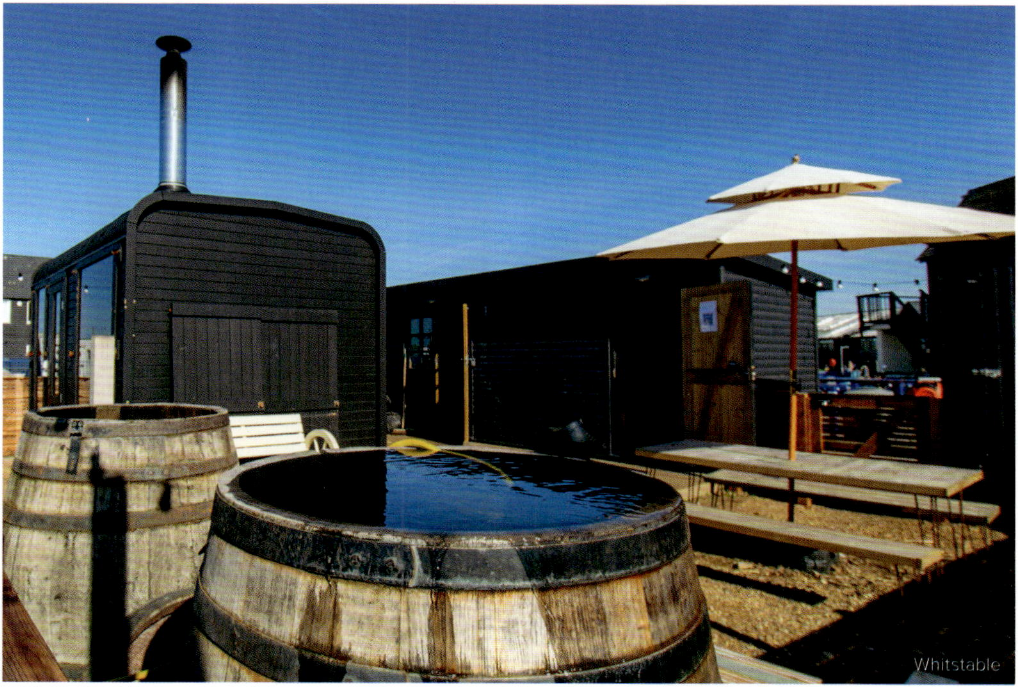

Whitstable

78

Haeckels® Sea Bathing Machine

MARGATE ❦ KENT

When the Sea Bathing Machine sauna opened, for free, on Walpole Beach in Margate in 2014, it was revolutionary. Its founder, Dom Bridges, had already created Haeckels® skincare using hand-picked seaweed, and he was hailed as a visionary. And so he is, for almost a decade on, hundreds of others have created community saunas – although few of them are free and manned by volunteers. Despite a stream of new saunas along the Kent coast, the Sea Bathing Machine still has a loyal following. Haeckels® funds it and oversees volunteers who help to run it. It's not open all the time, and its open-door policy means queues form at weekends. On Christmas Day, loyal followers bring mince pies and champagne.

➔ haeckels.co.uk/blogs/news/community-sauna
❄ Sea 📍 51.3921, 1.4025

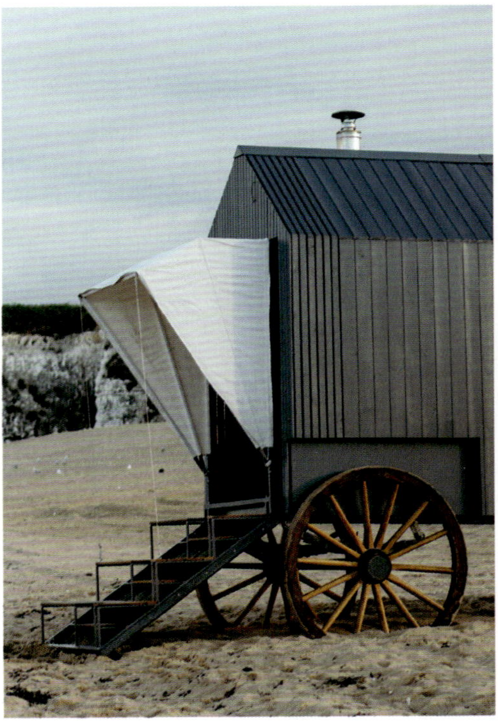

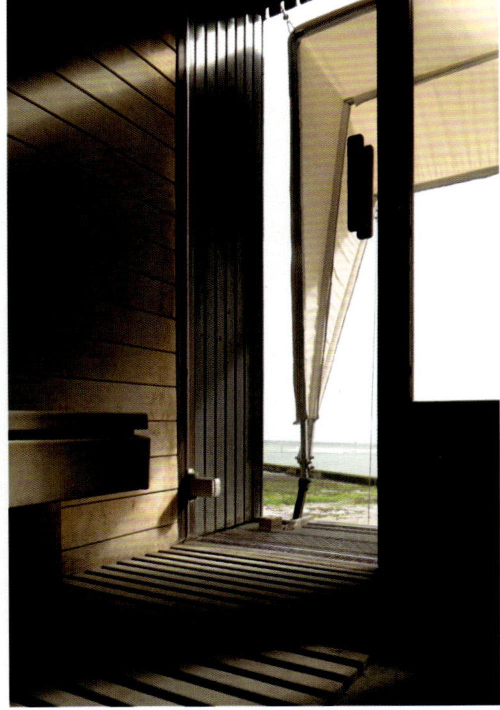

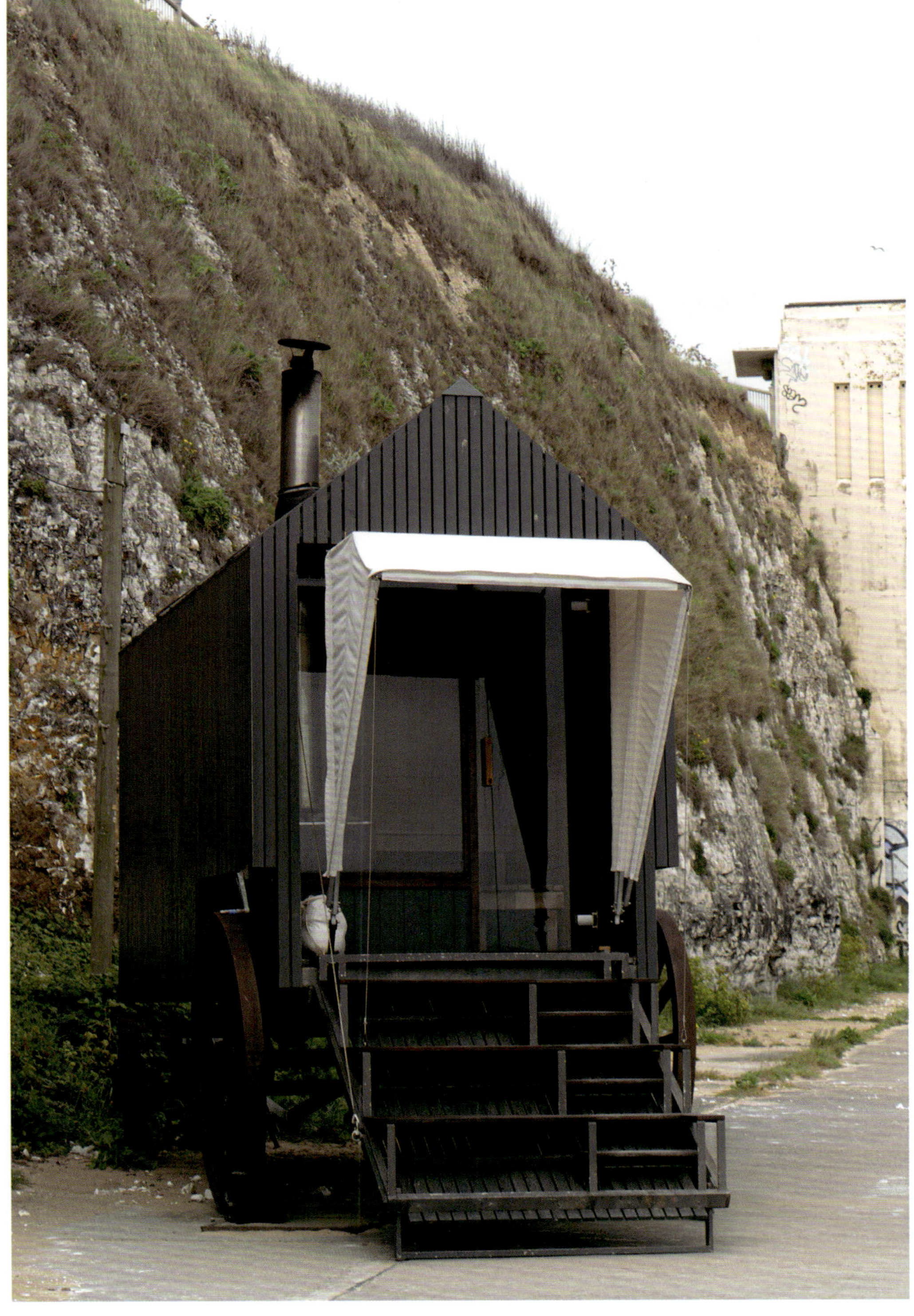

79

Secret Sauna

BUNGAY ❦ SUFFOLK

The location of the Secret Sauna is only revealed 24 hours before you book. Until then, all you need to know is that it's on an island, in the middle of the River Waveney on the Norfolk/Suffolk border.

Should you be staying at Wainford Mill House, a former riverside maltings in Bungay, you might have a head start, for both the sauna and the mill house are owned by Alex, Toby and Anna Hammond, a local entrepreneurial family who, in 2017, bought a derelict silo and a scrappy, uninhabited island. They didn't know what to do with the latter, so Anna suggested they build a sauna on it. The house sleeps 12 and has a garden and a small boat, so you can row a few minutes downstream to the island where the secret sauna sits.

If you're not a guest, you can still book the sauna, with a bridge over the river and a path guiding you to the spot. In Finland, the sauna path, or sauna polku is part of the ritual, a journey through nature towards purification, almost like walking down the aisle of a church. Secret Sauna's path, with its fairy lights, fire pit and glimpses of the snaking river, lives up to the Finnish ideal. So romantic is the setting, it's a popular spot for marriage proposals.

The sauna holds two to six people, and in summer, a willow weeps in front of its entrance and shrouds its secrecy. Cows graze in the fields along the banks and paddle boarders, kayakers and kingfishers glide past. The Waveney is a tidal river – the North Sea is 15 miles away – and between October and March it's high and fast flowing; it's sensible to use the steps into it from the sauna.

Sauna snacks are plentiful. You can order picnics from The Silo, where the Etude café and roastery on the ground floor serves coffee and kombucha, alcohol and pastries, including sell-out vegan brownies. The Silo is open seven days a week and the plan is to open a restaurant and bar on the roof, which at 25 metres high, offers splendid views over the Waveney Valley.

Anna had never built a sauna, but 'with a bit of ingenuity, a bit of imagination and a bit of research', she approached two local carpenters, and together they followed Finnish design standards to create something with a Nordic, rustic look. What was intended to be an add-on to the B&B and an asset to the scrubby island has taken on a life of its own. Regulars, locals and tourists love it. Lots of people have discovered it by paddling past (it's on a popular route within the Broads National Park), and since it opened in 2019, more than 8,000 people have enjoyed a session in the now not-so-secret sauna.

➔ wainford.co.uk/secret-sauna

❄ River ⚲ 52.4584, 1.4587

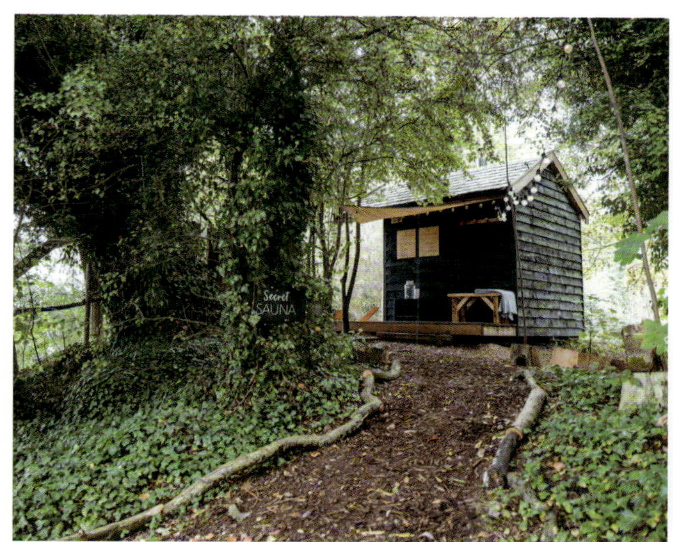
Secret
SAUNA

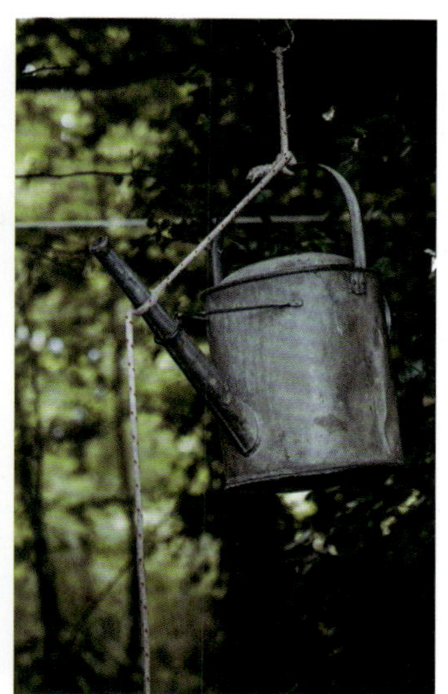

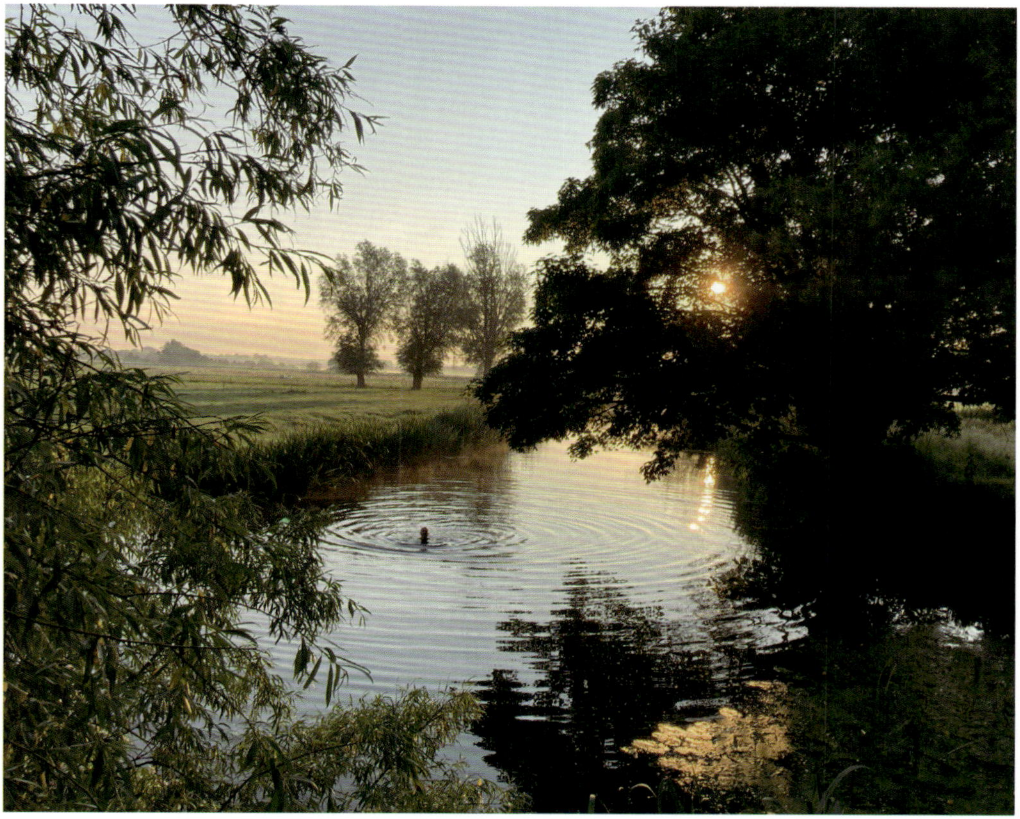

80

Sauna in the Woods

RACKHEATH ❦ NORFOLK

Maybe it's the freshwater pond dotted with tadpoles, or the forest of silver birch, or the chunky, hand-hewn cabin doors and frames, but Sauna in the Woods near Norwich feels as Nordic as it gets in the flatlands of East Anglia.

Built by Larry Campion, a self-confessed 'Heath Robinson' character who lives off-grid in a house he built next door, it's nestled in the private 40-acre woodlands of Pig's Park.

The sauna is made with fallen trees from the forest (mostly Scot's pine), cracks are filled with sawdust and clay, and insulation is a bird-nest mix: lamb's wool, foil, bits and pieces of everything. 'I just bang it together,' says Larry, 'and if you start a project, you end up having to finish it. It wasn't something I was planning to do commercially, but it's taken off.'

He has lots of couples using the sauna – the silence and privacy of the setting is magical – and locals and those who appreciate Larry's home-spun artistry come too. 'Making can be quite organic. Lots of people put things together with whatever they've salvaged,' says Larry. 'Brand new and shiny is not always what people want.'

An old bus that was once Larry's home is now a changing room, a former hot tub is a cold plunge, and there's a cold outdoor shower. A zip wire runs over the lake from his daughter's bedroom; Larry added it as his young family grew.

A compost toilet doubles as the store for firewood and Larry's beekeeping gear; from the sauna window, you can see two hives. The plan is to offer honey sauna scrubs. Guests can help themselves to herbal tea and Larry makes birch sap too; birch is a pioneer tree, said to have been the first to return after the Ice Age. In Celtic mythology, birch marks new beginnings and symbolises renewal and purification – and Pig's Park is filled with them. Birch trees only live for around 60 years, and Larry's are reaching their end of life, to be superseded by sycamore and ash.

Larry now has a sauna and a cold plunge every day, and in winter has to crack the ice on the pond. He's noticing benefits: 'I feel more focused, and deeply relaxed afterwards.' It's a superb combination, and one that's not easy to achieve. Larry, and his intuitive connection to the nature around him, has made it happen.

➔ saunainthewoods.co.uk ❄ Pond/shower
📍 52.6598, 1.3651

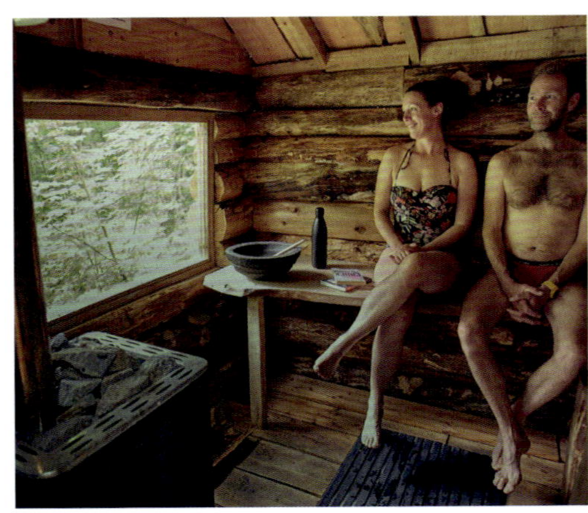

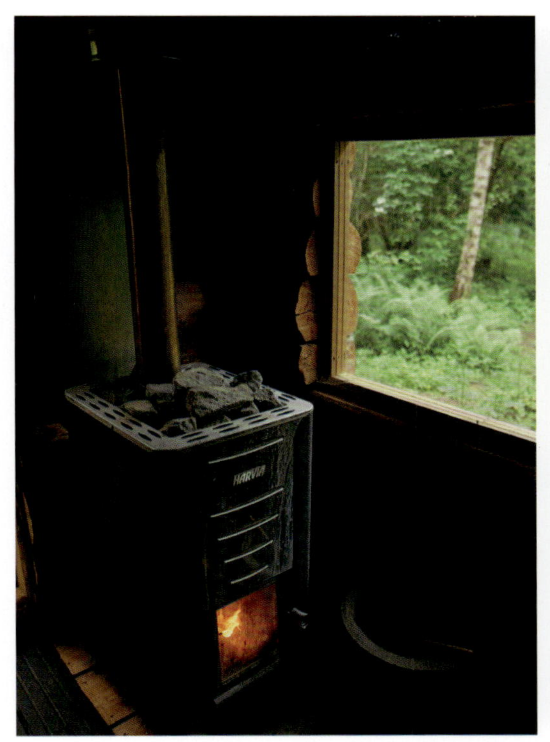
HARVIA

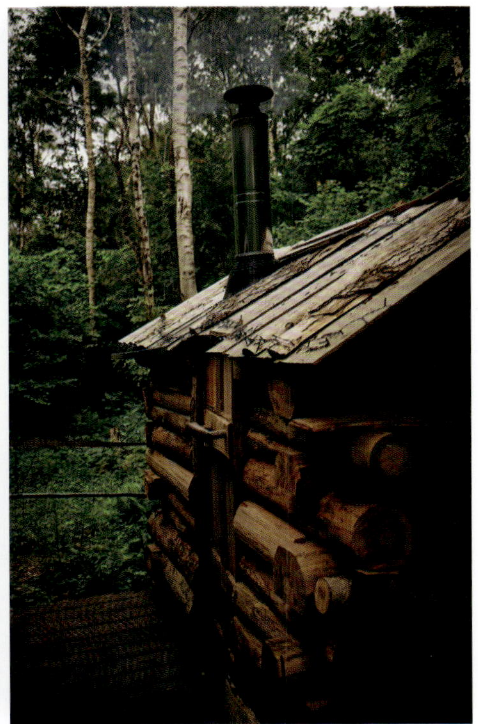

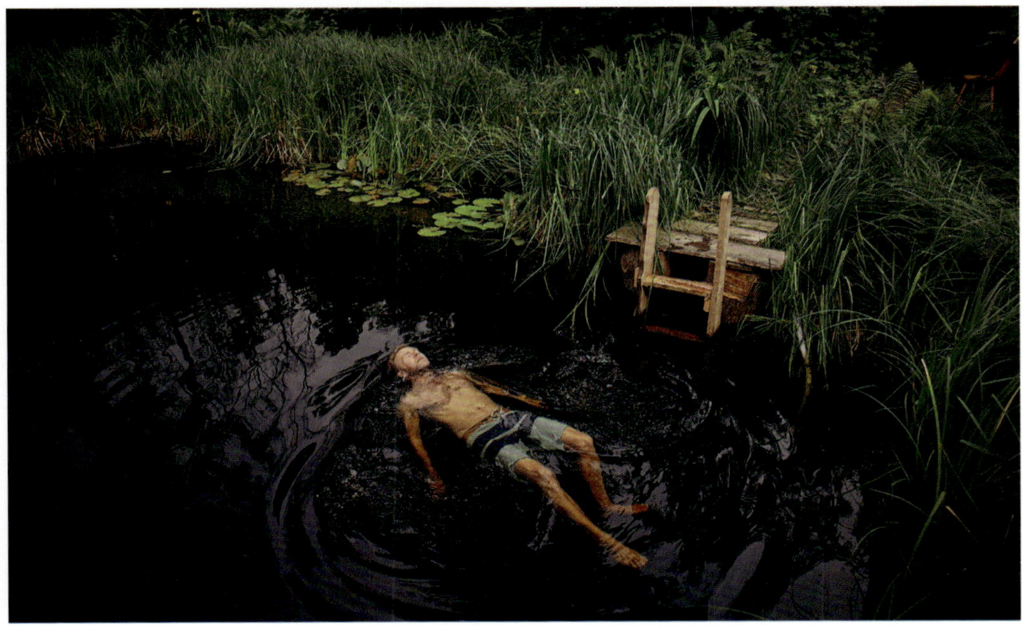

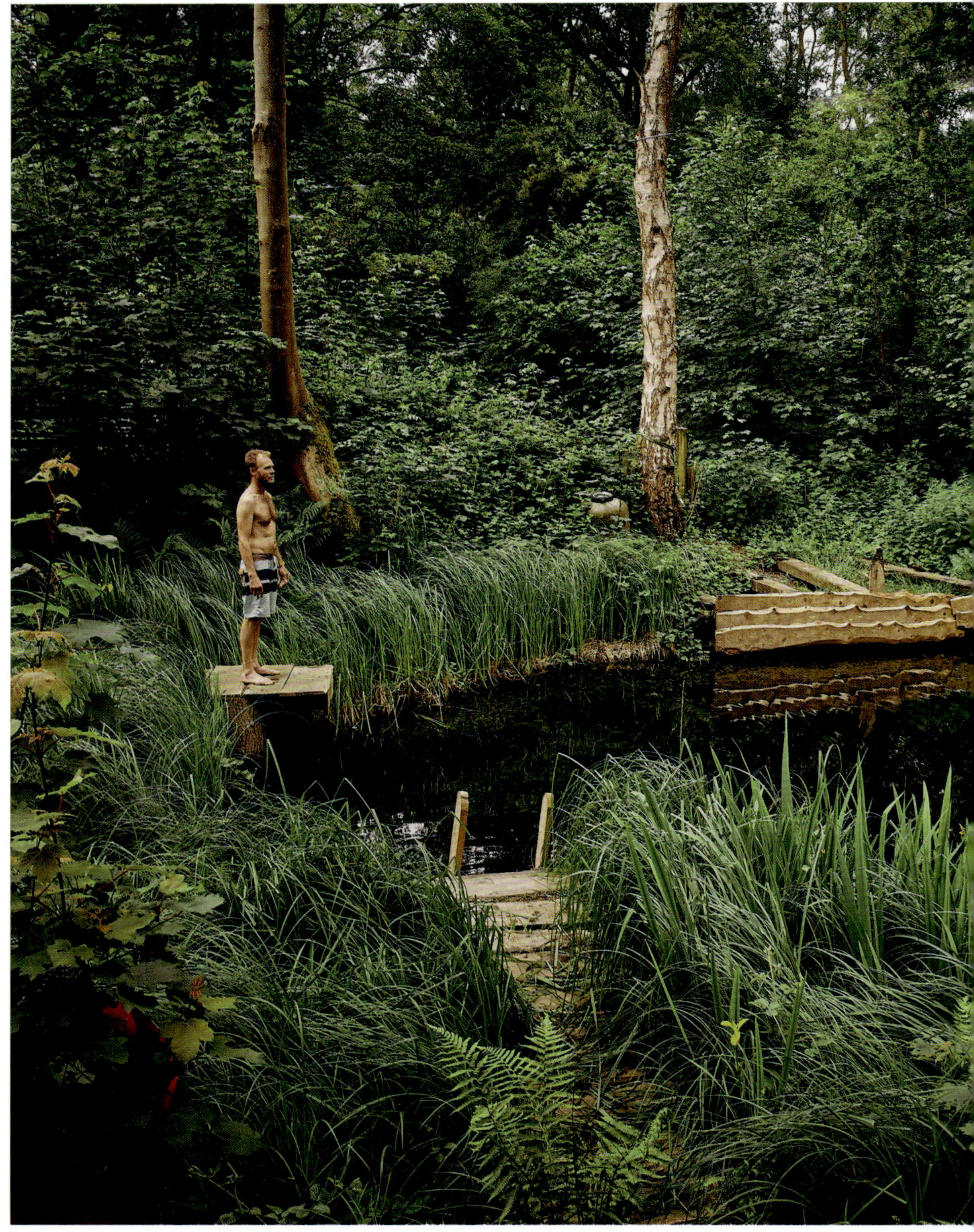

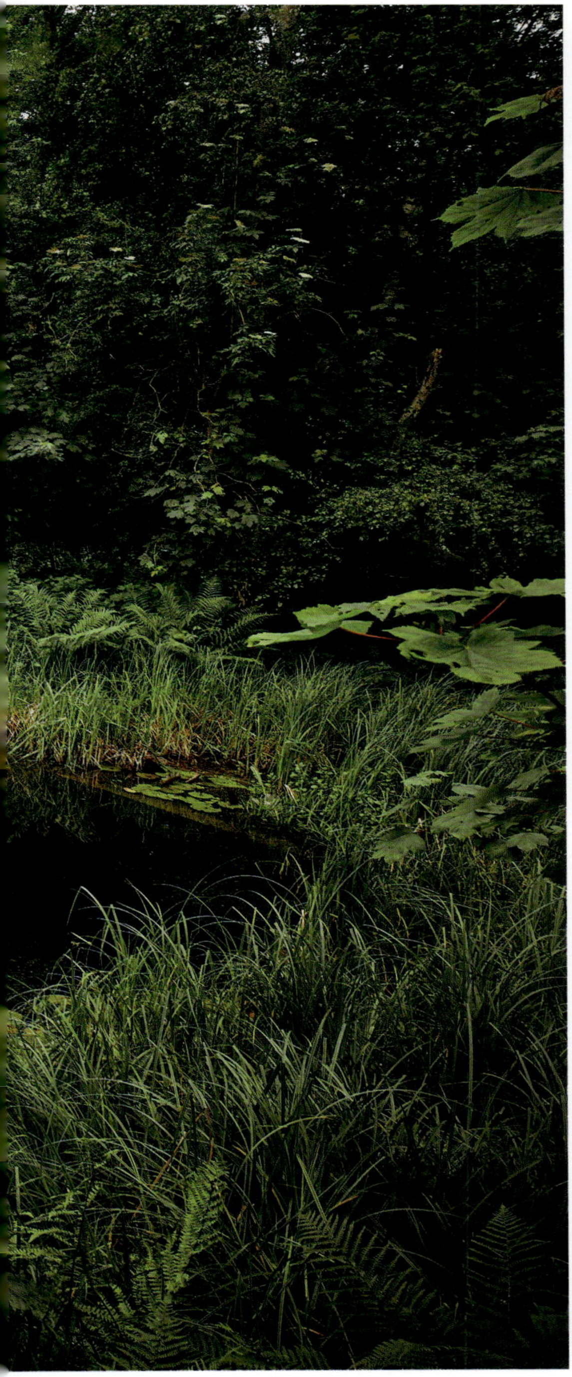

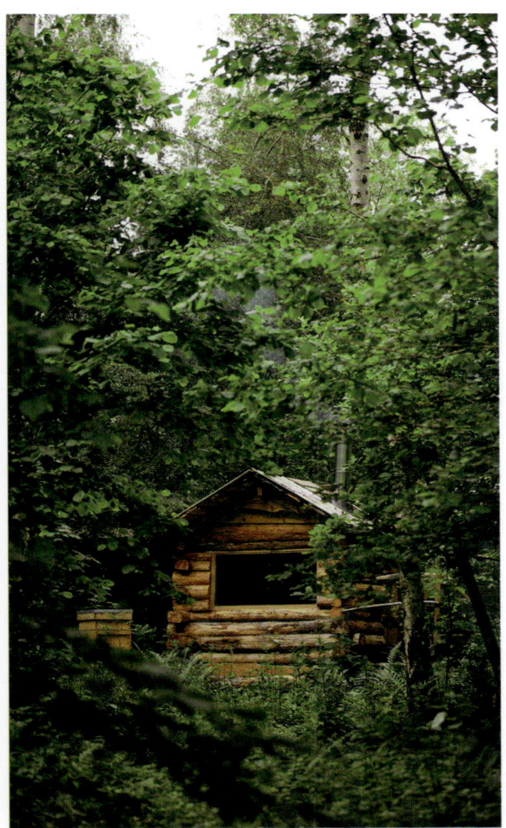

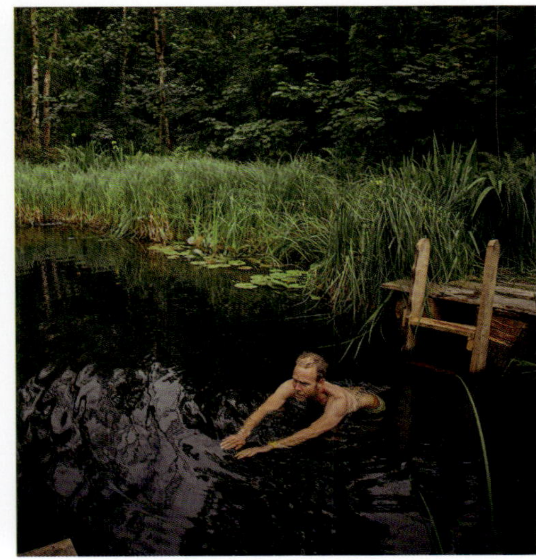

81

Salty Sauna

PAKEFIELD, LOWESTOFT ❦ SUFFOLK

Located in Pakefield on the south side of Lowestoft, the bijou Salty Sauna is greater than the sum of its parts. This is partly because Hannah, its owner, chats to everyone who passes, be they children, retirees, dog walkers. Situated on a busy coastal path, the sauna is serviced by two car parks and has access to the sea down some stairs (being right on the beach was a no-go due to the North Sea tides). Deans Beans coffee hut, a minute's stroll along the path, serves sausage rolls, coffee and cakes, along with famously good Bakewell tarts.

➔ instagram.com/saltysauna
Sea 52.4496, 1.7336

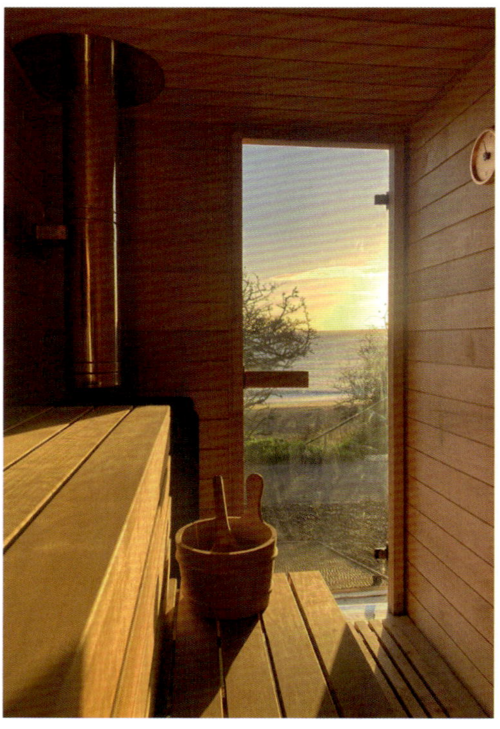

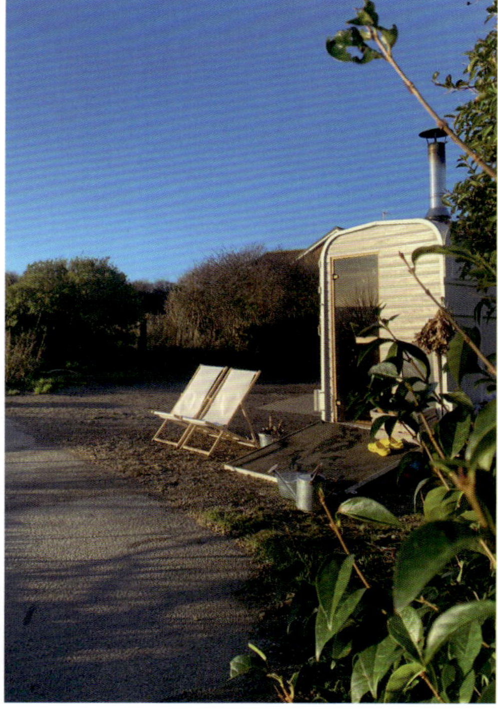

82

Sauna Box

SHERINGHAM & DUNWICH ❦ NORFOLK & SUFFOLK

If you're into saunas, chances are you've sweated it out in a Sauna Box somewhere. Since converting an old horsebox in his garden with his dad during lockdown, Tom Sutton has created around 20 of his signature black Sauna Boxes. Many are on the Norfolk and Suffolk coast, including two of his own at Sheringham and Dunwich respectively. A third Sauna Box moves around Norwich, stopping at like-minded sites, such as The Yoga Tree and West Lexham and can cater to pop-ups and events pretty much anywhere in the UK.

saunabox.co.uk Sea
52.9454, 1.2134 Sheringham
52.2793, 1.6335 Dunwich

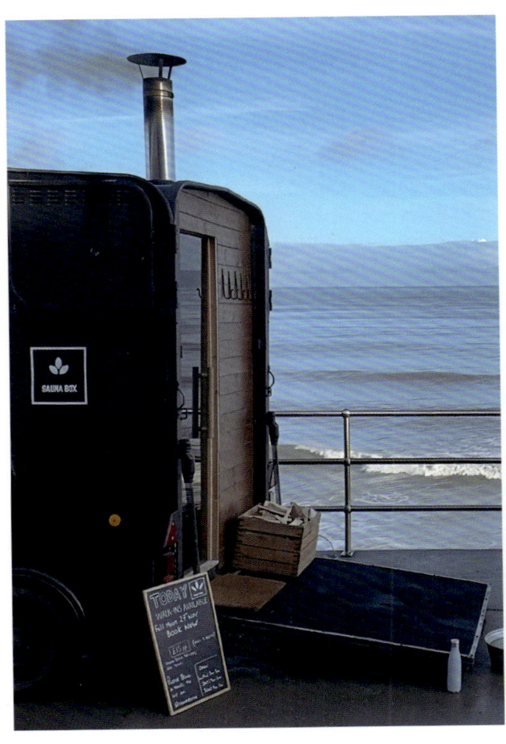

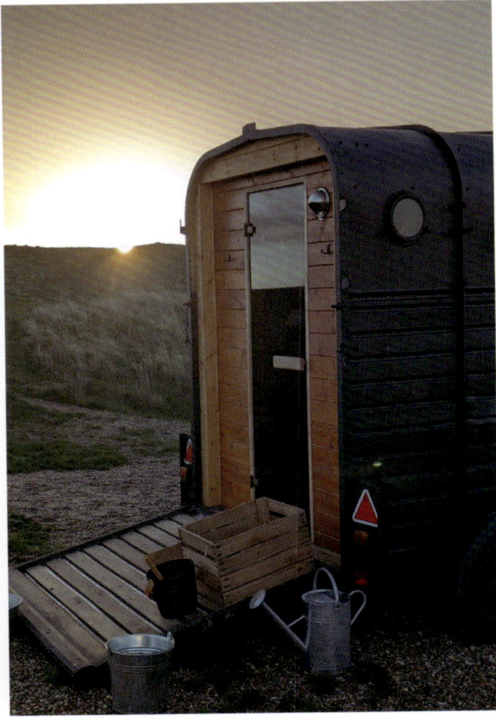

More

83 The Solent Sauna

LEE-ON-THE-SOLENT ✤ HAMPSHIRE

This barrel sauna on the beach at Lee-on-the-Solent sits on the seafront above a pebble beach and has parking and toilets.

➔ thesolentsauna.co.uk
❄ Sea ⚲ 50.8047, -1.2075

84 Mirror Houses Kirtlington

KIRTLINGTON, OXFORDSHIRE

Estonian company ÖÖD House and Hötels has built chic mirrored cabins in stunning nature all over the world – think Mexican jungle, Norwegian fjords, Icelandic volcanoes, and Estonian pine forests. And they are popping up in hidden corners of the UK too – farms, distilleries, private estates – where peace and quiet, privacy and a healthy dose of nature are in plentiful supply.

Park Farm in Oxfordshire is a large stud farm and home to the Kirtlington Park Polo Club. It has seven ÖÖD Mirror houses located in remote woodland next to an 18th-century lake designed by Capability Brown. Designed for two, each cabin comes with a king-sized bed, a kitchen with basic provisions, wifi, air conditioning, heating and a bathroom. On the private outside decks, guests will find a BBQ and either a hot tub, outside bath or a ready stacked sauna.

➔ themirrorhouseskirtlington.co.uk
❄ Shower ⚲ 51.8803, -1.2529

85 Saunagus

BERINSFIELD ✤ OXFORDSHIRE

Stephen Thomas runs sessions in his tent sauna around Oxfordshire. He's usually at Queenford Lake in Wallingford, where he'll do a guided session for groups of up to ten, but the tent can travel.

➔ saunagus.co.uk
❄ Lake ⚲ 51.6567, -1.1654

86 Seaside Sauna

LANCING ✤ SUSSEX

Kitesurfing teacher Frazer Stewart set up a wood-fired barrel sauna on the pebbles at Lancing beach for post-exercise muscle recovery and more.

➔ seasidesauna.com
❄ Sea/cold plunge ⚲ 50.8204, -0.3220

87 Widewater Sauna

LANCING ✤ WEST SUSSEX

Another spot on the Sussex coast sauna map, this horsebox sits on the shingle at Widewate r Lagoon in Lancing, where dippers can plunge in the sea.

➔ widewatersauna.com
❄ Sea ⚲ 50.8242, -0.2980

88 Lovebrook Farm

KINGSTON ✤ SUSSEX

Lovebrook Farm in the South Downs focuses on ecological, regenerative farming methods, and runs retreats incorporating yoga, organic food and sauna. A barrel sauna next to the barn comes with a shower and a cold plunge.

➔ lovebrook.org/sauna ❄ Cold plunge/shower
⚲ 50.8563, -0.0209

89 Savu Sauna

REIGATE ✤ SURREY

James and Ian Daly run Savu Sauna at Buckland Park Lake, a private estate with woodland trails, yoga, paddle-boarding and cold-water swimming. There are two cold showers and two plunge baths, warm showers, changing rooms and toilets.

➔ saunawithsavu.co.uk
❄ Cold plunge/shower ⚲ 51.2429, -0.2452

90 FLÖ Wellbeing

SILVERSTONE ❋ BUCKINGHAMSHIRE

Blackpit Farm, part of the Grade 1 listed Stowe Estate, is home to FLÖ Wellbeing, a tranquil wild spa offering a 16-person sauna built from a former shipping container, three hot tubs, a cold plunge, shower block and toilet which huddle round Blackpit's picturesque lake. With a jetty, two floats, and lifeguards, it is also a popular spot for wild swimmers.

➔ flowellbeing.co.uk
❄ Lake/ice bath ⊙ 52.0540, -1.0141

91 Forest Sauna

BATTLE ❋ SUSSEX

At this wild spa in Sussex, a wood-fired barrel Set in woodland, this small sister sauna to Beach Box is available for private hire only on Saturdays and Sundays for groups of up to ten people. It has parking, a toilet, a changing facility, and a plunge bath and cold tank are fed from a forest spring..

➔ beachboxspa.co.uk
❄ Cold plunge ⊙ 50.8847, 0.4569

92 St Andrews Lakes

HALLING ❋ KENT

A converted shepherd's hut, the sauna at St Andrews Lakes seats 12. It has wood-fired hot tubs and steps down into the small natural lagoon cold plunge. Included in the price of the sauna is an open-water swim, although swimmers have to complete a paid induction course before they can enter the water.

➔ standrewswatersports.co.uk
❄ Lagoon ⊙ 51.3597, 0.4385

93 Folkestone Sea Sauna

FOLKESTONE ❋ KENT

The Folkestone Sea Sauna is open in the winter months and is operated on a members-only basis. It is an electrically fired automated sauna, with access via waterproof wrist fob. Popular with sea swimmers, it has an open day for the public on the first Sunday of every month.

➔ folkestoneseasauna.com
❄ Sea ⊙ 51.0733, 1.1460

94 Ember pop up sauna

HERNE BAY ❋ KENT

Holly Triggs runs a pop-up sauna business around Herne Bay in East Kent. Hiring both the tent sauna and ice bath enable hot/cold therapies.

➔ ember-popupsauna.com
❄ Cold plunge ⊙ 51.3700, 1.1336

95 Phoenix Sauna

BURY ST EDMUNDS ❋ SUFFOLK

Painted blue with a red Phoenix emblazoned on its side, Toto Fenwick crafted her beautiful mobile sauna from salvaged wood in East Anglia. It has a removable bench and shower on the side. An easy ramp makes it wheelchair accessible, and an ice bath travels with it too.

➔ phoenixsaunas.com
❄ Cold plunge ⊙ 52.3046, 0.6605

96 The Little Heat Retreat

NORWICH ❋ NORFOLK

It's not easy to make a sauna in a back garden on the outskirts of Norwich feel like a wild spa, but The Little Heat Retreat's founder Amy has done just that. *Aufguss*, essential oils, fire pit, scrubs, showers and mocktails enhance the experience.

➔ thelittleheatretreat.co.uk
❄ Shower ⊙ 52.6123, 1.3006

97 The Enchanted Glade

ARDINGLY ❋ SUSSEX

At this wild spa in Sussex, a wood-fired barrel sauna with shower and cold plunge, plus a hot tub, form part of the retreat's activities that have nature at their core.

➔ enchantedglade.co.uk
❄ Cold plunge/shower ⊙ 51.0425, -0.0582

WALES & BORDERS

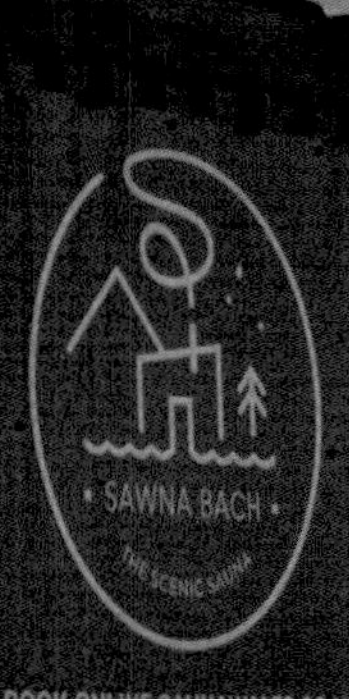

103 Sawna Bach, Porth Tyn Tywyn

98

Wildwater Sauna

NEWGALE ❦ PEMBROKESHIRE

The Pembrokeshire Coast National Park is one of the smallest national parks in the UK and the only completely coastal one. Wildwater Sauna moves around all 610 square miles of the park every four weeks, maximising everything the diverse landscape offers. It has gained a cult following among swimmers, surfers and locals in the process.

Popular spots are Newgale, Nolton Haven, Little Haven, Whitesands and Porthclais. It was at the latter, on the day the lifeboats were being launched for the summer season, that I had the pleasure of a sauna. Porthclais is a postcard-pretty inlet with a shingle slipway that leads to the harbour where the lifeboats dock until September. They are busy, thanks to the freezing, swirling waters of Ramsey Sound, a treacherous tidal sea passage that separates Ramsey Island from the mainland and draws thrill-seeking kayakers and canoeists.

Many of these adventurers make it into the sauna, along with surfers, swimmers, tourists and locals. Among them is Jules King, an award-winning CrossFit athlete who has early-onset Parkinson's disease, and uses sauna for pain relief and insomnia (see Jules' story overleaf).

Wildwater founders Scott Chalmers and Richard Lynch are documentary filmmakers who set up the sauna as a side hustle after travels to Estonia. They had the six-seater trailer made in Denmark, and they often pitch up in spots with no phone signal, which fits with their 'primal' approach. Wild by name, wild by nature, offering a truly immersive experience within the rugged landscape of Pembrokeshire. On full moon evenings, when it's calm and crystal clear, Scott and Richard organise special sauna, swim and meditation sessions under the light of the moon. And in a bid to leave each destination in a better place, beach cleans happen when the sauna is open.

Buoyed by Wildwater's popularity, Scott and Richard are currently seeking planning permission for a permanent location with their second sauna.

➔ wildwatersauna.com
Sea · 51.8454, -5.1179

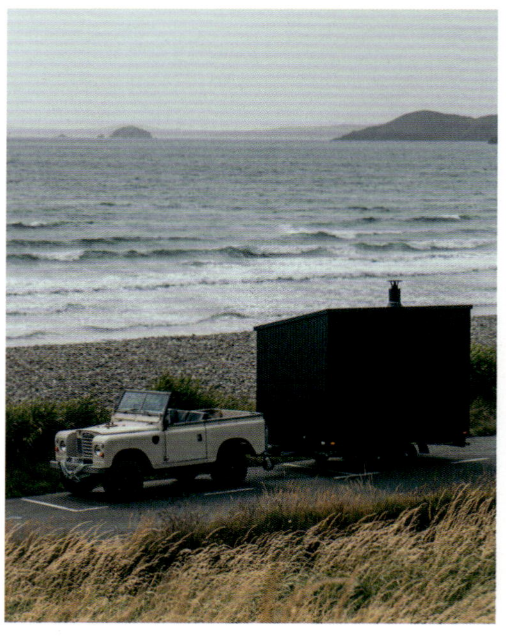

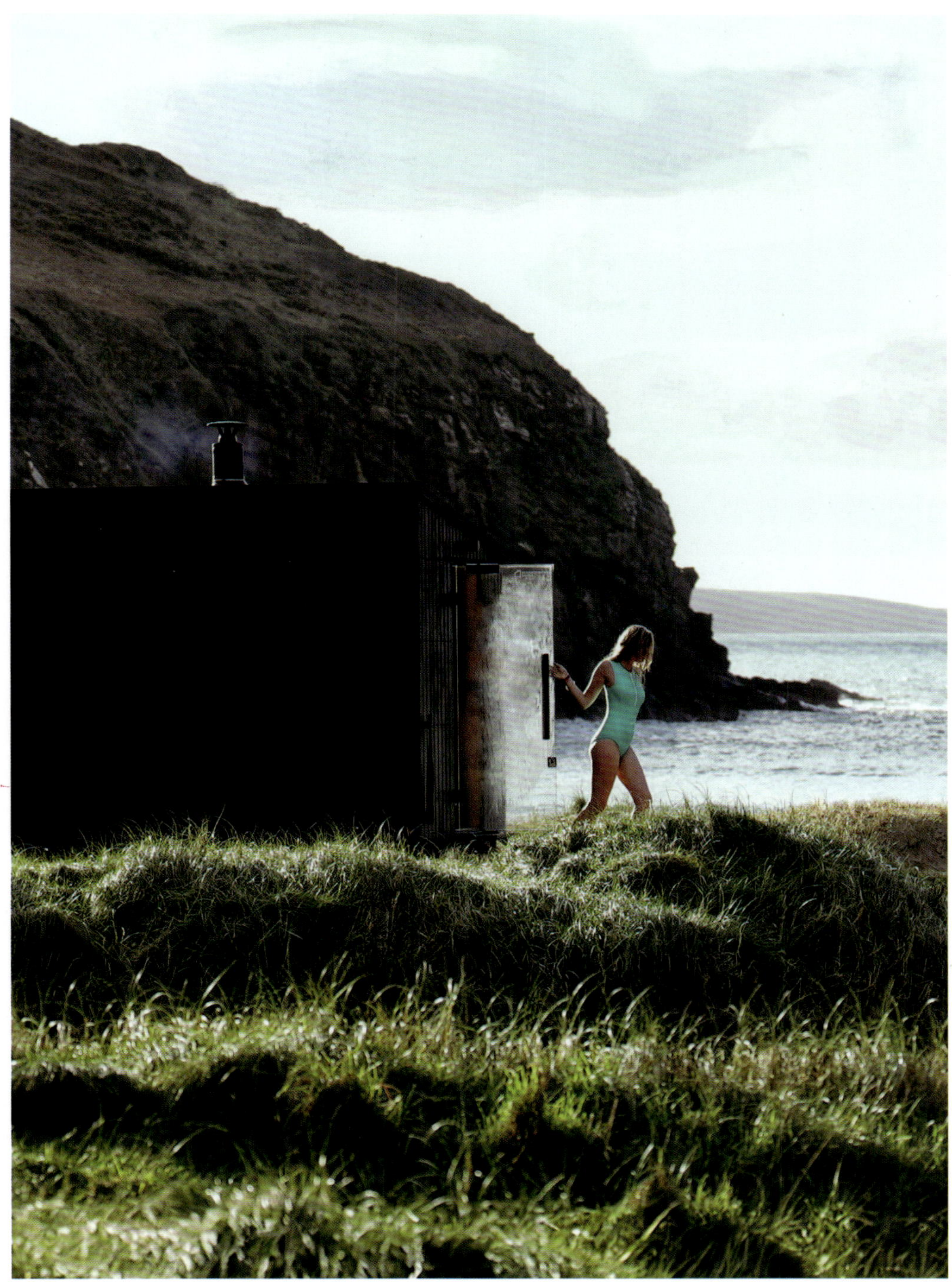

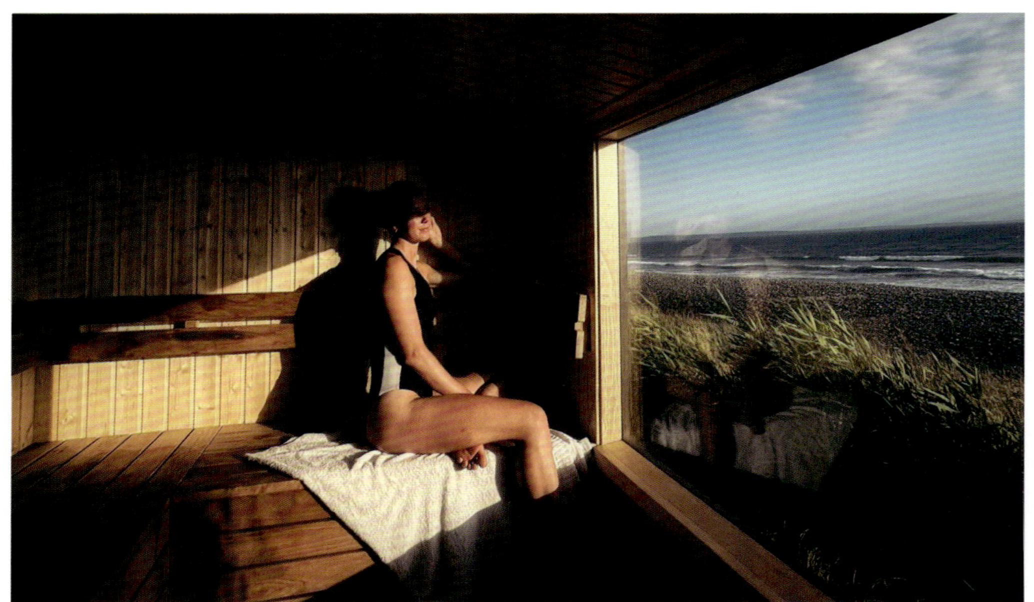

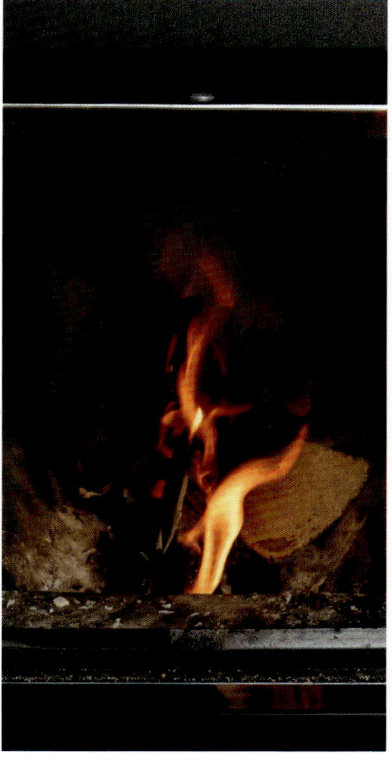

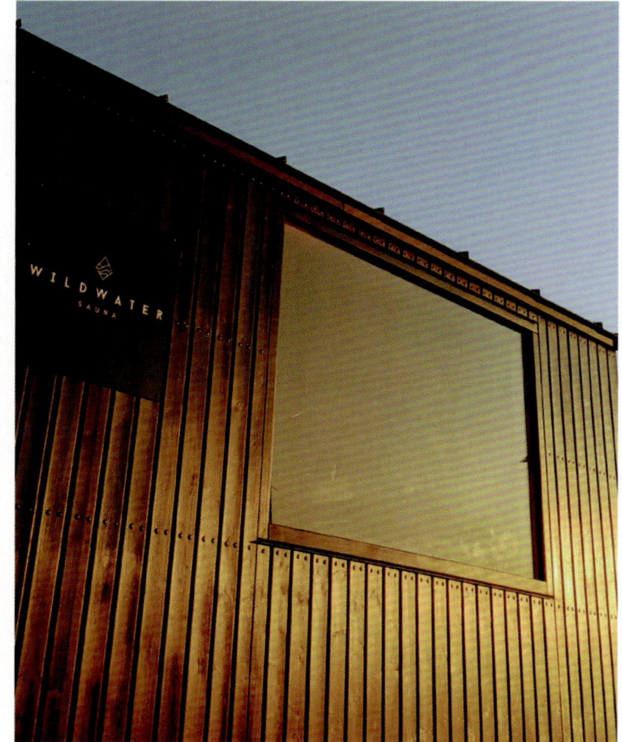
WILDWATER
SAUNA

Jules' Story

Jules King suffers with Parkinson's and was wheelchair-bound for 16 years before a correct diagnosis saw her turn her life around and reclaim her mobility. She is a regular at Pembrokeshire's Wildwater sauna and an award-winning Adaptive CrossFit athlete and she sees ice baths and saunas as central to her self-care routine.

'I had my first sauna at Wildwater in October 2023. I had already started cold water therapy as I had been given a barrel by Brass Monkey. It helps so much with pain relief, but it only lasts a few hours. When I combine the cold with sauna, the pain relief lasts all day. I pop pills every two hours for the Parkinson's so I don't want to take painkillers as well.

'No one's really ever explained why the hot works, but I think it's the relaxation. It loosens my muscles and I have more control, less rigidity. The effect of hot and cold depends on how my medication's working, but if it's working all day, I have no pain all day.

'I try to go to Wildwater three times a week and I'll dip in the sea as long as I have someone with me, the sauna has a real community around it. People with Parkinson's lack dopamine, and I presume I produce it when doing hot and cold. But I don't know how it works; it'd be so interesting to find out how – tap me into some wires. I would encourage anyone with Parkinson's to try hot and cold. All this medication doctors give me and all the money spent on it, when they could be sending people to cold water and sauna! I want to be an advocate for it.'

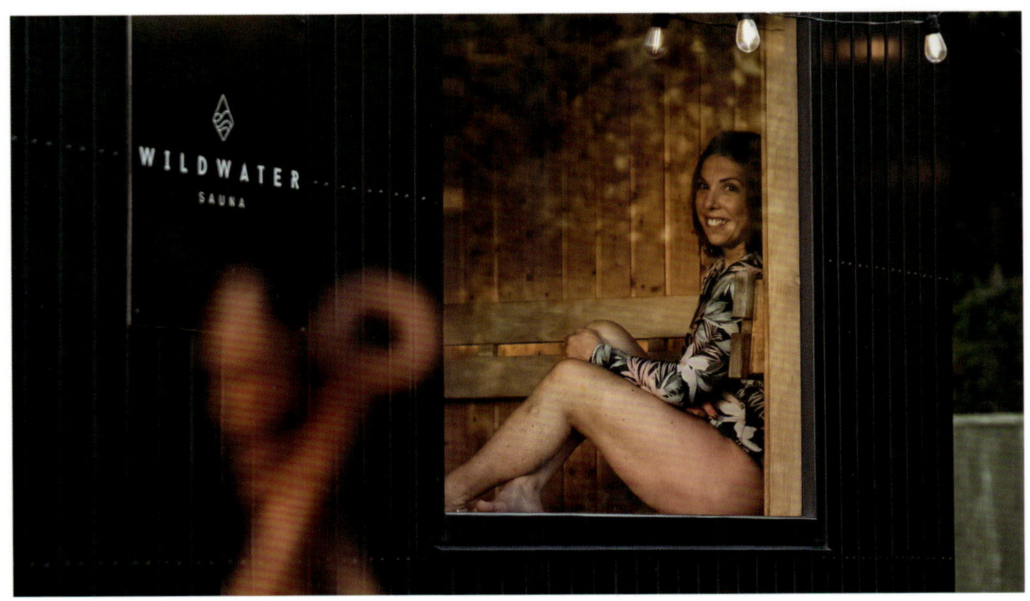

99

Sea + Steam

SAUNDERSFOOT ✤ PEMBROKESHIRE

Sea + Steam, in the village of Saundersfoot, is one of the few saunas in the Pembrokeshire Coast National Park to have a permanent site. It sits on the promenade above the beach and has a large viewing window and a bespoke changing area with six booths. The sauna is open seven days a week, with sessions from early in the morning until late in the evening.

Saundersfoot is home to the largest New Year's Day Swim in the UK, which has been held for 39 years and has raised over £800,000 for local charities. Sea + Steam's founders, Bryony and Kerry, aim to complement the thriving swimming community while connecting people to the coastline, promoting physical and mental health through sauna use, and supporting biodiversity projects in the harbour.

The lighting is solar-powered, the logs are sourced from just 0.2 miles away, and the ash is disposed of in the adjacent community sensory garden, creating a full circular economy.

→ seaandsteam.co.uk
Sea 51.7114, -4.6978

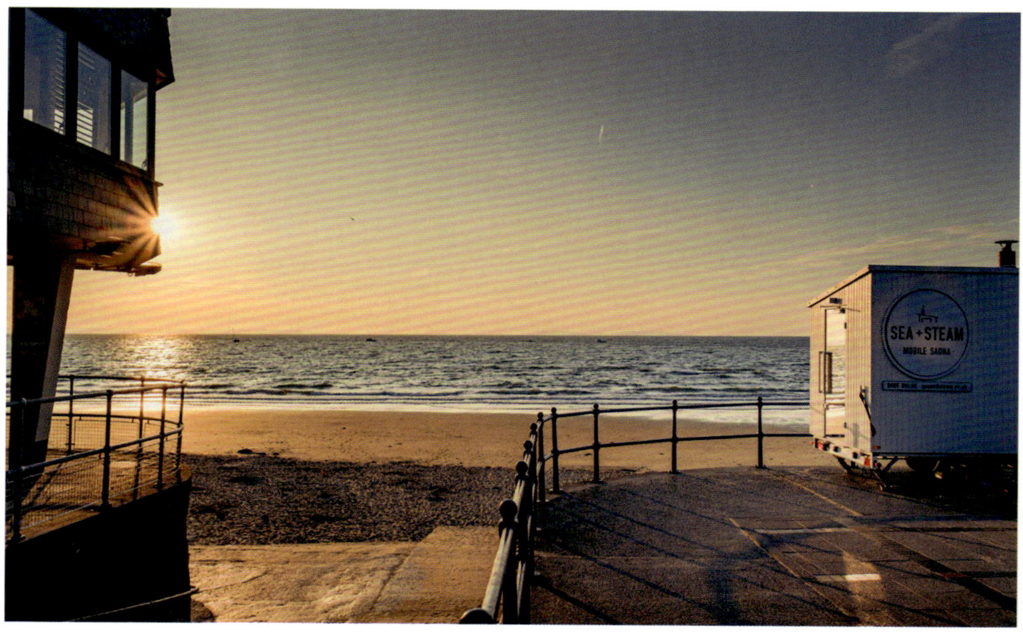

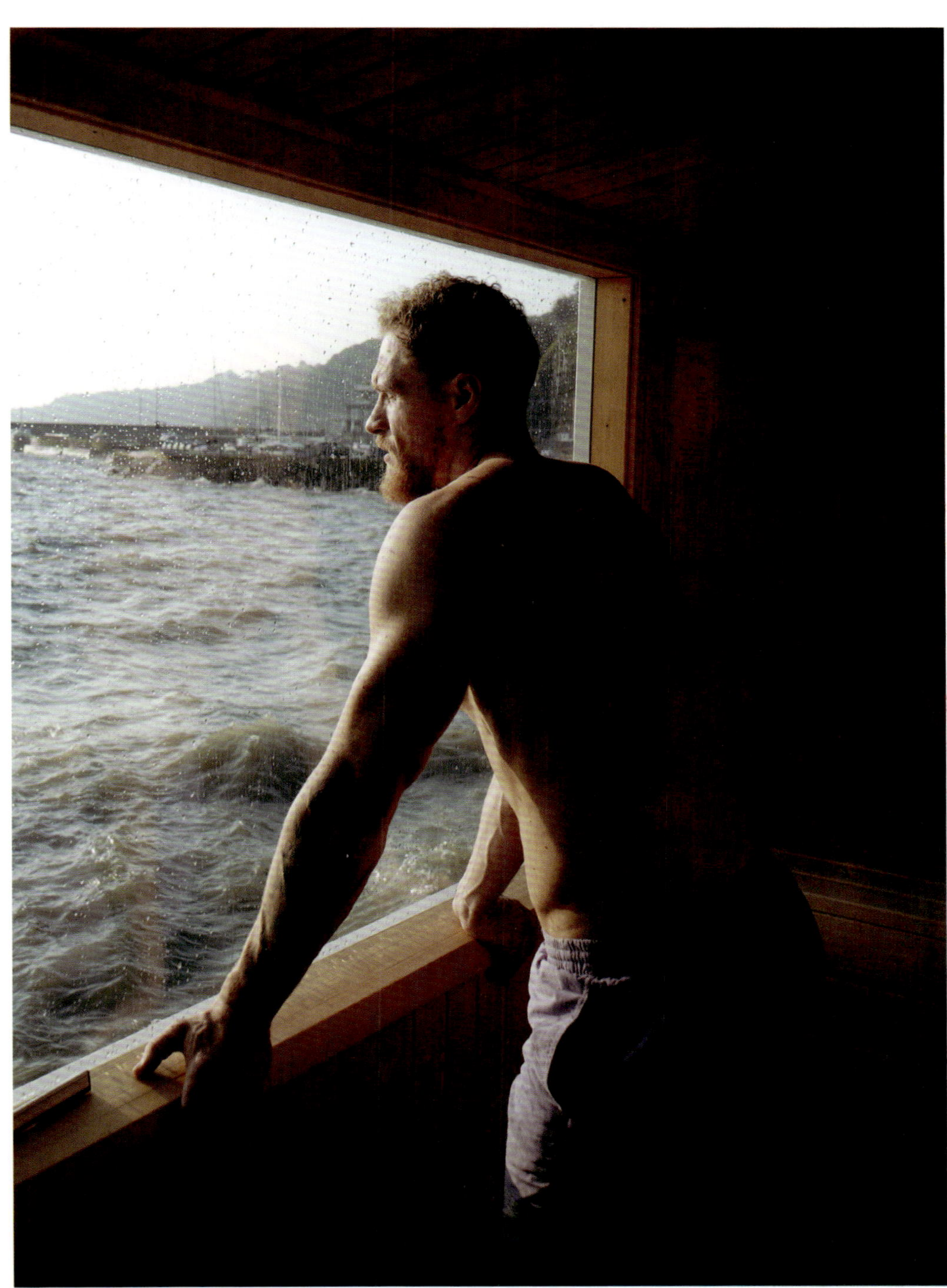

100

Ty Sawna

OXWICH BAY ❦ SWANSEA

Oxwich Bay is a pure pleasure beach, offering water sports, hotels, cafés, a Michelin-starred restaurant and, courtesy of Ty Sawna (which translates as Sauna House in English), two saunas. Folks from Swansea come to have picnics, light fires and swim and bathe on this much-loved spot on the Gower Peninsula. Thanks to being privately owned, Oxwich was one of the first beaches in Wales to allow a sauna on its sands.

Its founder, Harri, discovered sauna on a trip to Ireland. She lived in her camper van for six months on Oxwich Bay, getting to know the lay of the land and the locals. There's a toilet block, parking, changing rooms and running water, and Harri offers body scrubs, breathwork, yoga, sauna ceremonies, tea, and Thursday club socials. At high tide, the sea comes close; at low tide, freshwater buckets are on hand for rinsing off.

➔ tysawna.co.uk
❄ Sea/watering can ⌖ 51.5587, -4.1600

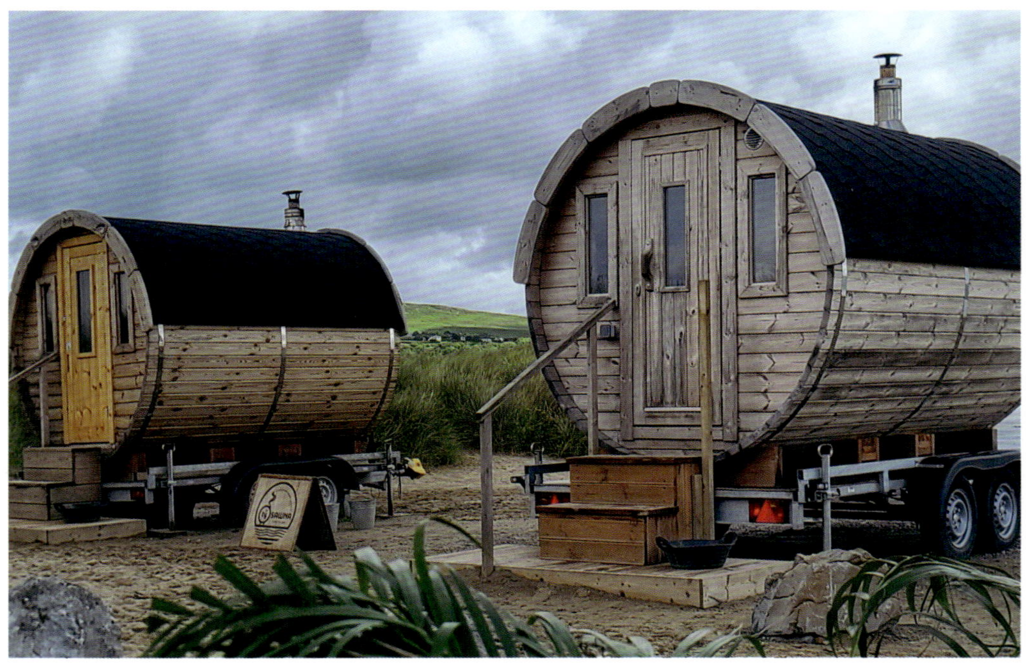

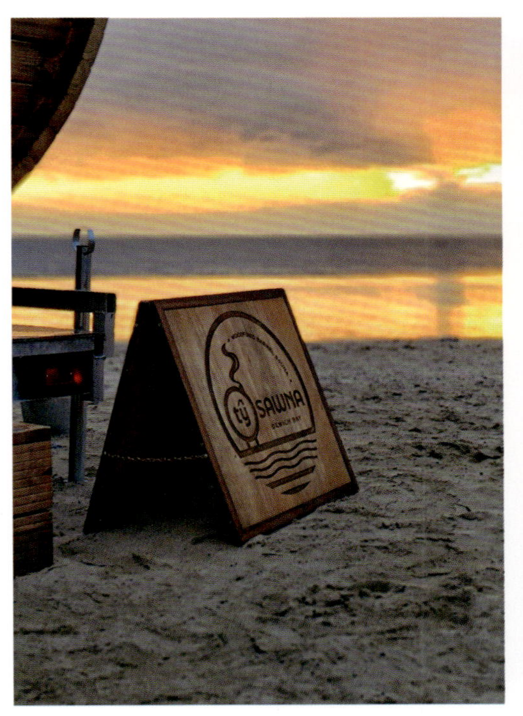
tŷ SAWNA

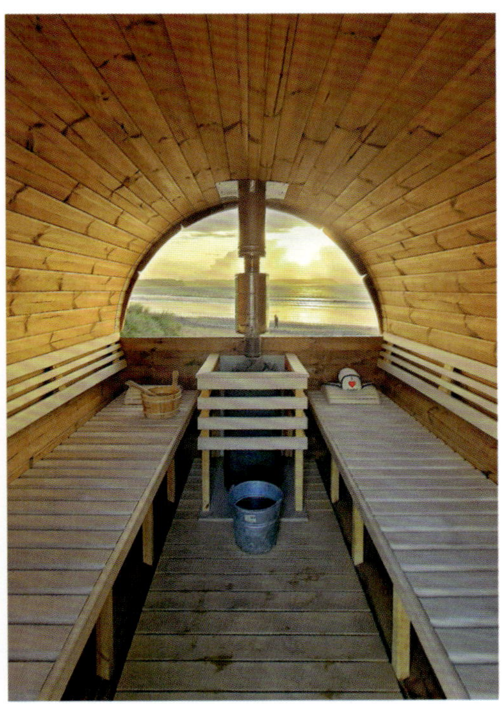

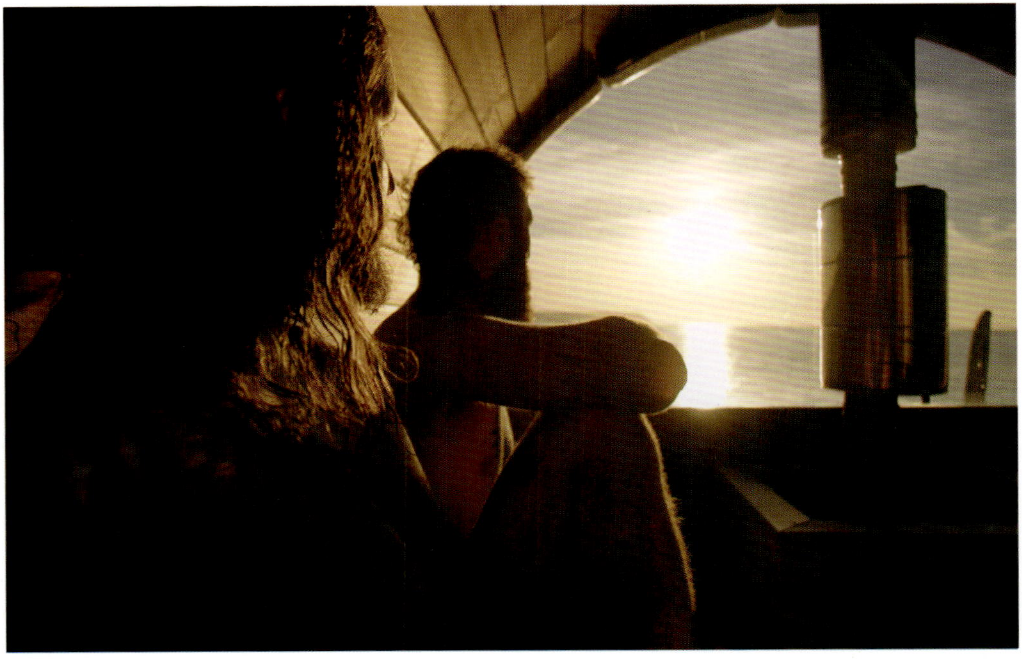

101

Sawna Llosgi

LLANGRANNOG ❦ CEREDIGION

After experimenting with building their own makeshift saunas, local lifeguards and surfers Sam and Vinny imported Sawna Llosgi from Scandinavian Sauna, a Danish company with a workshop in Krakow . It sits in a permanent location just above the beach in Llangrannog, where the sea can be tranquil or tempestuous depending on the weather, and the sunsets are legendary.

Llosgi is Welsh for 'burning', and Sawna Llosgi has a loyal and regular customer base. They offer a five sauna package and the pair have worked with a local aromatherapist to develop their own essential oils. Sawna Llosgi has become a social hub – so much so that they have even received a couple of complaints from bathers who have turned up and been on their own in a session, and thus missed the chat. Families are welcome.

sawnallosgi.co.uk
Sea/cold plunge 52.1600, -4.4709

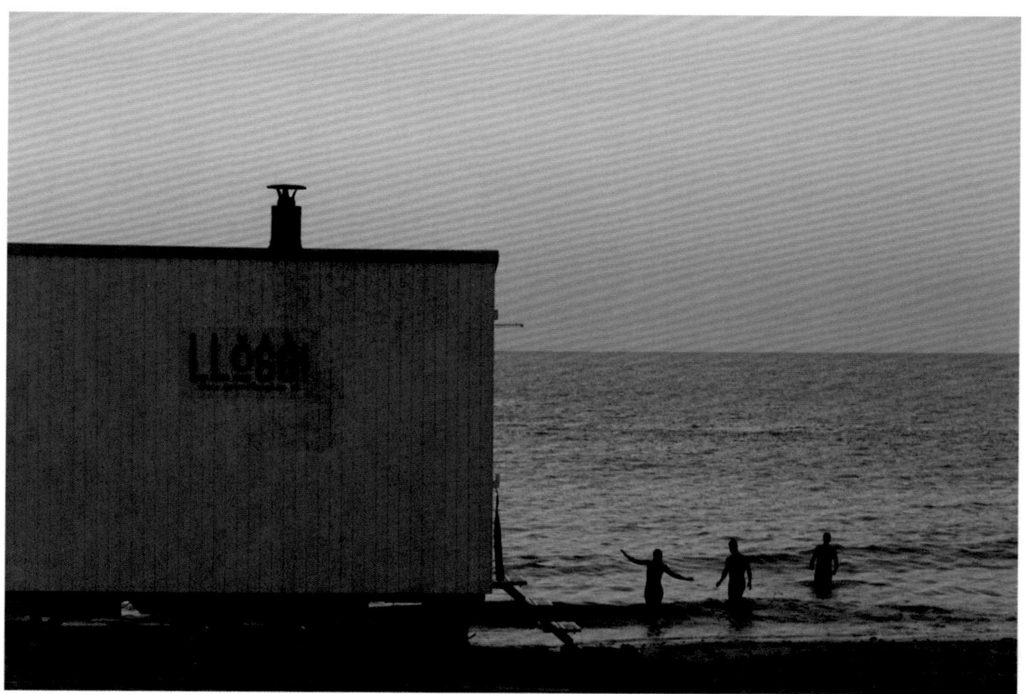

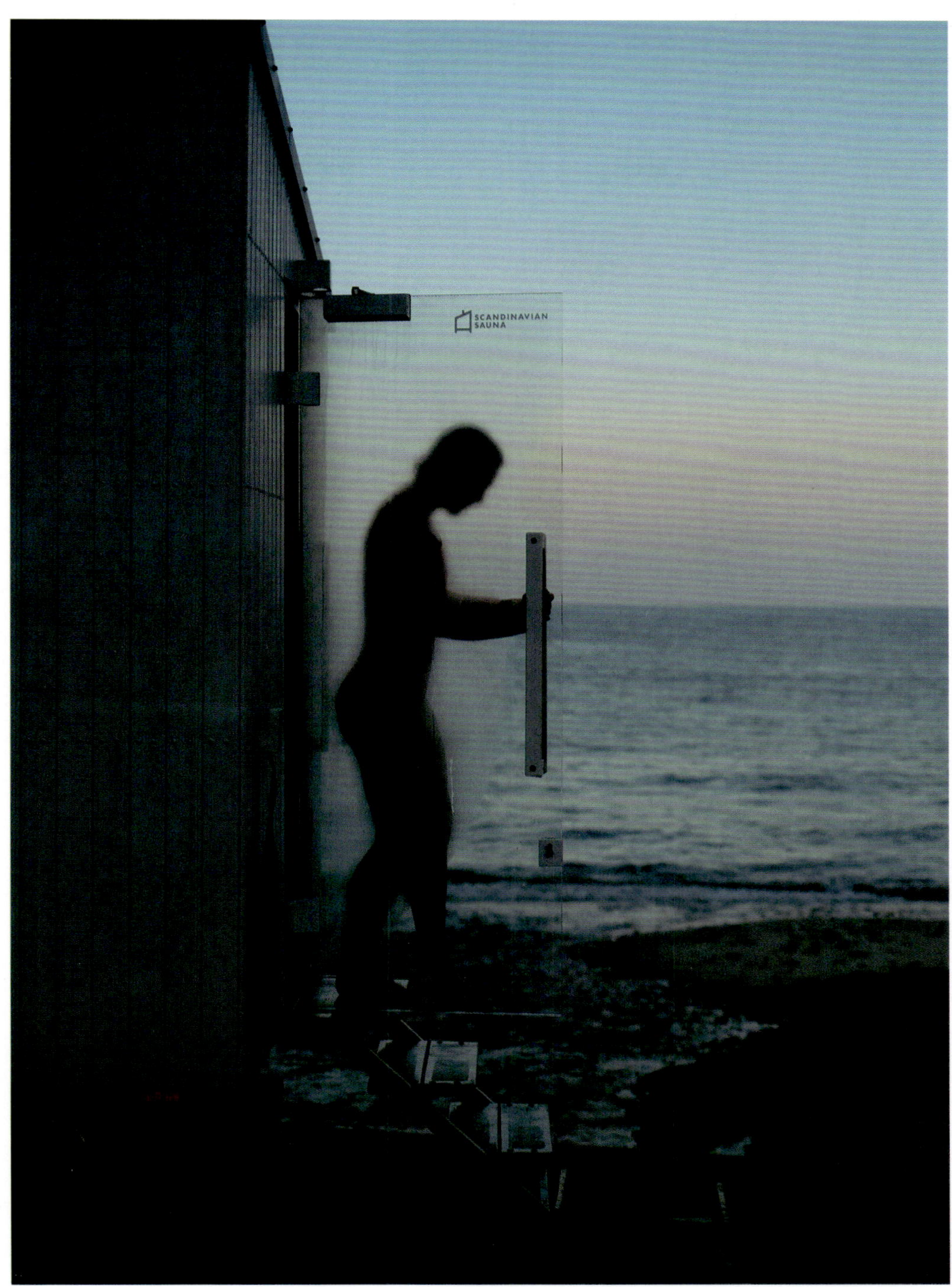
SCANDINAVIAN
SAUNA

102

Hikitalo

PORTHCAWL ❦ BRIDGEND

William Jenkins' sweat-bathing odyssey lasted 13 years, and took him through the saunas of Ireland, to the *aufguss* of Germany via the *temazcals* of South America. This autumn it brought him back home to Wales – to Porthcawl, where he surfed during school holidays when he was a kid. He called on Sauna Craft in Bristol to create a 10-seater trailer sauna and christened it Hikitalo, which means 'sweathouse' in Finnish, as a nod to his Finnish sweat-bathing partner in South America.

Along the way, William has faced his own mental health challenges but found immense healing in cold and sauna therapy. To this end, he's committed to using sauna as a tool to combat loneliness and promote mental wellbeing. 'In Wales, loneliness is a significant issue, impacting both mental and physical health. The social aspect of sauna can play a key role in reducing these numbers and fostering a sense of community,' says William.

hikitalo.com

Sea 51.4786, -3.6924

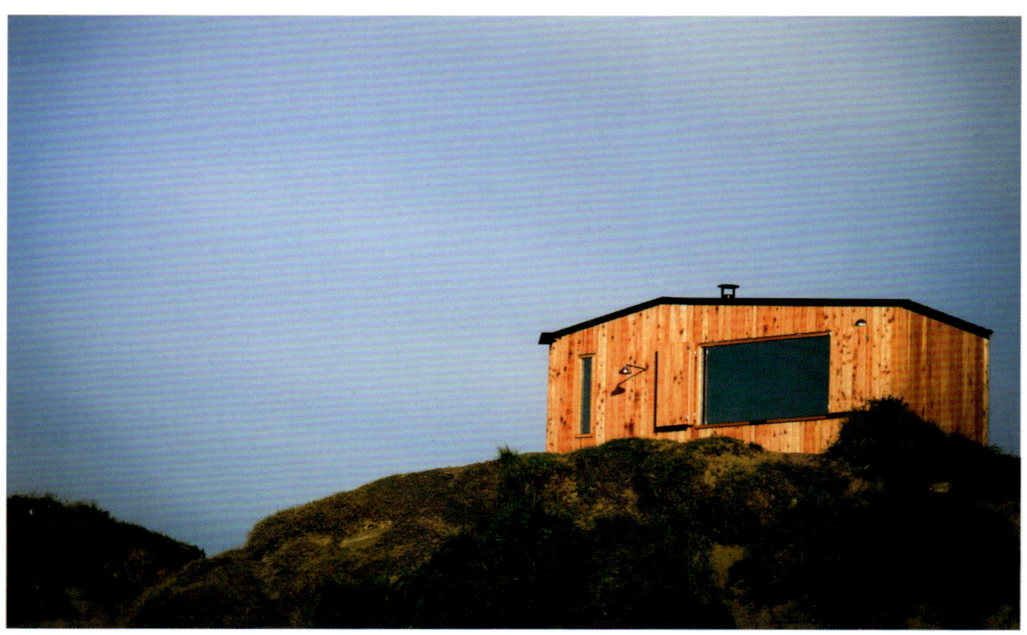

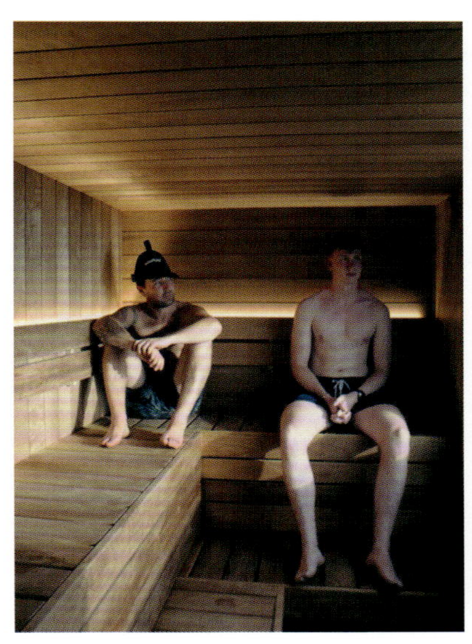
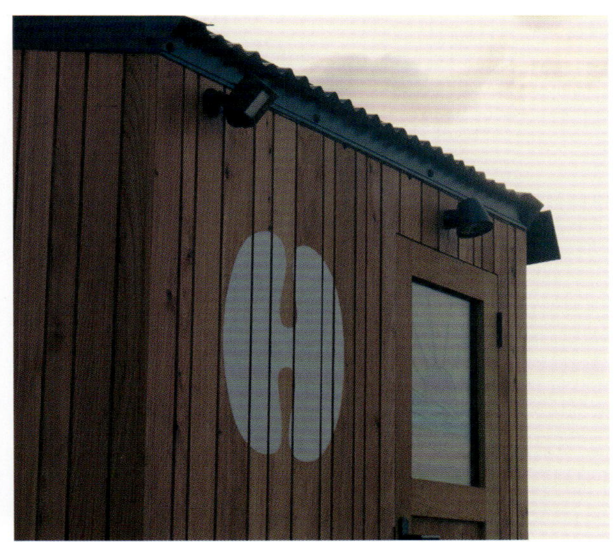
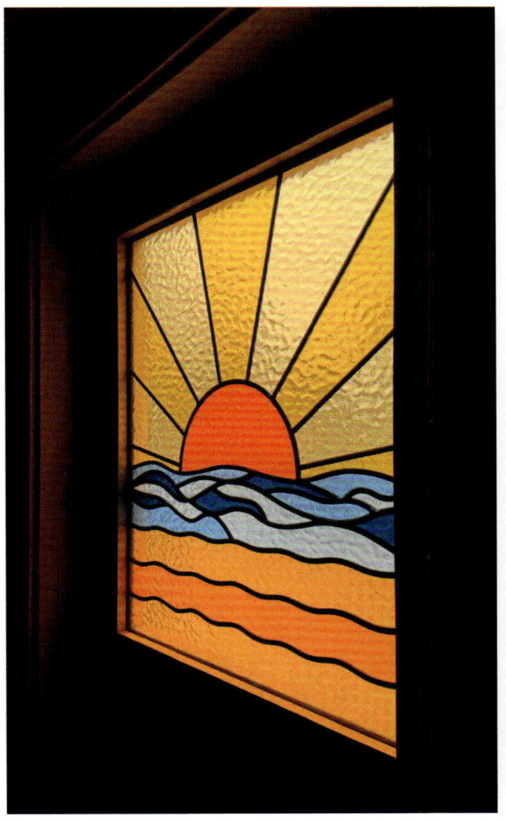

103

Sawna Bach - The Scenic Sauna

PORTH TYN TYWYN & LLYN PADARN

The emphasis at Sawna Bach is to slow down, relax and connect with nature and yourself. Given this little eight-seater sauna's location among the dunes next to white sands and clear seas at Porth Tyn Tywyn on Anglesey, this is not such a challenge. *Bach* means 'small' in Welsh, and given the scale of its setting, it perfectly suits this sauna.

Sawna Bach was founded by friends Caroline Coch, Jen Holloway and Alex Zalewski as a side hustle. Caro is a German polar researcher who lived in Iceland and Sweden before moving to Anglesey with her husband, so she is well-versed in sauna culture. Jen's husband, Alex, is an ocean scientist and a wood enthusiast, and he spent 700 hours building the sauna in his spare time.

A second sauna, in a magnificent setting on the shores of Llyn Padarn in Llanberis, is discreetly nestled next to the National Slate Museum, at the base of Snowdon in the Snowdonia National Park.

Both saunas offer induction courses for safe cold water immersion, guided sessions for men, sauna ceremonies, yoga, and sound baths. For anyone hiking the 135-mile Anglesey Coastal Path that circuits the island, the sauna at Porth Tyn Tywyn provides some welcome respite. Certain sessions are specifically aimed at Welsh speakers and social media posts are written in English and Welsh, offering nuggets of local history.

Sawna Bach's founders are collaborating with Bangor University to research the physiological response of the body to sauna bathing. The bathers here are predominantly local, active, and outdoorsy, though the number of athletes in the 30-60 age bracket visiting for post-exercise muscle recovery is on the rise.

saunawales.co.uk Sea/lake/shower/hose
53.2156, -4.5027 Porth Tyn Tywyn, Anglesey
53.1222, -4.1174 Llyn Padarn, Llanberis

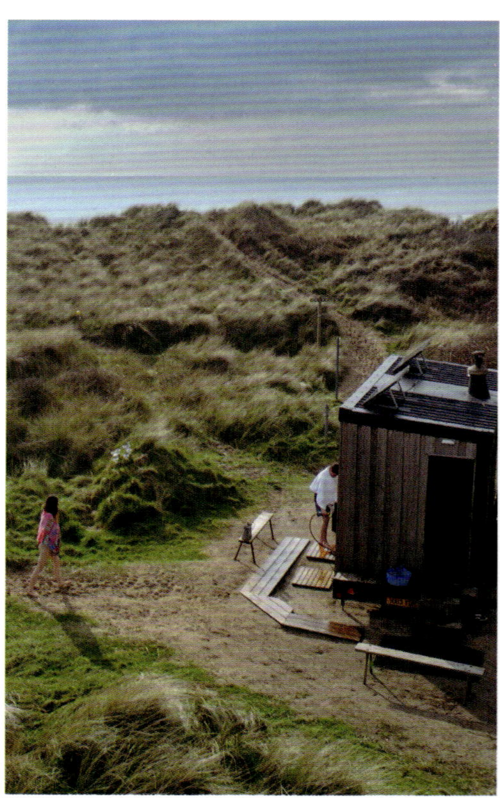

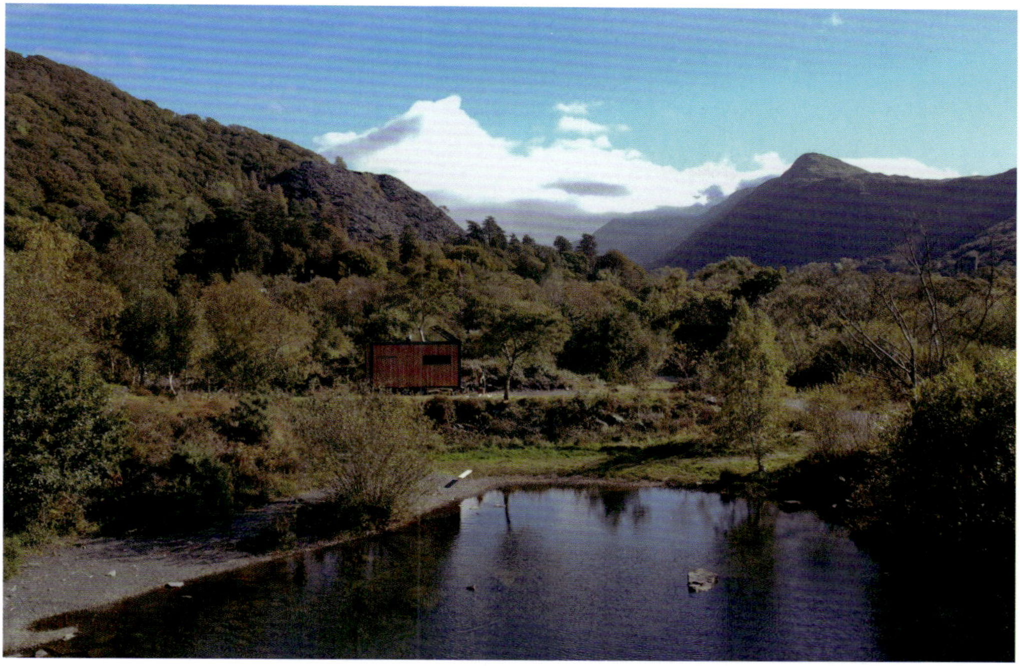

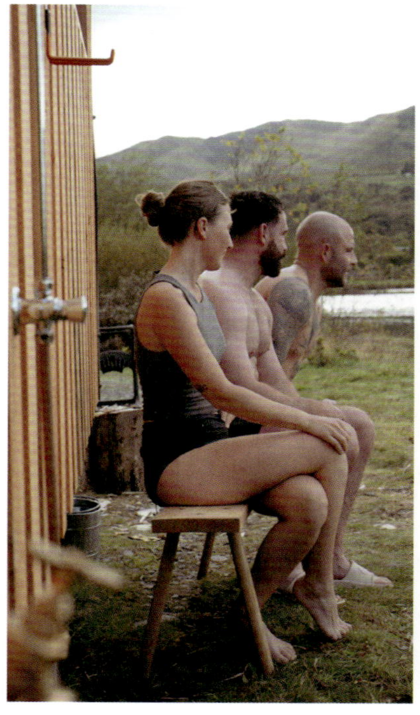

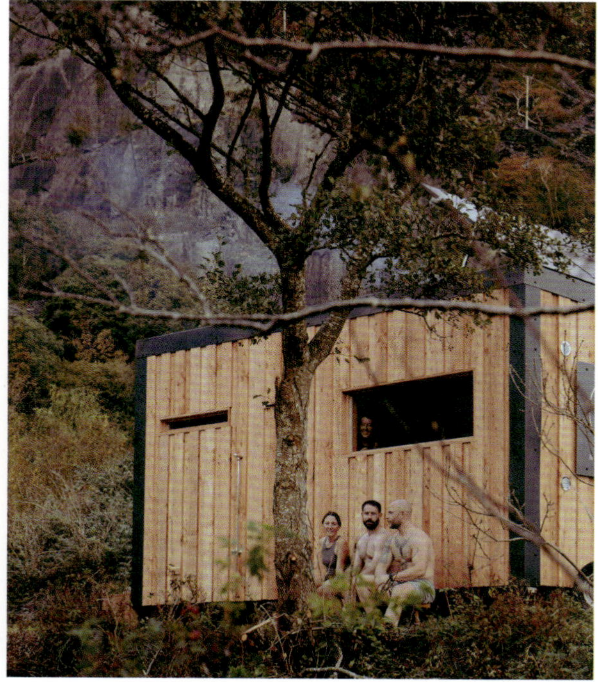

104

Wern Derys

HAY-ON-WYE ❦ HEREFORD

Artist, Jim Ursell started doing sweat lodges in Wales when he was in his 20s, making them himself from willow, hazel and firebricks. Experiments included throwing lemon juice on the fire (not recommended) and combining the sweating with moonlight plunges in remote waterfalls and gorges.

During the Covid-19 lockdowns, Jim decided to convert a former barn building at his home near Hay-on-Wye into 'a serious temple space' in which to take refuge and sweat. He sourced local reclaimed cedar, charred it, and oiled it in linseed following a Japanese technique called Shou Sugi Ban. He paired the wood with 450-million-year-old sandstone, taken from what was an ancient sea lagoon less than a mile away, and a year later his sweat house was complete.

The sweat house is part of the guest offering at Wern Derys, the homestead he and his wife Georgie, a painter, have spent 12 years creating. Their artworks decorate a cottage and cabin; Georgie's handmade quilts line the beds, and on one wall is a wooden sea kayak that Jim made and then paddled from Kimmeridge Bay in Dorset to Falmouth in Cornwall. Hens cluck around underfoot, and a 500-year-old oak tree is the perfect spot to sit after a sauna and take in the rolling views.

This is Tolkien country; the writer came to Herefordshire on holiday and its influence can be felt in The Hobbit and The Lord of the Rings: Archenfield, Bredwardine (Brandywine), Rivendell. *Wern Derys* is Welsh for 'oak grove', and a 5,000-year-old standing stone marks the entrance across a field. A picture window in the sauna faces west over the Black Mountains, and in summer the sun sets over Hay Bluff. Behind an acid-green hedgerow, horses twitch their ears.

The sauna gets seriously hot. Jim often cranks it up to 105°C. He makes whisks from birch and mint, and oak and nettle, and between sauna rounds, likes to snack on gherkins and local cider. At night, when the sauna is lit, the earliest invertebrate fossils show up in the sandstone panels.

The tiled cold plunge is fed by a borehole and is always cool, but there are plenty of other local swimming spots nearby. Georgie swims in The Warren in Hay-on-Wye, and Bredwardine is a 20-minute drive away; further still is Llangynidr on the River Usk and Wolf's Leap on the River Irfon – the site of Jim's sweat lodges of yesteryear.

There are castles too, built in the time of the Marcher Lords and the Norman invasion. 'The ideas of the Green Man originate from this time when everyone – aristocracy and peasantry – hid in the Welsh woods in a societal utopia,' says Jim, 'It's still the vibe.' To feel a little piece of it, head no further than Wern Derys.

➔ canopyandstars.co.uk/britain/england/herefordshire/wern-derys
❄ Cold plunge 📍 52.0254, -3.0157

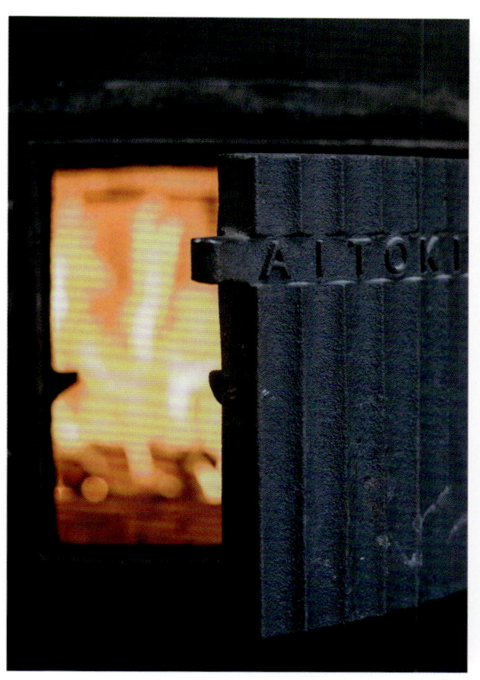
AITOKI

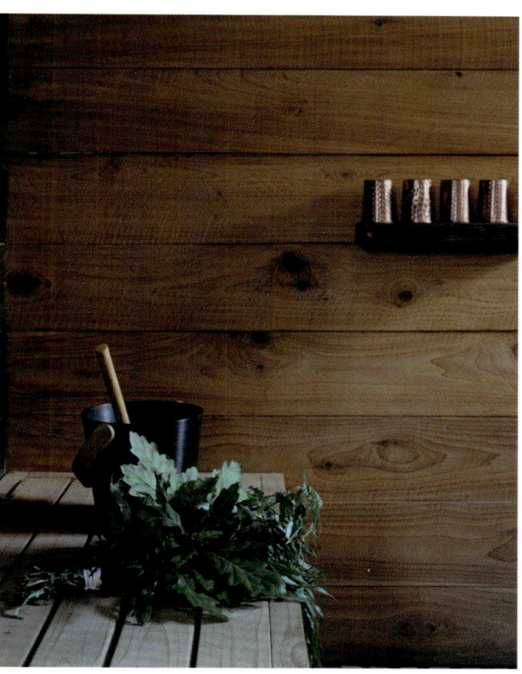

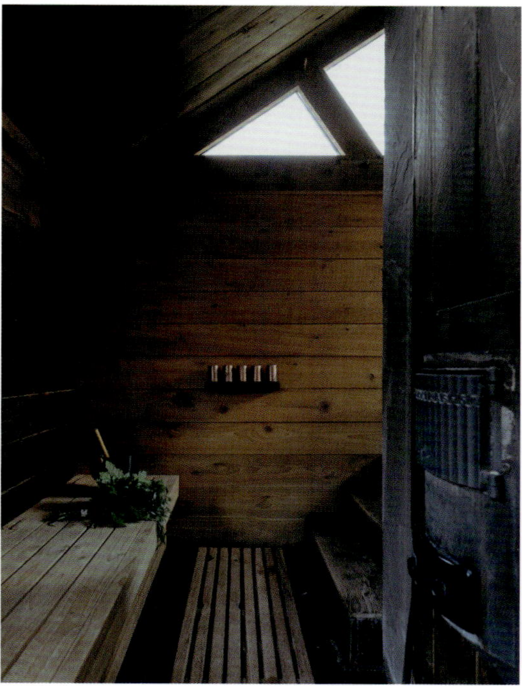

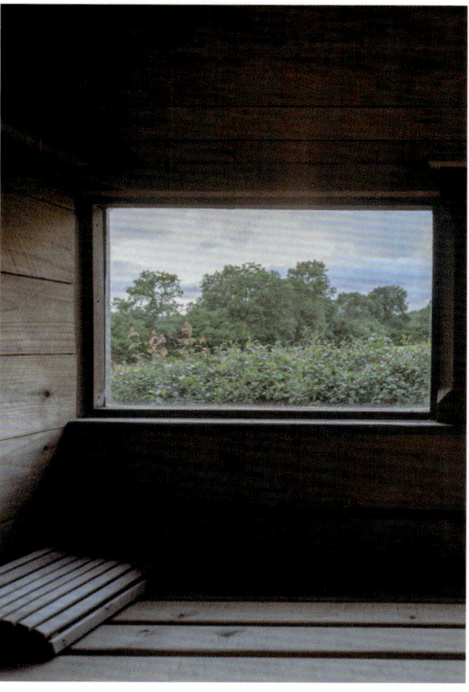

105

Casgen Sawna

COLWYN BAY ❦ COUNTY CONWAY

Porth Eirias in Colwyn Bay is a top tourist spot; its Waterfront Complex houses a top-quality restaurant, café and water sports centre, along with changing rooms, toilets and two outdoor showers. Casgen Sawna is the latest arrival.

It's owned and run by friends, David and Tom, who were inspired to bring sauna to their hometown beach after a visit to Ireland where they met Donie McAuliffe, a legendary singing sauna operator who moves between beaches. David and Tom commissioned Donie's builder in Skibbereen to build them a sauna for ten and towed it back to North Wales.

Word of the sauna quickly spread among the various sports, exercise and cold-water swimming groups in Colwyn Bay and further afield. Everyone agrees that a wood-fired barrel sauna with a great view of the beach and the chance to cool off in the sea is vastly superior to a gym sauna, which is often pokey, smelly and not very hot.

Operating a sauna in a busy, touristy spot means fielding lots of questions. There's so much curiosity and trepidation – and many misconceptions – about what a proper sauna is, that David and Tom are educators too. They see many converts, among them the dad who arrived with his wife and adult kids and declared it wasn't for him. He sat on the wall outside while they went in for their session, but after seeing how much fun his family were having, he joined them for the last half hour. He emerged transformed and is now a sauna evangelist.

instagram.com/casgensawna
Sea 53.2953, -3.7181

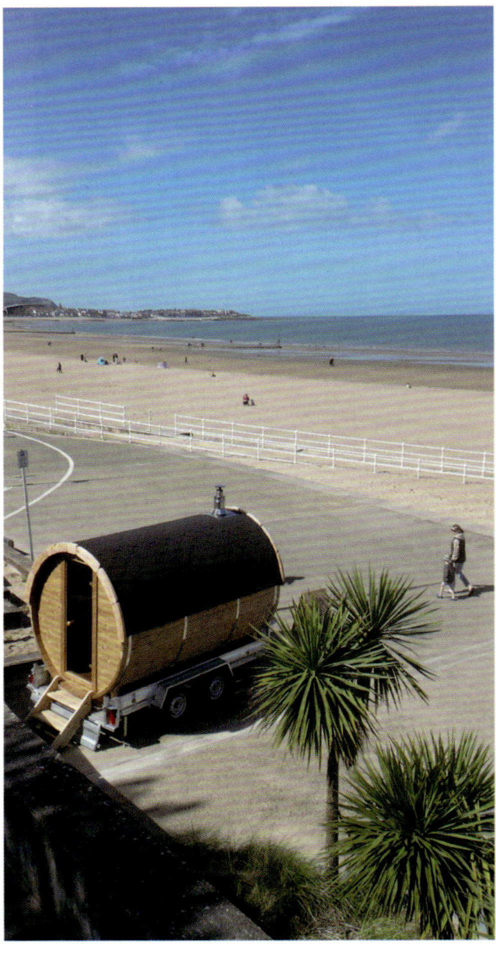

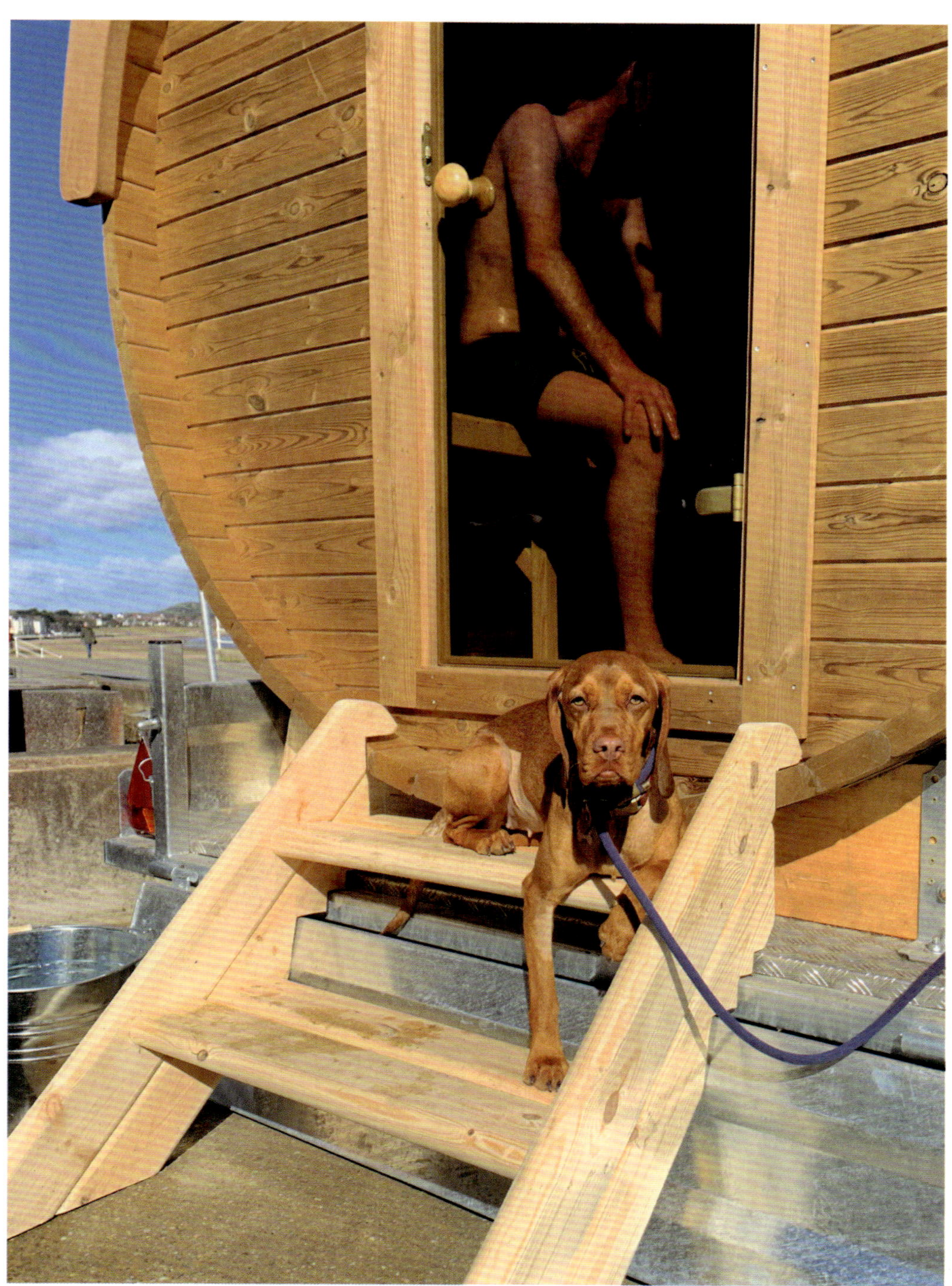

106

Secret Sauna at Penguin Pool

LLANDEGLA ❦ DENBIGHSHIRE

So popular is the Secret Sauna at Penguin Pool, that as soon as it opened word quickly spread among the Bersham Bathers, the Wirral Bluetits and the Colwyn Bay Blue Bits. These groups of cold-water swimmers come from as far away as Manchester and Liverpool to sweat and swim at the nature-soaked spot. It's part of Faraway Follies – a hideaway in Llandegla in North Wales that draws a wellness-loving crowd.

Faraway Follies belongs to Jenny and Margaret, a pair of committed contrast-therapy addicts who each morning, regardless of the weather, dunk in the freshwater pool for 90 seconds before heading to the sauna. The couple met 40-odd years ago when Margaret, a single mother with three children, dialled Jen's number by mistake. An 18-year-old Jen came to say hi with her girlfriend, both on horseback, and the rest is history. Margaret is in now in her 80s but looks 20 years younger, and Jen in her 60s.

Jen dug and dredged the pool that had been created long ago to measure the flow in the stream, assessing its suitability to supply the local village with water. She also commissioned the two wooden penguins who watch over the bathers as they clamber in and out.

'It's colder going into running water than an ice bath, because in stationary water your body makes a little warm wetsuit – a thermal layer – round itself,' says Jen, who bought the sauna after the Covid-19 pandemic.

The sauna sits next to the pool, and to get there you climb a wooden log path past a treehouse and gypsy caravans that sleep eight. Self-catering lodges, a tipi, outdoor kitchens, fire pits, barbecues, cast iron pans, griddles and a Dutch oven for cooking over the fire complete the scene. When it's full, Faraway Follies accommodates 26 people.

The sauna is now open to the public and is also part of the mix for those on foraging and yoga retreats, and Jen combines it with her sound baths, the passive nature of which complements sitting still in a sauna. She has played gongs, rattles, drums and crystal bowls for 20 years and is now qualified with The British Academy of Sound Therapy. Sound baths have been used for millennia to bring about altered states of consciousness and encourage relaxation and a restorative, meditative state.

➔ mindfulretreats.fitness
❄ Pond 📍 53.0402, -3.1974

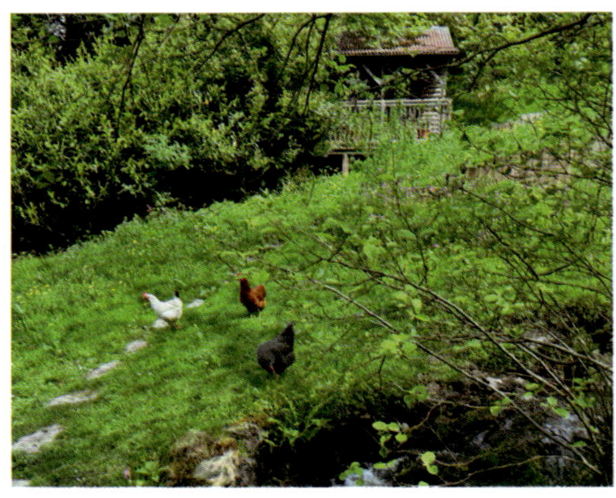

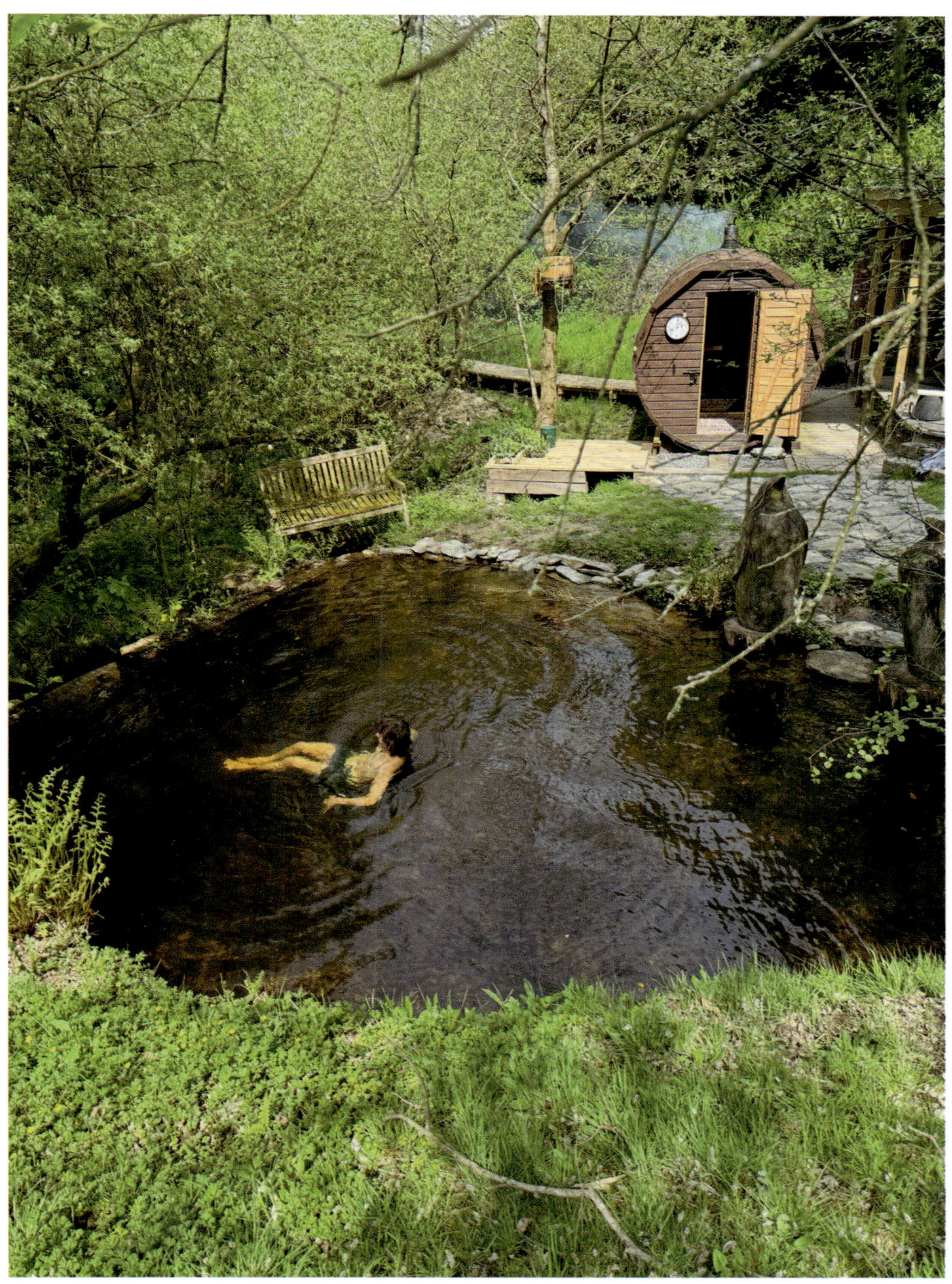

More

107 Logi Sauna

MARTLETWY ❦ PEMBROKESHIRE

Logi offers communal sessions at the sport-focused Wild Lakes at Martletwy. It can also be rented for private events and parties.

➔ logisaunas.co.uk
❄ Lake ⌖ 51.7749, -4.8101

108 Sauna Y Coed

SWISS VALLEY ❦ CARMARTHENSHIRE

Sauna Y Coed operates as part of Live Free Adventures, which manages a reservoir and woodland in Swiss Valley, Carmarthenshire. Nestled in the woodland, it's a contrast therapy centre with a woodfired horsebox sauna, cold plunge tanks, cold showers, firepits and Haitus coffee shop. Sessions can hold up to eight and there are separate 'bros' and 'sisters' sessions too.

➔ livefreeadventures.co.uk/sauna-new-1
❄ Three cold tubs ⌖ 51.7081, -4.1447

109 FForest

CARDIGAN ❦ CEREDIGION

Tucked away in woodland above the Teifi Gorge, enjoy 1 hour and 45 minutes at the natural spa, featuring a wood-fired hot tub, cedar barrel sauna, and cold plunge. Complimentary herbal tea is available in the spa lounge. Before you depart, you have the option to spend time relaxing in front of the fire at Fforest Lodge, where delicious homemade snacks and drinks are available.

➔ coldatnight.co.uk/natural-spa
❄ Cold tubs ⌖ 52.0635, -4.6430

110 Aberpoeth Sawna

ABERPOETH ❦ ABERYSTWYTH

This sleek 10-seater sauna is the Arbor X designed by high-end Welsh sauna makers Heartwood. It was founded by local friends Gethin and Lolo and sits on the Aberystwyth promenade, offering stunning sea views and easy access to the beach via a jetty. It offers tailored group sessions for sports teams and clubs. Gwesty Cymru nearby provides drinks and snacks.

➔ aberpoethsawna.as.me
❄ Sea with access to a jetty.
⌖ 52.41632, -4.08555

111 Sauna Hut Wales

GOWER ❦ WALES

Barney O'Kane built his mobile Sauna Hut Wales on the back of a Fiat Ducato flatbed van. It often pops up at the Gower Heritage Centre. For those who don't want to dip in the running water next to the mill, there are plenty of buckets of water and a cold plunge.

➔ saunahutwales.co.uk
❄ Leat/bucket/cold plunge ⌖ 51.5838, -4.1033

112 Hälsa Sauna

CASWELL BAY ❦ SWANSEA

Caswell Bay in the Gower Peninsula is a picture-postcard beach, framed by white sands, gentle rollers, rock pools and a couple of retro cafés. If you bag a bench at Hälsa Sauna, you can soak all this up, along with the spectacular views across the Bristol Channel to North Devon. Located along a private road five minutes from the beach (where it's advisable to park), it's too far to walk into the sea between rounds, so this small sauna complex has cold plunge barrels and cold showers.

➔ halsasaunacaswell.com
❄ Barrel/shower/sea (5-minute walk)
⌖ 51.5699, -4.0315

113 The Outdoor Sauna

CANDLESTON WOODS ❋ BRIDGEND

There is a lot going on in Candleston Woods on the Merthyr Mawr Estate. You can combine your sauna, hidden deep in the trees, with various outdoor activities, and a shower and drench bucket are close at hand.

➡ theoutdoorsauna.co.uk
❄ Shower/bucket/immersion pod
📍 51.4828, -3.6215

114 Môr a Sawna

BARRY ❋ GLAMORGAN

Kathryn Donovan is applying her career in mental health to her new venture, Môr a Sawna, in Barry. Getting people to connect with friends, strangers and nature, without tech, is Kathryn's mantra. The sauna seats 10 and sits in a private area just above Jacksons Bay, a quiet cove with high cliffs. A slip path provides easy access down to the sandy beach and sea for a cold dip.

Kathryn is a sea swimmer who enjoys hot/cold therapy for her own health needs, and she combines yoga, dance and sound baths with the sauna and holds a two-and-a-half-hour sacred sisterhood session.

➡ môrasawna.com
❄ Sea/Shower/Cold plunge 📍 51.3925, -3.2637

115 Alive Sauna & Ice Baths

SULLY ❋ VALE OF GLAMORGAN

Alive is a barrel sauna and four filtered ice baths on the grounds of Sully Sports and Social Club. It is open all day from Tuesday to Sunday and affords a great view across the fields to the Bristol Channel. Owners James Abbott and Dan Tucker are really keen advocates of contrast therapy treatments.

➡ instagram.com/alive_bp
❄ 4 filtered cold plunges 📍 51.4035, -3.2077

116 Penpont Sauna

BRECON ❋ POWYS

Perched on the banks of the River Usk near a riverside campsite and house you can rent, the sauna is crafted from cedar, Douglas fir, and larch from their woods. It is insulated with sheep's wool and heated by an Estonian wood stove. The Usk provides an exhilarating cold plunge, and there are water buckets available. They run regular communal sauna sessions year-round.

➡ penpont.com/sauna
❄ River/bucket 📍 51.9475, -3.4954

117 Tân a Rhew

BLACKWOOD ❋ MONMOUTHSHIRE

Tân a Rhew means 'fire and ice' in Welsh, and at Pencoed Fach Farm in the southern valleys, you can experience both. The Davies family has owned the farm since 1912, and it has diversified to survive. Organic milk, coffee, and treats are sold from The Littlest Dairy, and the farm hosts various wellness events. The main focus is contrast therapy, featuring a wood-burning sauna, four cold plunges, changing rooms, and composting toilets.

Views extend over the Brecon Beacons, and the sounds of chickens, sheep, and cows fill the air. You might even spot the High Brown Fritillary, Britain's most endangered butterfly, which breeds on the farm.

➡ pencoedfachfarm.com/tan-a-rhew
❄ Cold plunge 📍 51.6826, -3.2095

118 Cosy Cask Sauna

WHITCHURCH ❋ SHROPSHIRE

Emma and Karen Plunkett, both massive sauna afficionados with infectious enthusiasm, run an eight-person barrel sauna on Alderford Lake water-sports centre in Shropshire. The lake is a perfect place for a dip or a swim.

➡ cosycask.com
❄ Lake 📍 52.9513, -2.6754

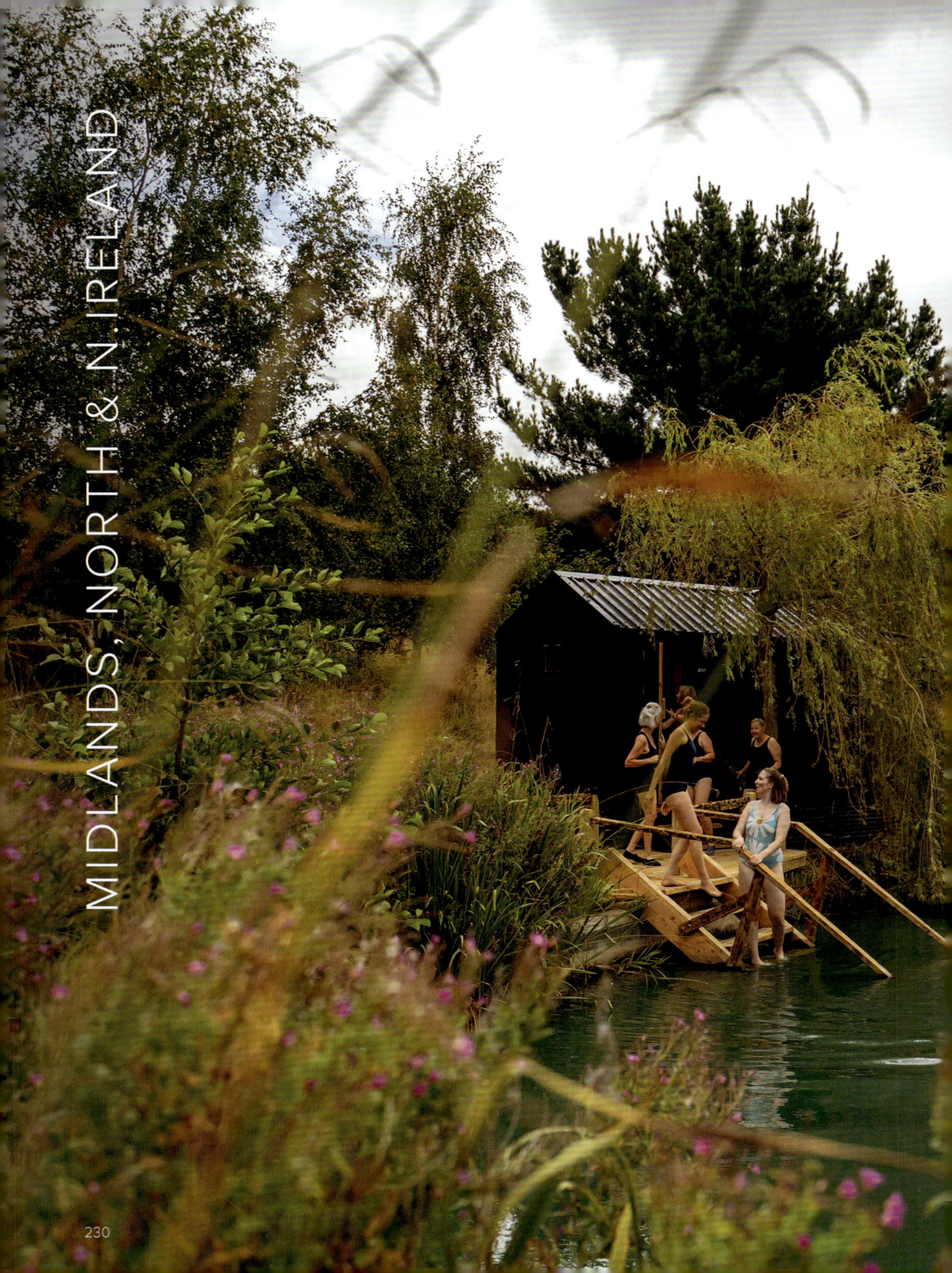

MIDLANDS, NORTH & N.IRELAND

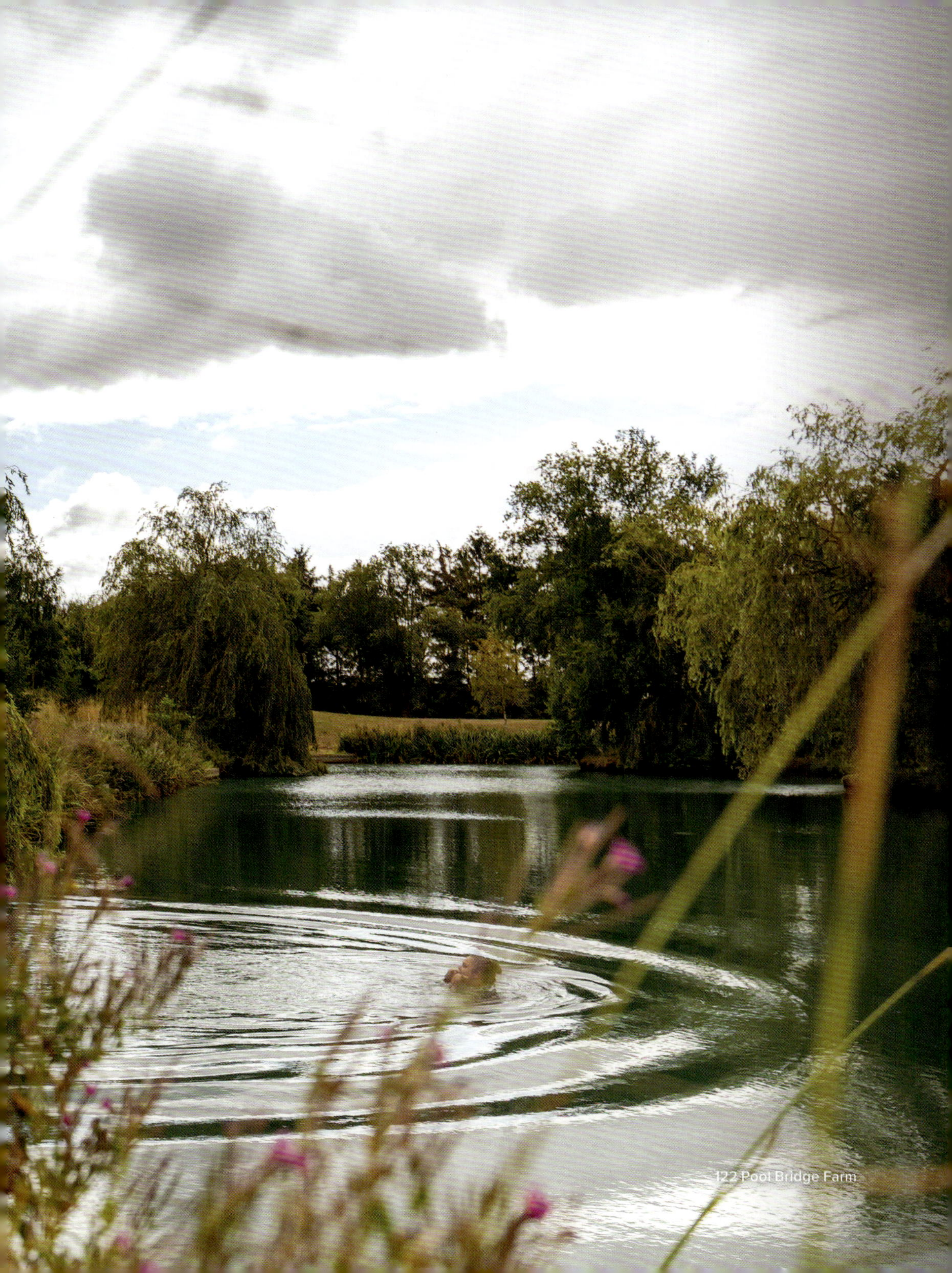

122 Pool Bridge Farm

119

WARMTH Community Sauna

SHEFFIELD ❦ YORKSHIRE

In 2011, a decade before any sauna boom, Bethany Wells built a tent sauna for an architectural research project while studying at the Royal College of Art. It was timber-framed and lined with felt, lit with a stove made from an old gas canister by an artist friend and fed with wood. It was borne of Bethany's fascination with 'the sensory and social conditions sauna presented, and the warming and anti-hierarchical effect it has on people.'

In 2016, she converted a horsebox into WARMTH Community Sauna commissioned by Compass Festival in Leeds, and funded by the Arts Council. It landed at the Brighton Fringe Festival, created a buzz, and has travelled to arts festivals ever since, offering sauna for free. In winter 2024, this OG horsebox sauna landed permanently at Nomad Maison in Sheffield. In keeping with its egalitarian ethos, a pay-it-forward option lets people contribute towards free community sessions, sound baths and other curated experiences. Bethany, who has worked as a theatre designer for many years, is planning to tap into the creative community of eager enthusiasts around her native Sheffield.

→ warmthsauna.co.uk
❄ Drench bucket ⌖ 53.3877, -1.4634

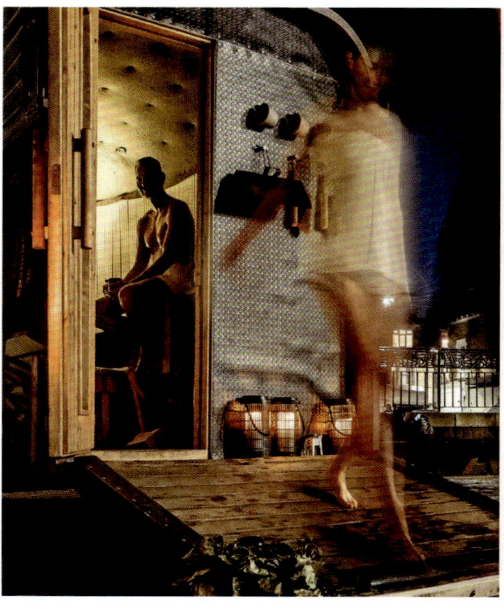

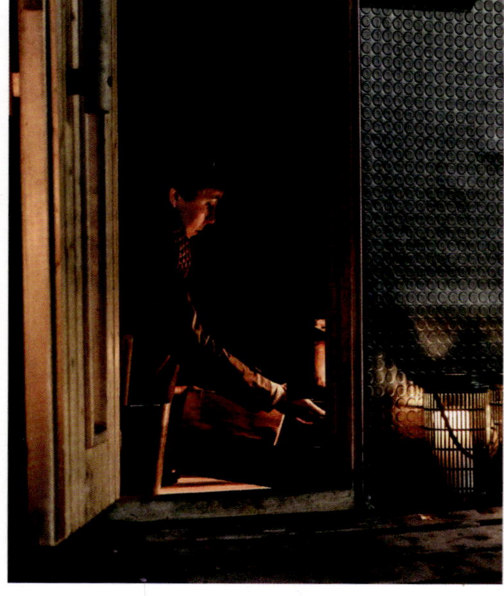

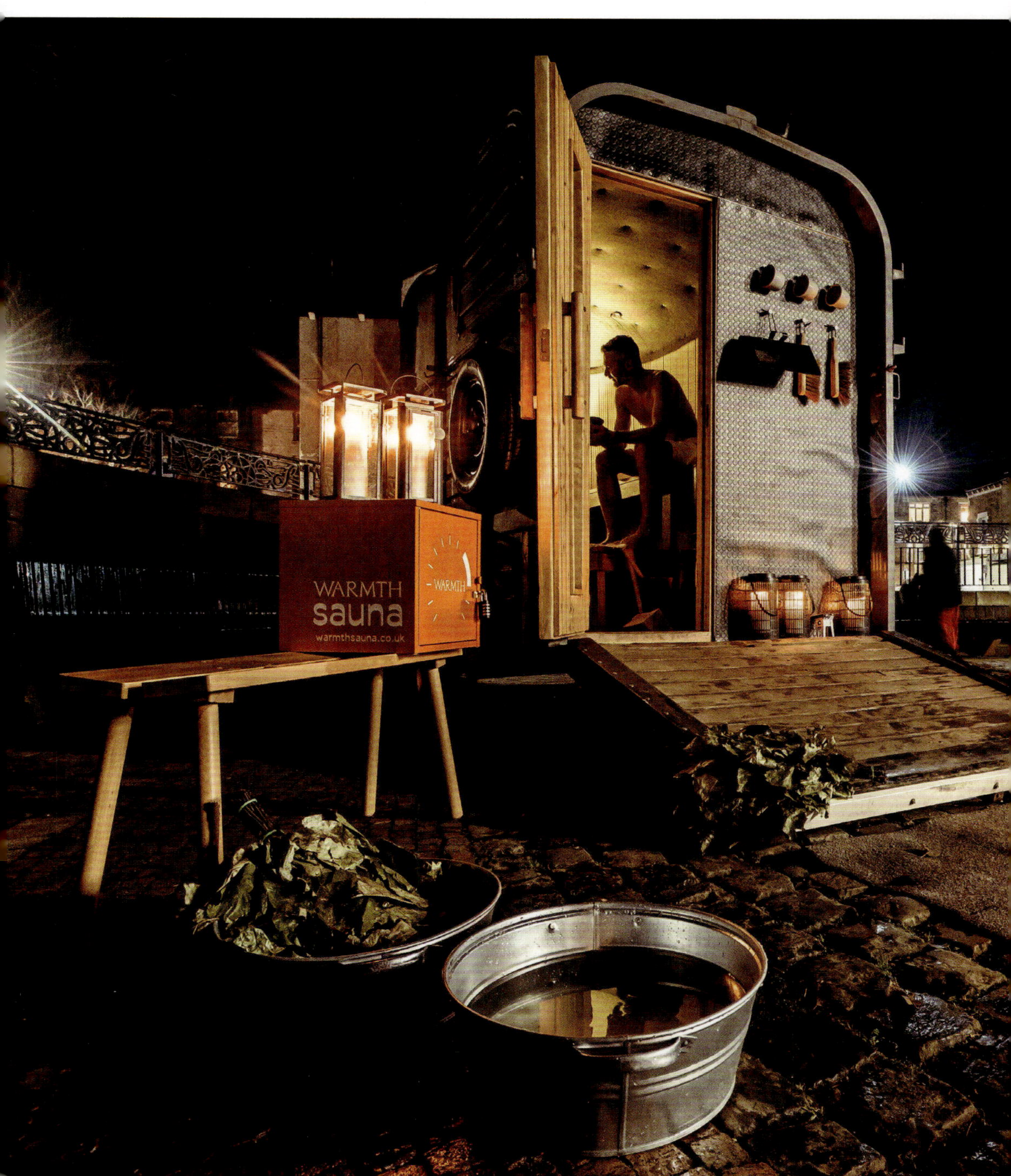
WARMTH
sauna
warmthsauna.co.uk
WARMTH

120

iglu sauna

HEBDEN BRIDGE ❦ YORKSHIRE

iglu is a sauna 'village' with a sauna, three urban ice baths, a horsebox changing room with four cubicles, a Portaloo, deckchairs, a firepit and a drinks van. It's the brainchild of Sam Popper, a local civil servant who visited his local leisure centre sauna every day. This passion for sauna, along with the dearth of wild saunas in the north of England, kick-started iglu, which opened in Hebden Bridge in the car park of the Birchcliffe Centre and the IOU Hebden Bridge Hostel, high above the town. It was an instant success, partly because there is a huge cold-water swimming community in the area.

Along with regular sessions, iglu holds two 'silent' sittings each week, and weekend spa sessions where bathers can apply Himalayan body salt scrubs and Rhassoul mud face masks.

➔ iglusauna.co.uk
❄ Cold plunge 📍 53.7434, -2.0081

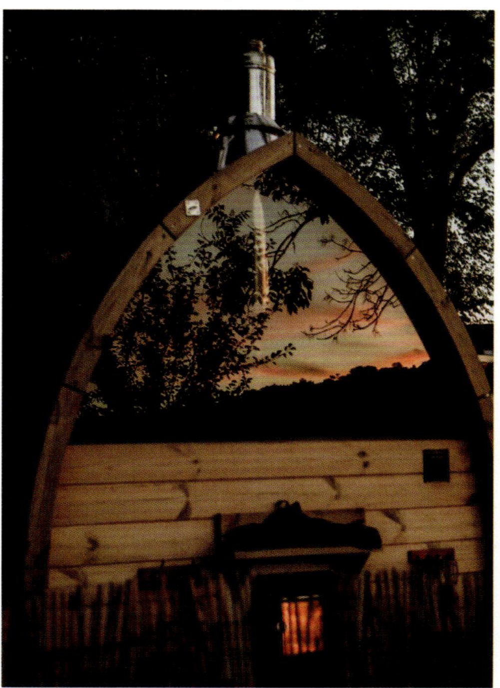

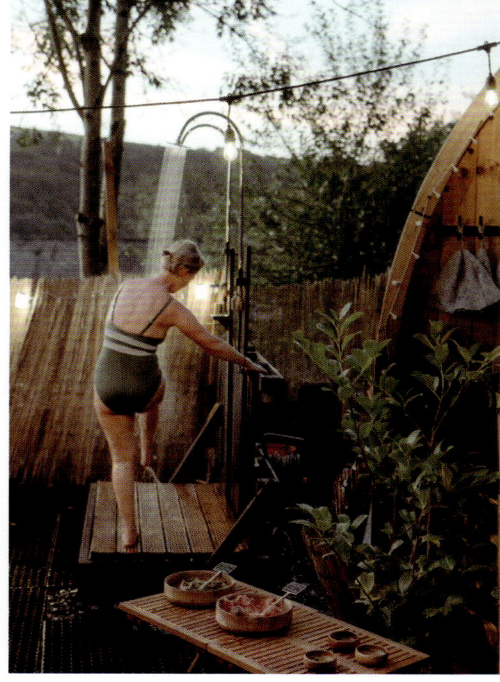

121

WholeHealth Sauna

COLWICK ❦ NOTTINGHAMSHIRE

There are few city centres with access to a spring-fed swimming lake, but Nottingham is one of them. WholeHealth is based in Colwick Lake and Country Park, 1.5 miles from the city centre, offering wild swimming in West Lake, including a 200m and 600m buoy-marked circuit for lap swimming. It's here too, that Whole Health operates three wood-fired lakeside saunas for their membership of swimmers and locals. Offerings include weekly mindfulness dips, full moon swims and saunas, Solstice sauna events and more. The Wired on Wheels cafe on site serves snacks and drinks, all set in the country park which also offers fishing and accessible walking/cycling paths.

➔ whollyhealthy.co.uk
❄ Lake ⌖ 52.9452, -1.0978

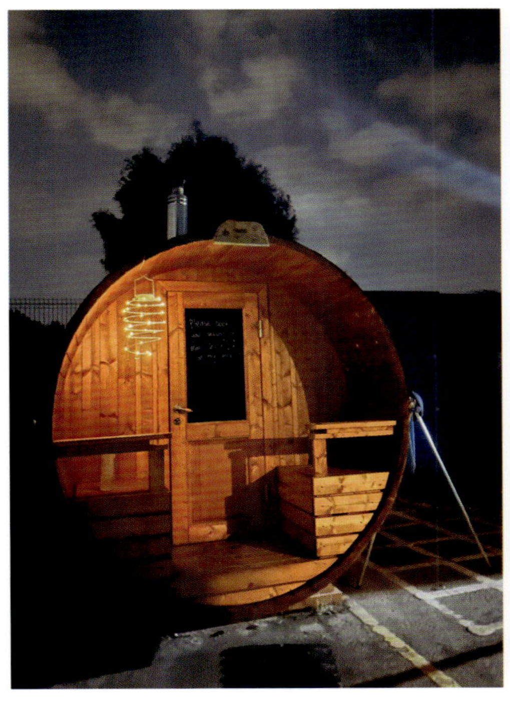

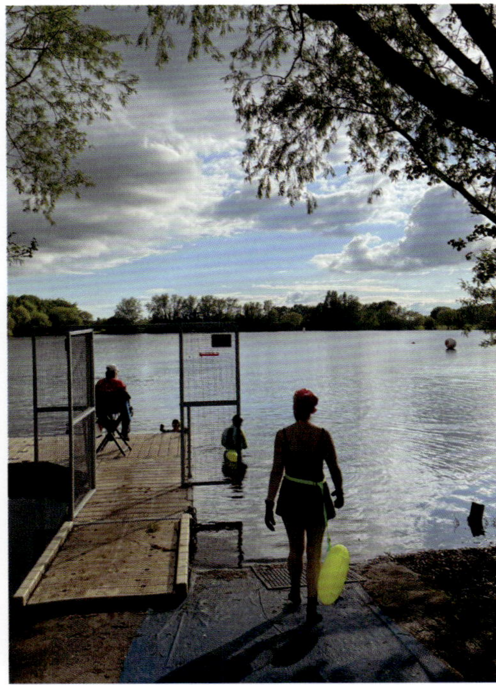

122

Pool Bridge Farm

YORK ❦ YORKSHIRE

For years, the lakes at Pool Bridge Farm were one of the best fisheries in the north of England. Today, these 137 acres of rewilded land outside York are one of the country's best wild swimming spots. Facebook group The Pool Bridge Farm Swimmers has more than 11,000 members, and to service them, discreetly situated around one of the four lakes, are four saunas.

One of them was a shepherd's hut with no roof that had been on the farm since 1911. It was converted by Pool Bridge Farm co-owner Mike Fletcher into a dark, intimate space that seats six. This was quickly followed by two larger saunas. Bathers pay for an hour's sauna session but can stay to swim and relax by the lakes all day. There is also a ten-acre campsite, ideal for tents and small campervans, while other areas offer paddleboarding and kayaking (you need to bring your own) and lessons for those who want them. One lake is lit for winter morning and evening swimming.

Mike does everything to benefit the Pool Bridge community while maintaining the natural, peaceful, wild environment. There are wellness weekends, sound bath sessions, meditation, moon swims with fire pits, yoga, breathwork, ladies' skinny-dipping sessions, and a café open Wednesday to Sunday. And a choir.

poolbridge.co.uk
Lake 53.9096, -1.0254

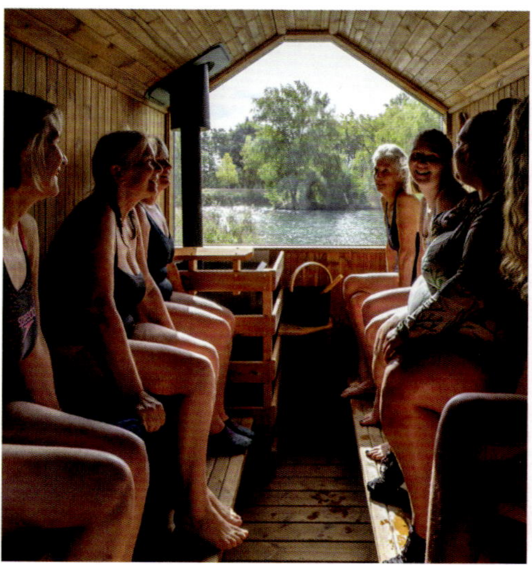

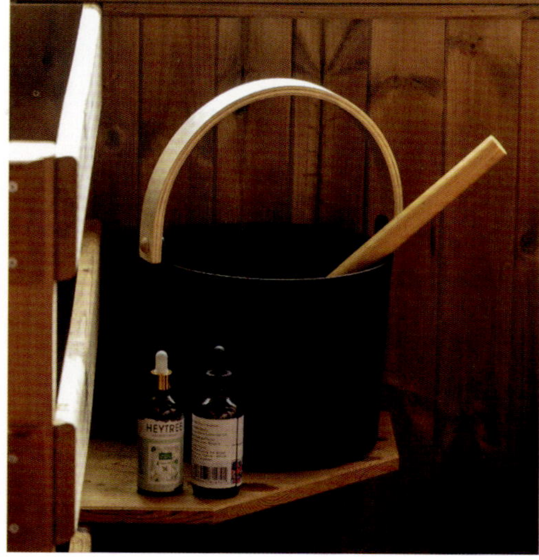

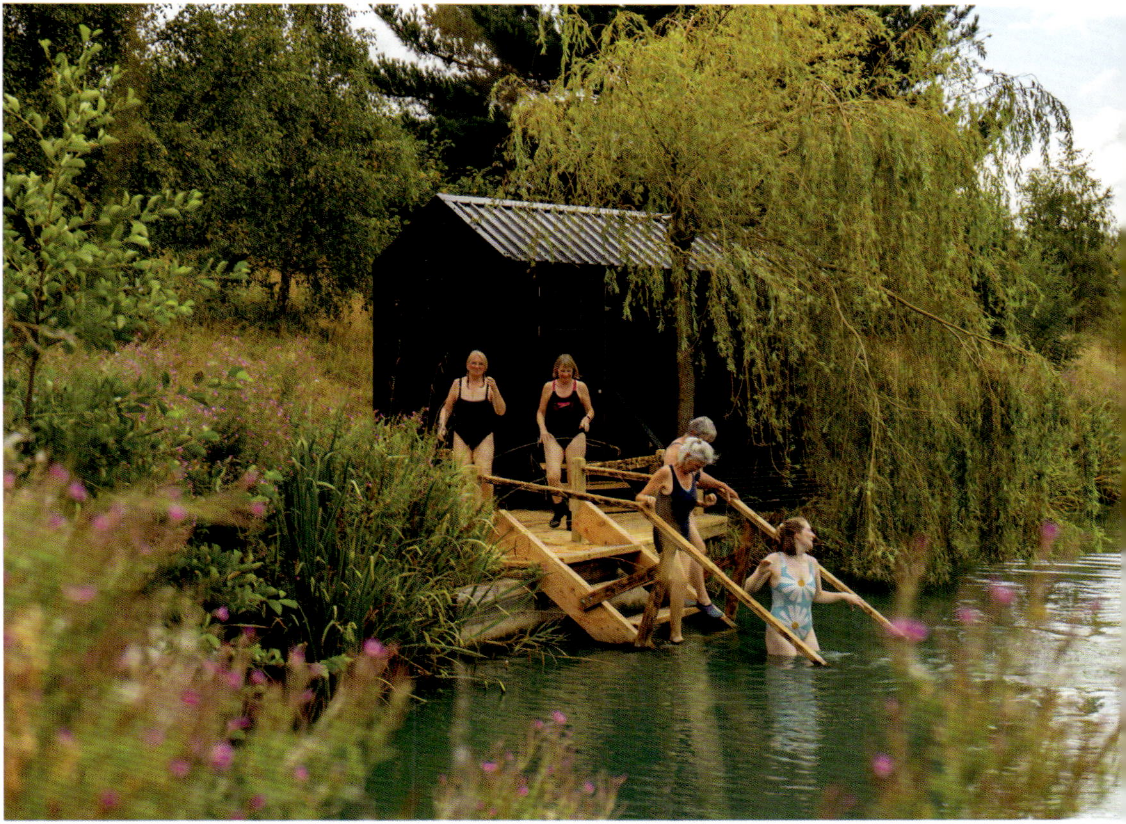

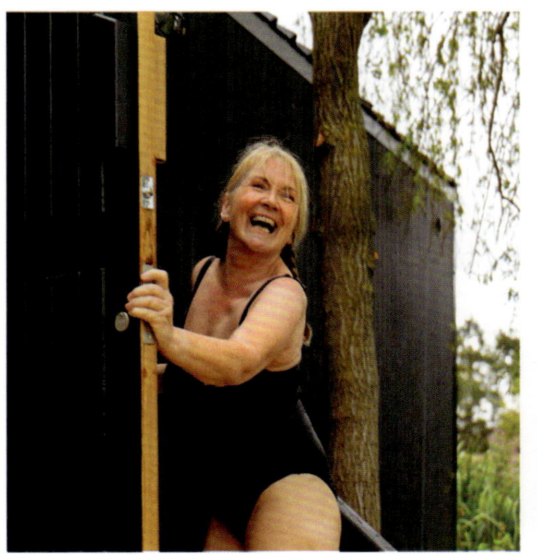

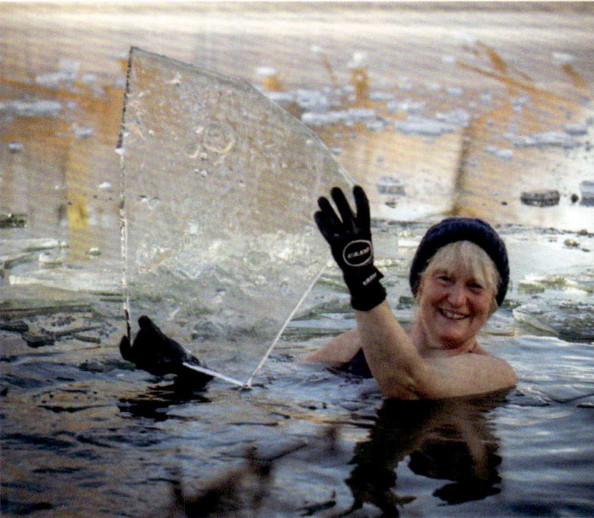

123

Steam and Salt

TYNEMOUTH ❦ TYNE AND WEAR

Nestled below the watchful gaze of the breath-taking ruins of the Medieval Tynemouth Priory and Castle on picturesque King Edward's Bay, Maggie's sauna tents, which she runs with her hammam-loving Turkish husband Sal, attract a diverse crowd. Hugely popular and always fully booked, Steam and Salt has become a cherished part of the community. It caters for large groups and plans are underway for a permanent structure on this stunning stretch of the North Tyneside coastline.

steamandsalt.co.uk
Sea 55.0190, -1.4206

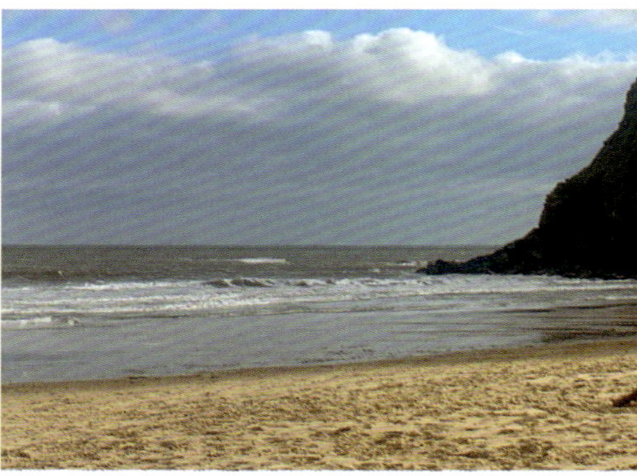

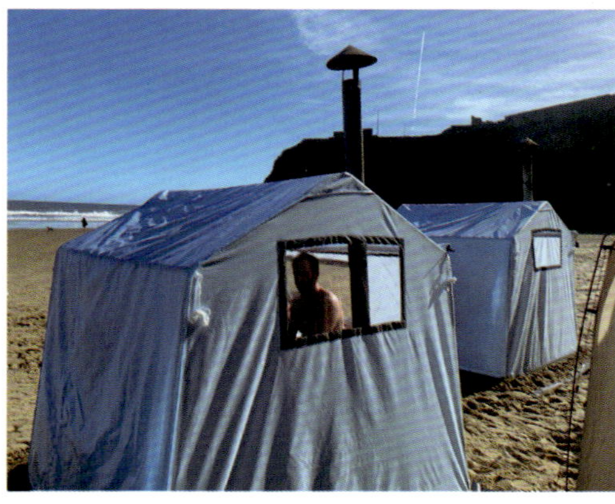

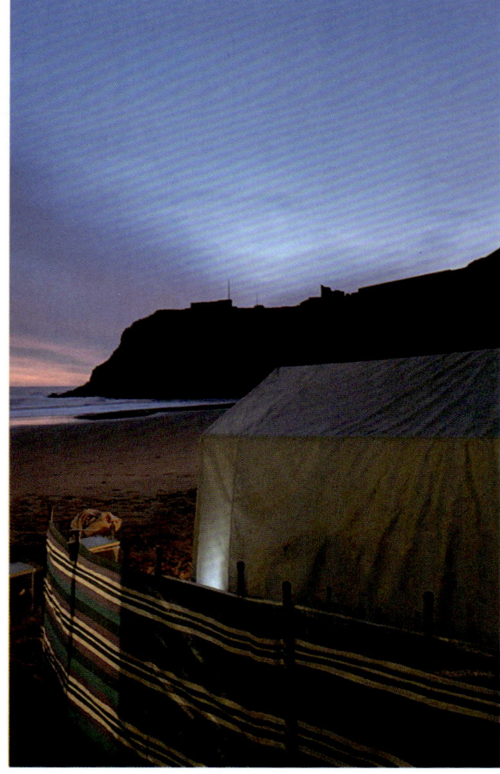

124

Earth Bond

LONGSANDS ❦ TYNE AND WEAR

A cold-water dipper, bored of being really cold on the way home, Laura Bond decided to spend £3,000 on a Finnish Arctinar sauna tent and pitched up on the beaches of Tyne and Wear, from Tynemouth Longsands and neighbouring Cullercoats Bay in North Shields, to Roker Beach and Sandhaven in South Shields. Laura quickly filled her benches and loves her tent sauna sidehustle (she has a managerial job in the NHS). She does it for her love of sea dipping and being outside in the elements. 'I prefer tent sauna to trailers, as I like having my feet on the sand,' says Laura.

So, what happens in her tent sauna? 'There's never a dull moment,' she says. 'The people of South Shields, the 'Sand Dancers' as they are known, are wild and not as reserved as the North Shields' crowd. But lots of people come alone, those who have no one to spend a Sunday with. There's something about sitting in your cozzie sweating that makes you feel like you can share. People who come are non-judgmental of bodies and accepting of the conditions, and they generally have a positive attitude. And if they don't have one when they arrive, they have one when they leave!'

➔ earthbond.uk
❄ Sea ⦿ 55.0307, -1.4296

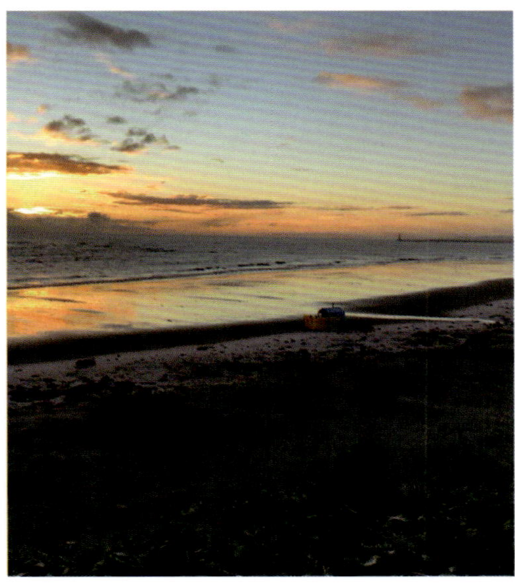

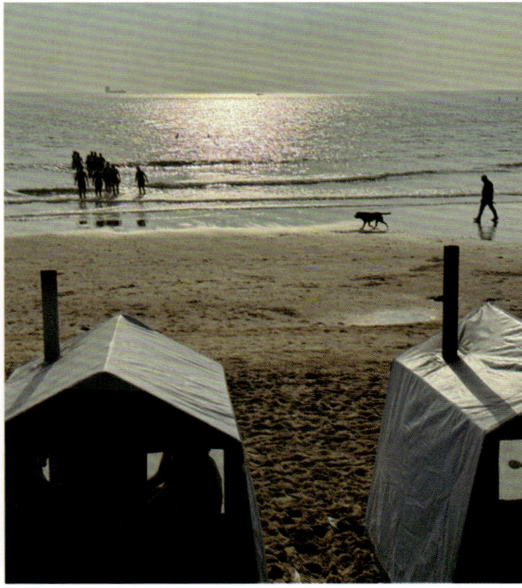

125

Whitby Wellbeing

WHITBY ❦ YORKSHIRE

Tent saunas are popping up all along the Yorkshire coast, and it's thanks in part to Daniel O'Connor, founder of Whitby Wellbeing. Danny got into sweat lodges, breathwork, meditation and cold water a decade ago, and he's on a mission to bring it to others, no matter what. His gung-ho, 'just do it anyway' attitude sees him sweating it out on 12 beaches, from Hornsea to Saltburn.

This 'guerrilla approach' has gathered pace in the wild sauna scene. Bathers from the River Tees to the Humber, from York and Leeds come to Whitby Wellbeing sessions, and many tent sauna operators around the country have been inspired by Danny's chutzpah.

Some Whitby Wellbeing sessions are reminiscent of the rave culture of the 1990s: an eager band of bathers receive a text and head to a secret location – a special spot in a forest or by a waterfall – where Danny will operate under the radar. Only with Whitby Wellbeing, it's about respecting nature and leaving no trace, and the only drugs in sight are endorphins, adrenaline and dopamine.

➔ whitbywellbeing.com
❄ Sea ⚲ 54.4917, -0.6191

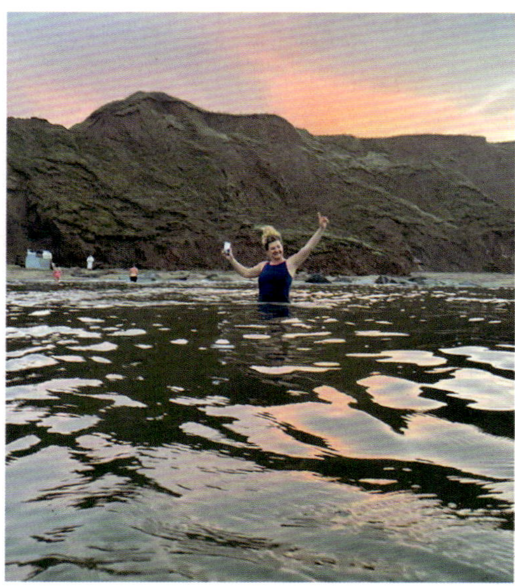

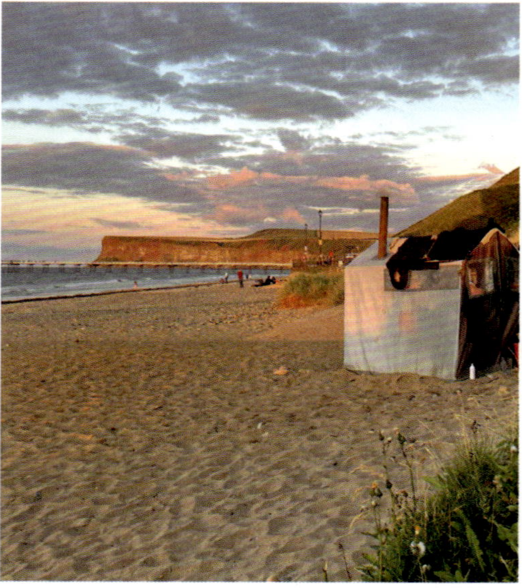

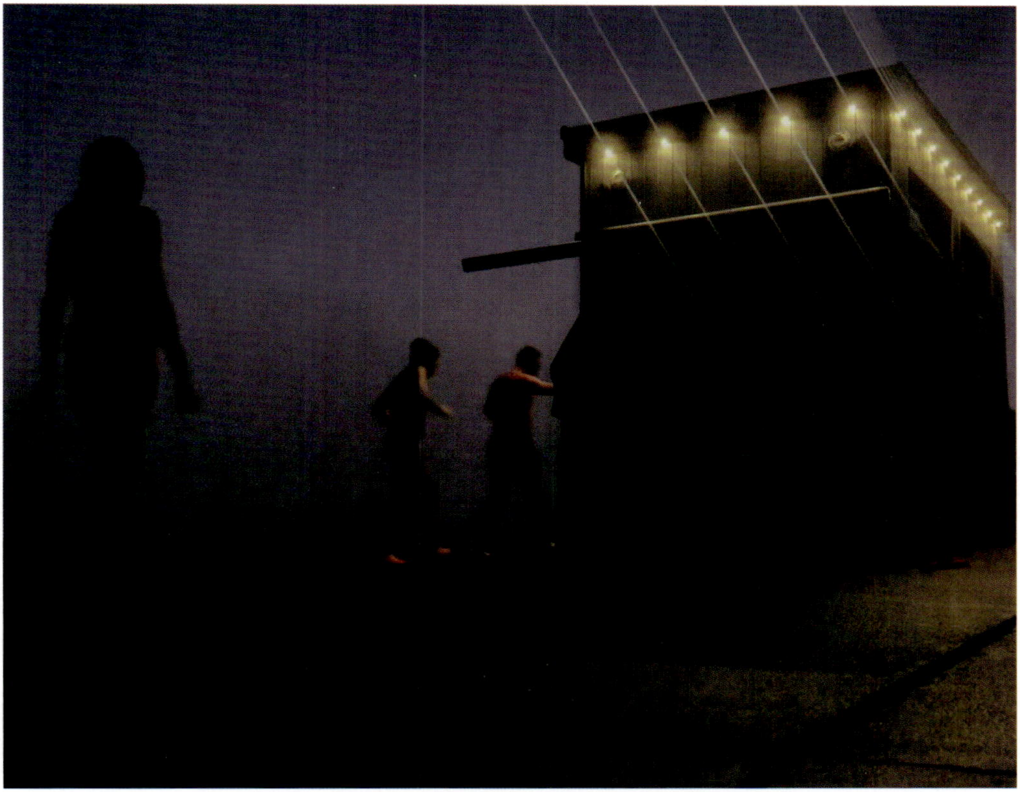

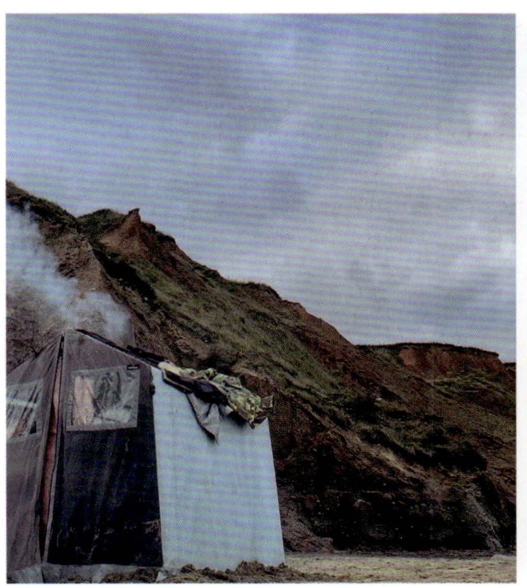

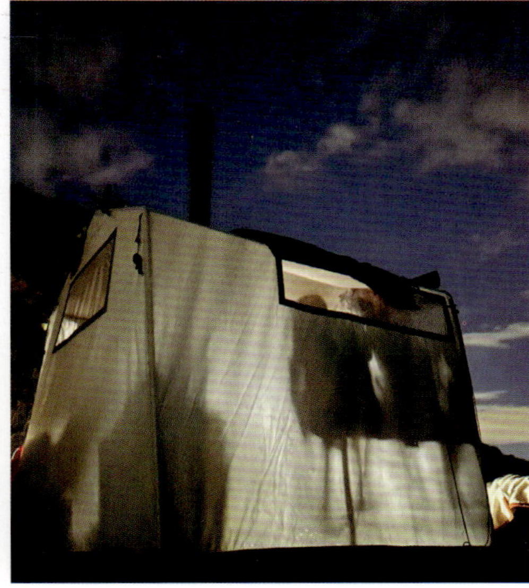

126

La'al Sauna

AMBLESIDE ❦ CUMBRIA

You have to have resilient, nimble and next-level multi-tasking skills to be a wild sauna operator. Debbie Noble of La'al is one such 'supertasker'. She built her sauna from a 1950s horsebox, alone, in a field, in the middle of winter. She spent months wrangling with the National Trust for permission to set it up somewhere in the Lake District – a national park and UNESCO World Heritage site – and all the while, she was going through breast cancer.

In winter, La'al (which means 'little' in Cumbrian dialect) operates from Fell Foot Park, a popular swimming spot located at the southern end of Lake Windermere, with views of snowcapped fells. In summer, Debbie plans to host sauna nights on the shoreline of Coniston Water. At La'al, she urges other bathers to adopt her Cumbrian mantra: 'whatever the weather'.

laalsauna.co.uk
Lake 54.4034, -2.9654

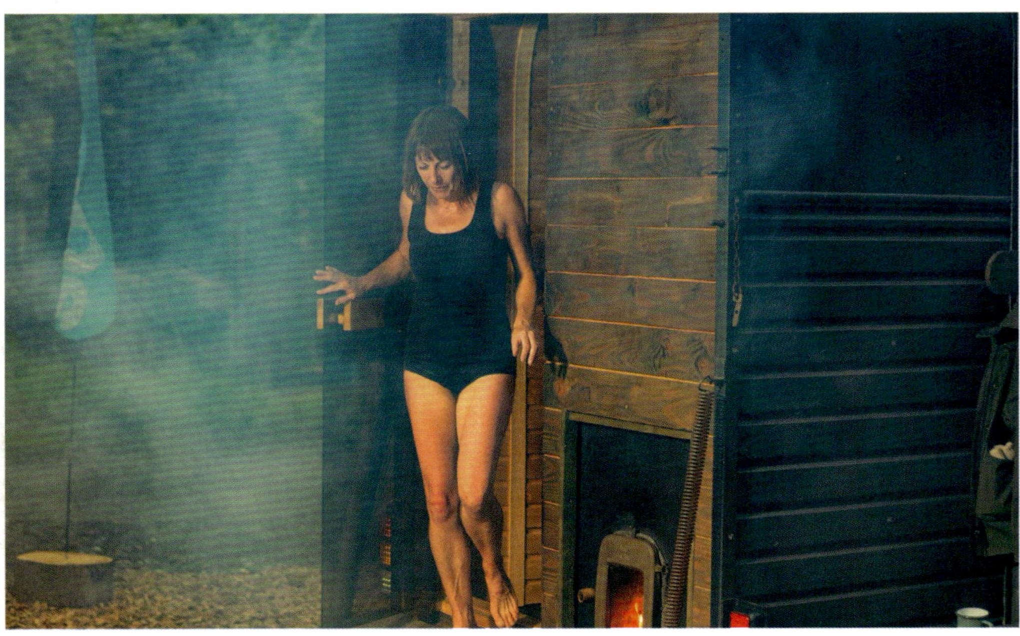

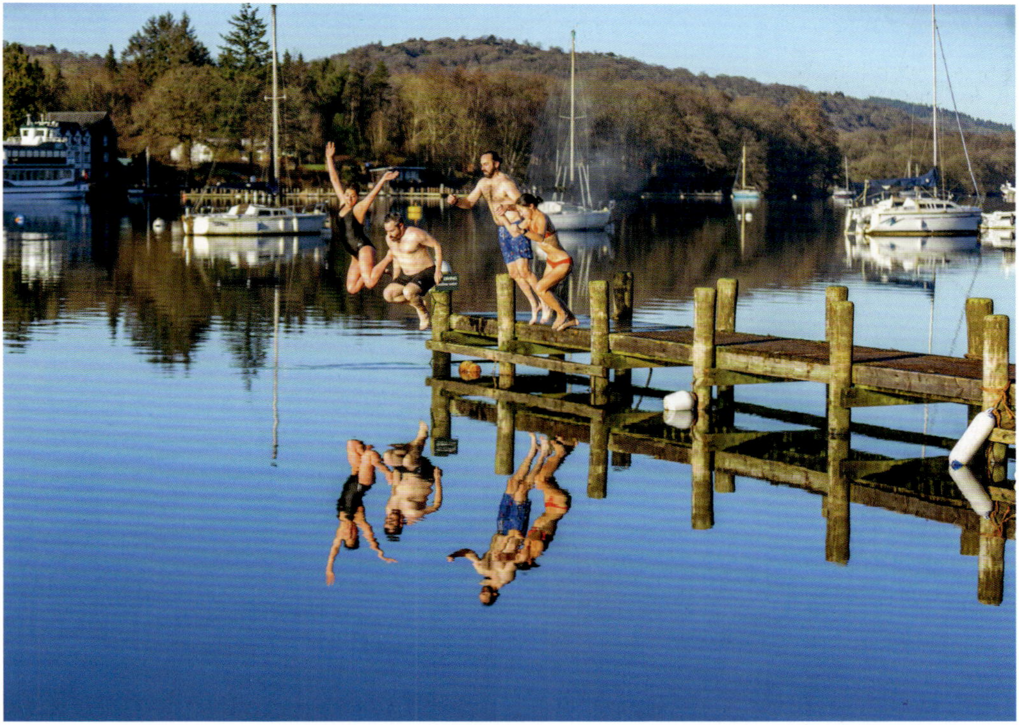

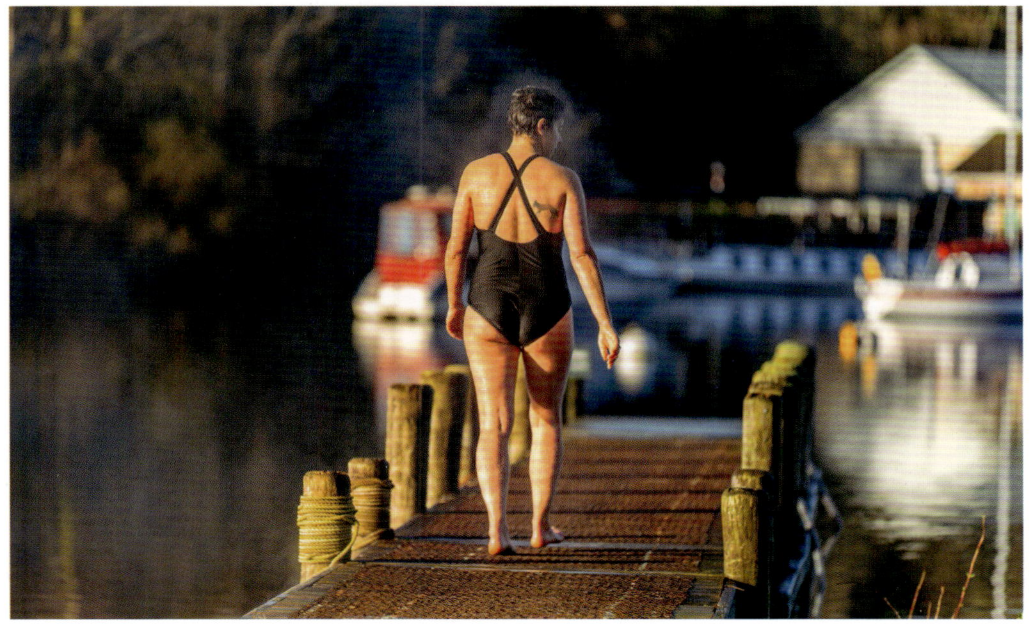

127

Finn Lough

ENNISKILLEN ❦ COUNTY FERMANAGH

Finn Lough is the kind of wild spa you might find in Finland or Japan. Occupying a 50 acre peninsula in the Fermanagh Lakelands of Northern Ireland, it has been offering quiet, nature-based luxury for more than 40 years. Guests come to switch off in River Cabins, Bubble Domes, Lake Villas and suites, as well as to enjoy the restaurant, bar and thermal spas.

You don't have to be checked in to enjoy the famous Elements Trail Spa – a two-hour wellness 'walk'. For those who enjoy contrast therapy, there's nowhere more idyllic. The self-guided journey starts with a magnesium float bath and herbal sauna, a lakeside hydropool and a Finnish sauna perched on the northern shores of Lower Lough Erne, two hours from Belfast and a stone's throw from Donegal.

Everything is designed to maximise the unspoiled beauty of the forest and the magnificent lough, and from March to September the additional Shoreline Spa offers a private hot tub, sauna and lakeside swimming. The 2025 launch of Awen Springs features a geodesic dome cocooning natural rainwater-fed pools, waterfalls and serene gardens that guide guests through natural hot and cold therapies.

finnlough.com
Lough 54.5150, -7.8908

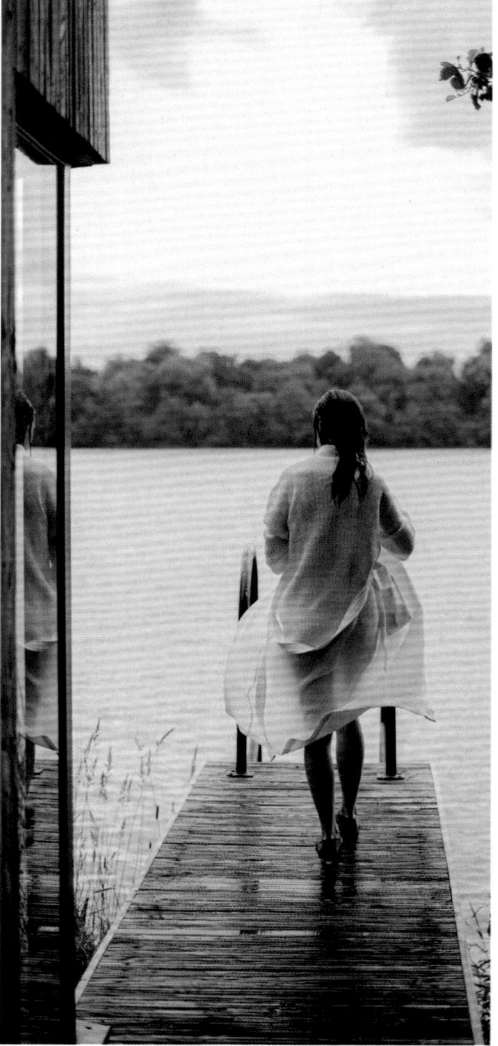

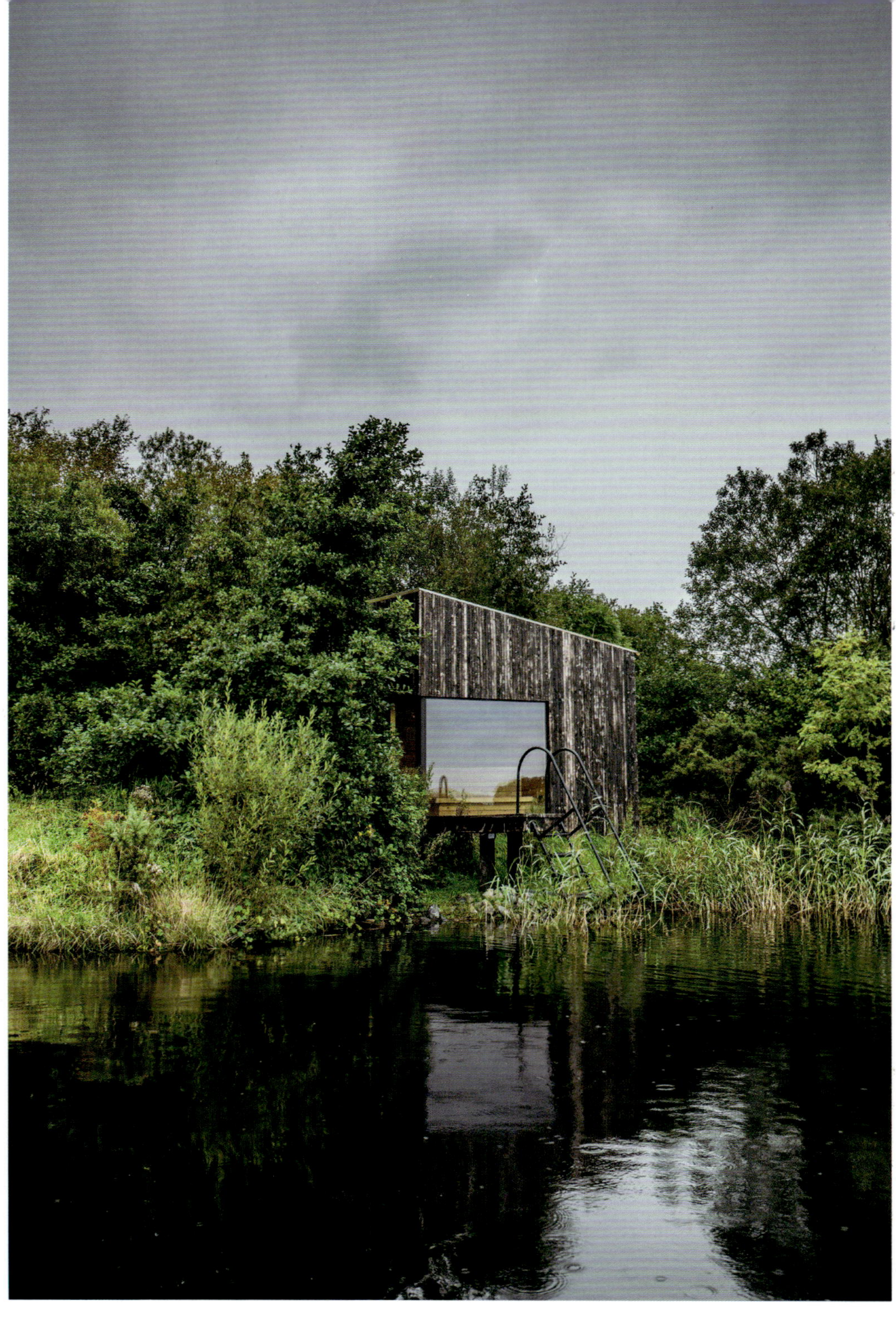

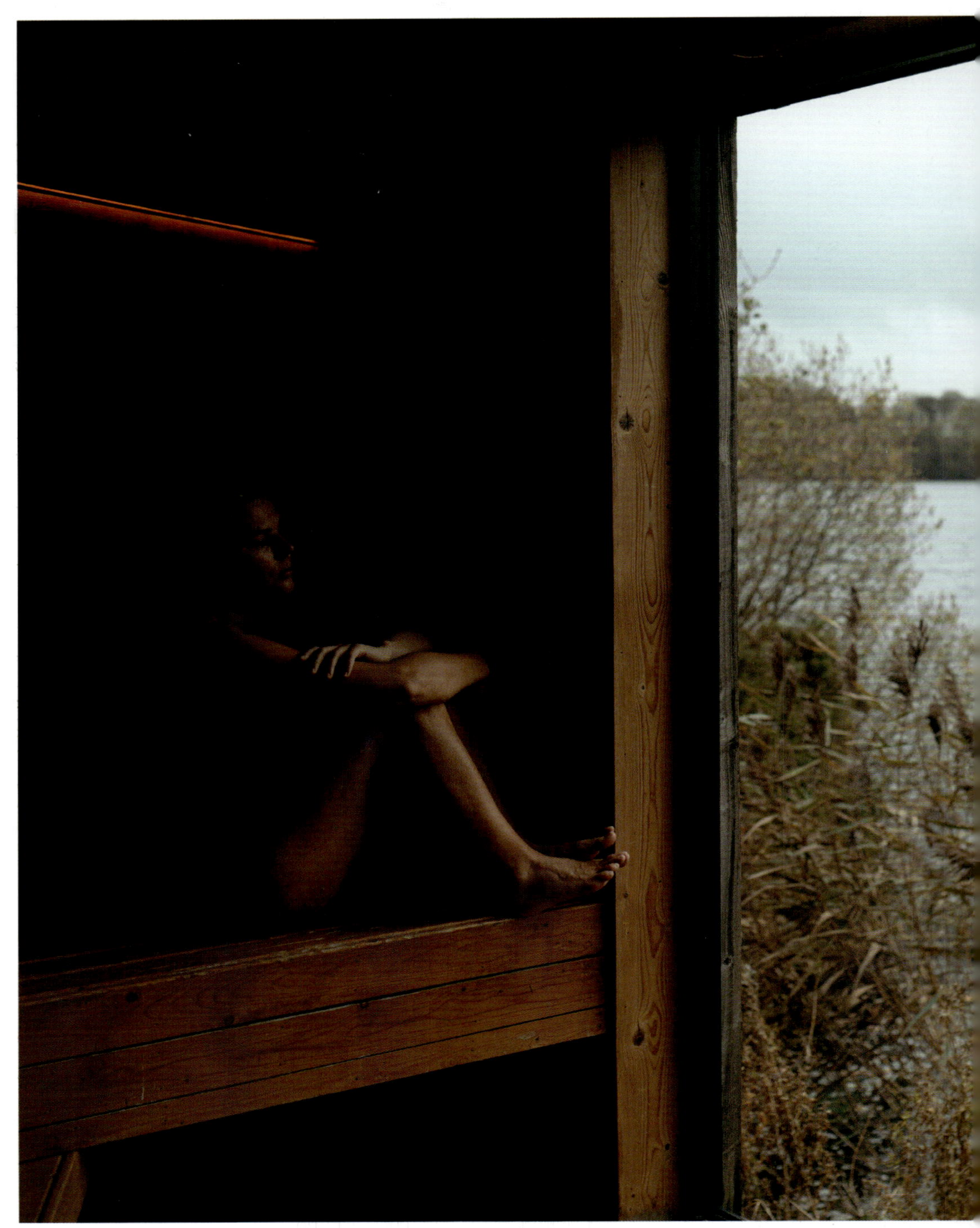

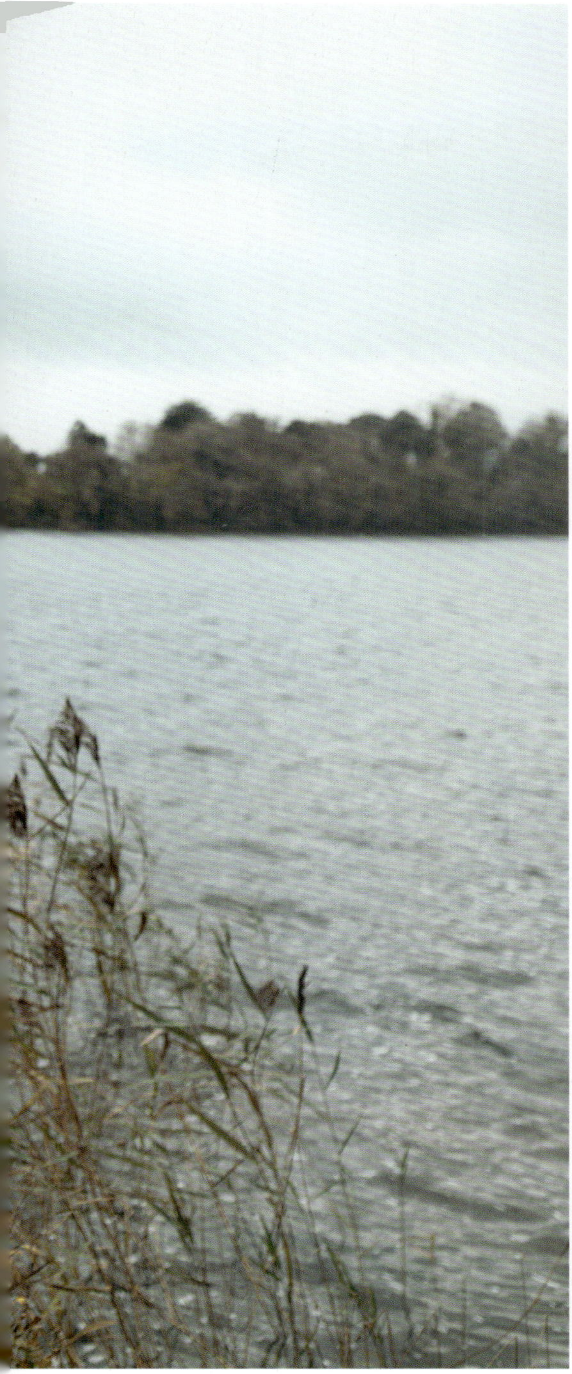

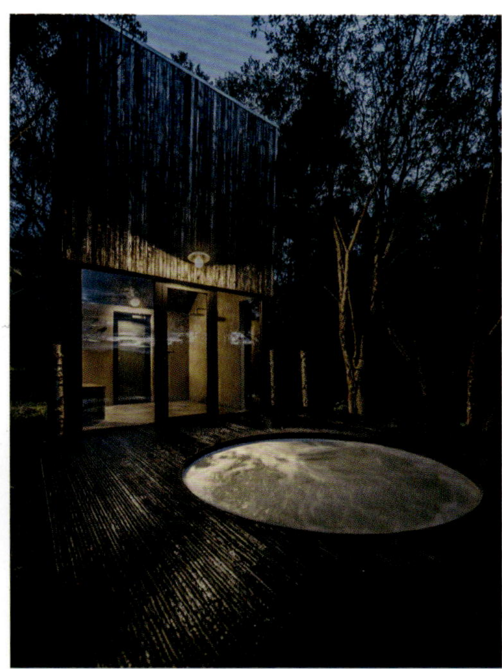

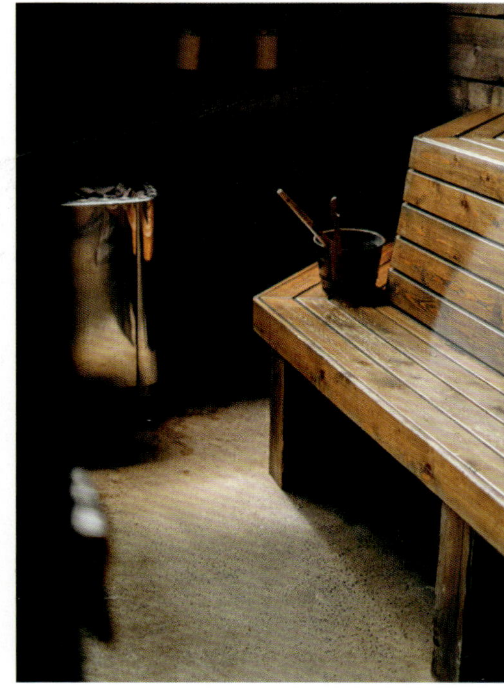

128

The Hot Rocks Sauna

AGHALEE ❦ COUNTY ARMAGH

Located at Gawley's Gate on Lough Neagh – the largest lake in the UK – is The Hot Rocks Sauna built by Andrea, an Armagh native, and her Polish husband, Jacek Remus. It' s part of a tourism development programme with Armagh, Banbridge and Craigavon councils, and the pair are developing a 'make your own whisk' experience called Whisk it Up. Visitors are shown how to make whisks which they take into the sauna for a guided session. A tie-in with the local Gate Inn has led to a sell-out Steak and Sauna night.

➔ thehotrockssauna.co.uk
❄ Lough/barrel/shower ◉ 54.5420, -6.3208

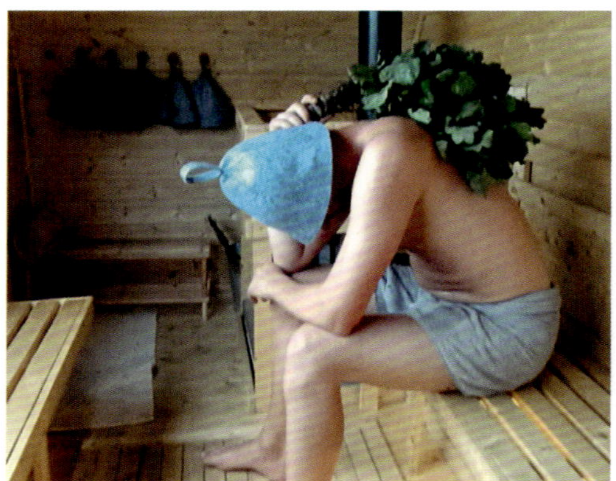

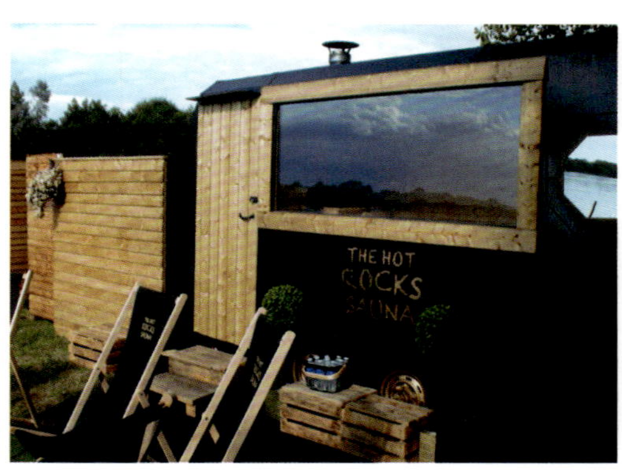

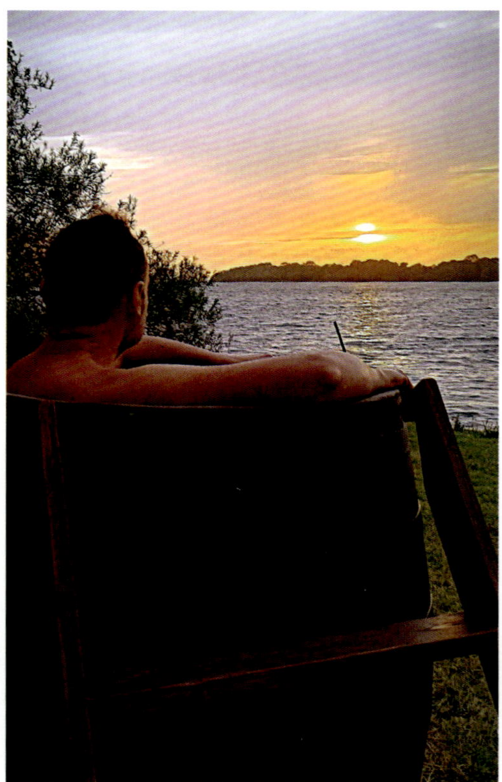

129

HotBox

BENONE STRAND ❦ LONDONDERRY

In 2020, Anna and Carl Isaksson decided they wanted to start a sauna business. They drove the whole Causeway Coastal Route, from Magilligan Point to Larne, scoping out every potential location and every beach. As it turns out, they came full circle and settled on Benone Strand, the beach of Anna's childhood. It had it all: a café, a surf school, toilets, showers, even wild ponies in the sand dunes. What's more, it was seven miles of unspoilt shoreline with stable sand, so they could drive their trailer sauna onto the beach every day.

Since landing on Benone, they haven't looked back. Now the only things that stop them are 50mph gales, rogue tides and swell, which have been known to lap against the sauna door.

Carl is Swedish and grew up with saunas, so he knew what was needed. For HotBox, they hired sauna maker Finnmark and fitted Thermo Aspen benches, a natural hemp exterior, and larch cladding which they burnt by hand to create a *shou sugi ban*/charred black finish. The sea is shallow at Benone, so you need to wade out a bit for a decent dip, and dolphins and porpoises are known to pass by. From the sauna window, views stretch over the hills of Donegal one way and the quirky Mussenden Temple the other. HotBox may seem like it's perched at the edge of nowhere, but it's actually a hotbed of activity and has pioneered many other saunas along the coast, as well as its own countryside sauna at Drumagosker.

hotboxseasauna.com · Sea
55.1676, -6.8732 Benone Strand
55.0165, -6.8845 Drumagosker

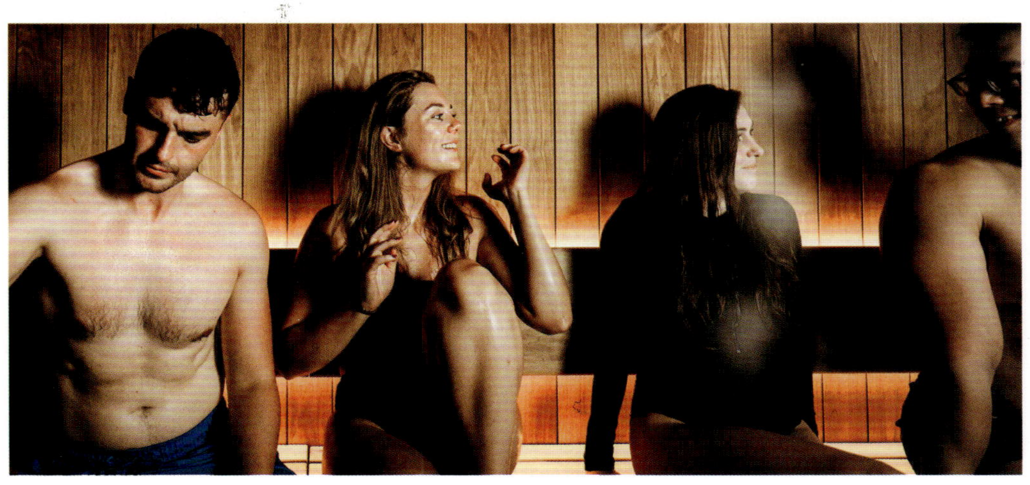

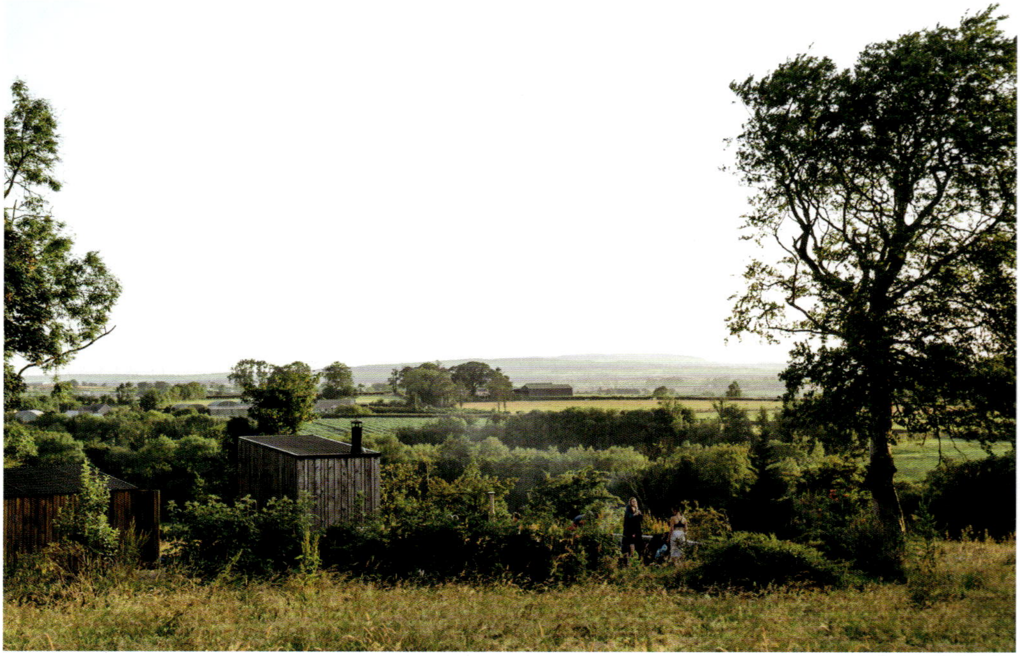

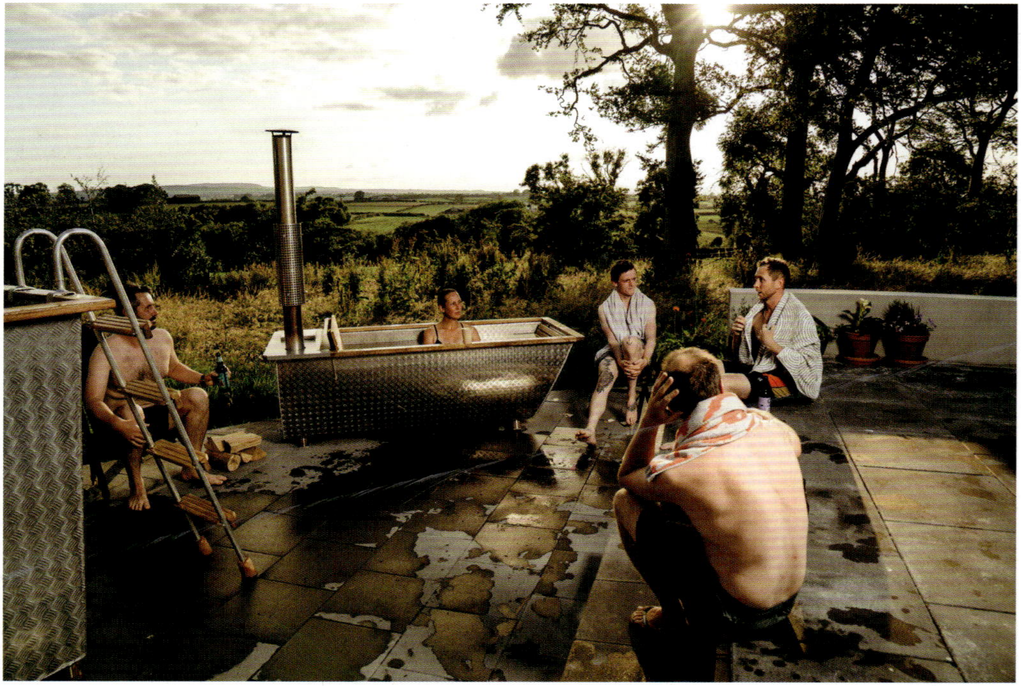

HotBox Drumagosker

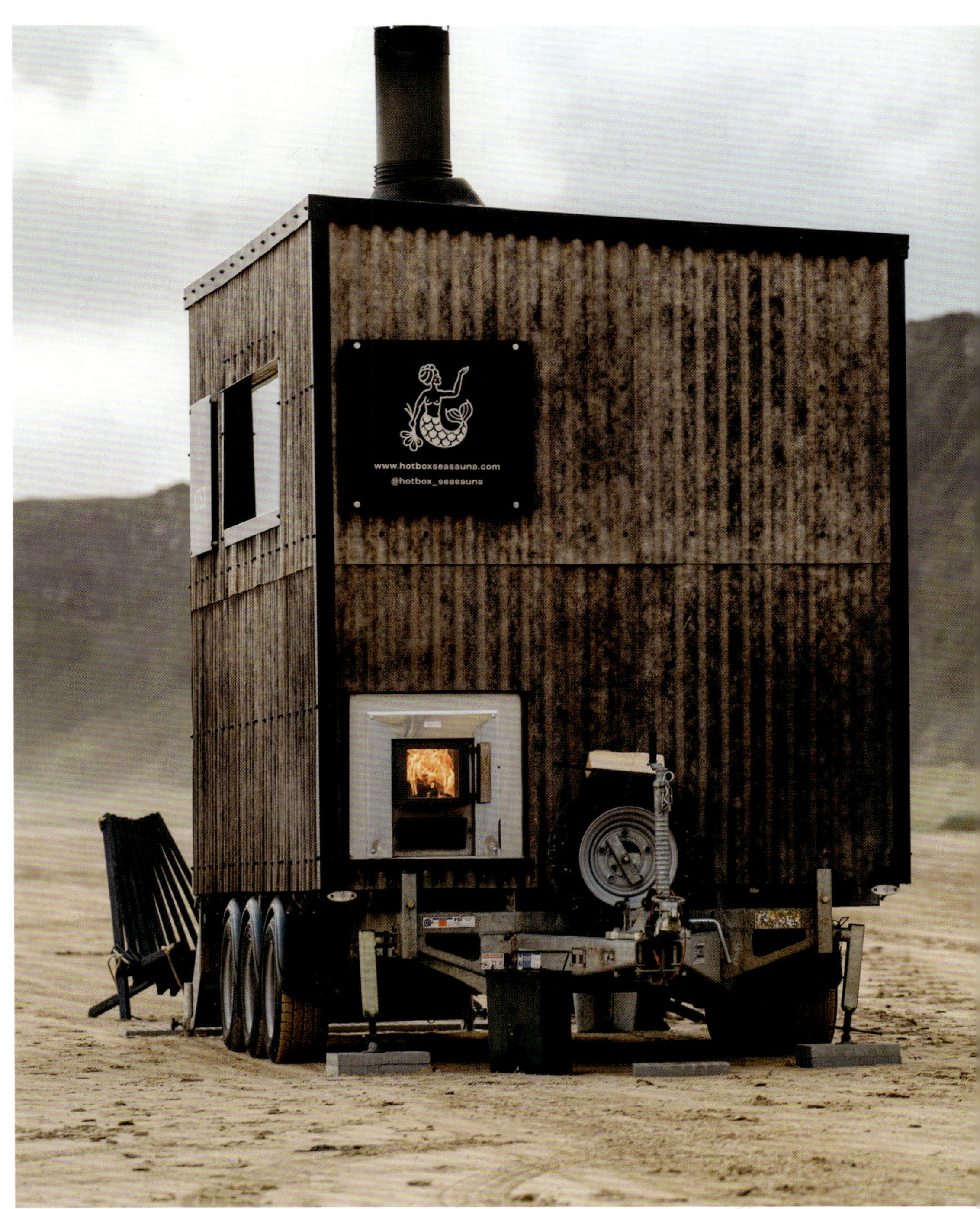

HotBox Benone Strand

130

Sauna & Sea

PORTSTEWART STRAND ❦ LONDONDERRY

'You need to learn about tides and sea, and the sauna and its benefits and dangers, and speak to people, and be able to drive a pick-up truck and tow a trailer... it's a massive skill set,' says Conor Neill of Sauna & Sea in Portstewart Strand. Conor has these skills, which is why the National Trust granted him a weekend spot on this popular family beach on Northern Ireland's Atlantic coast. He moves his sauna off the beach every night, 'in case it's underwater in the morning'.

The eight-seater sauna was built by Skotlanti in Scotland and has an awning for changing and keeping clothes dry, a water dispenser and lockers. The next stop across the open seas is Iceland.

Portstewart Strand is the starting point for the 33-mile-long Causeway Coastal Route, which takes in the Giant's Causeway. The beach has parking and toilets, and Harry's Shack is the perfect post-sauna pit stop.

saunaandsea.co.uk
Sea 55.1718, -6.7275

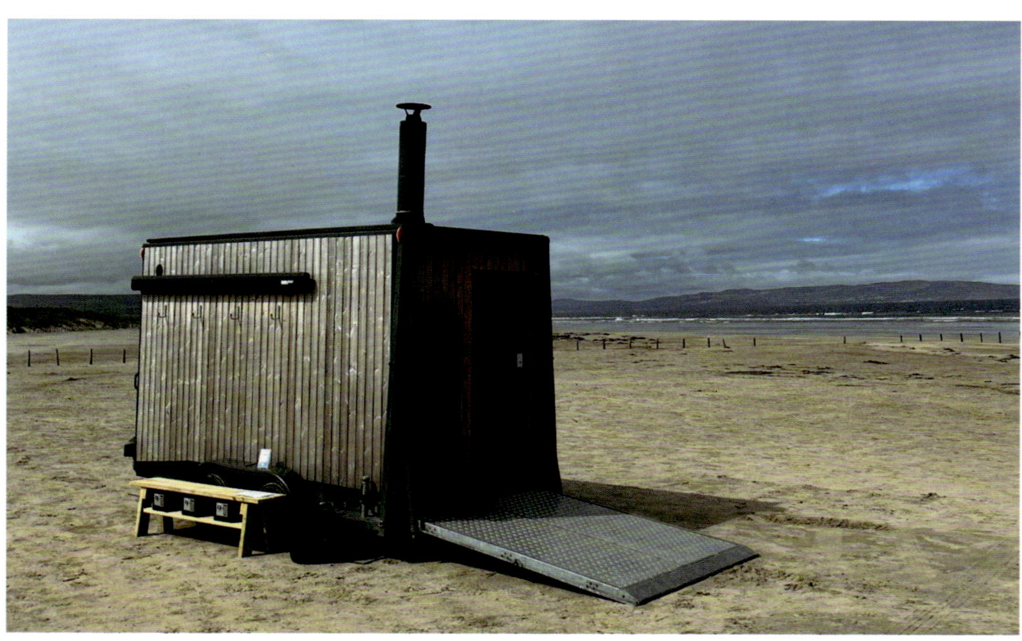

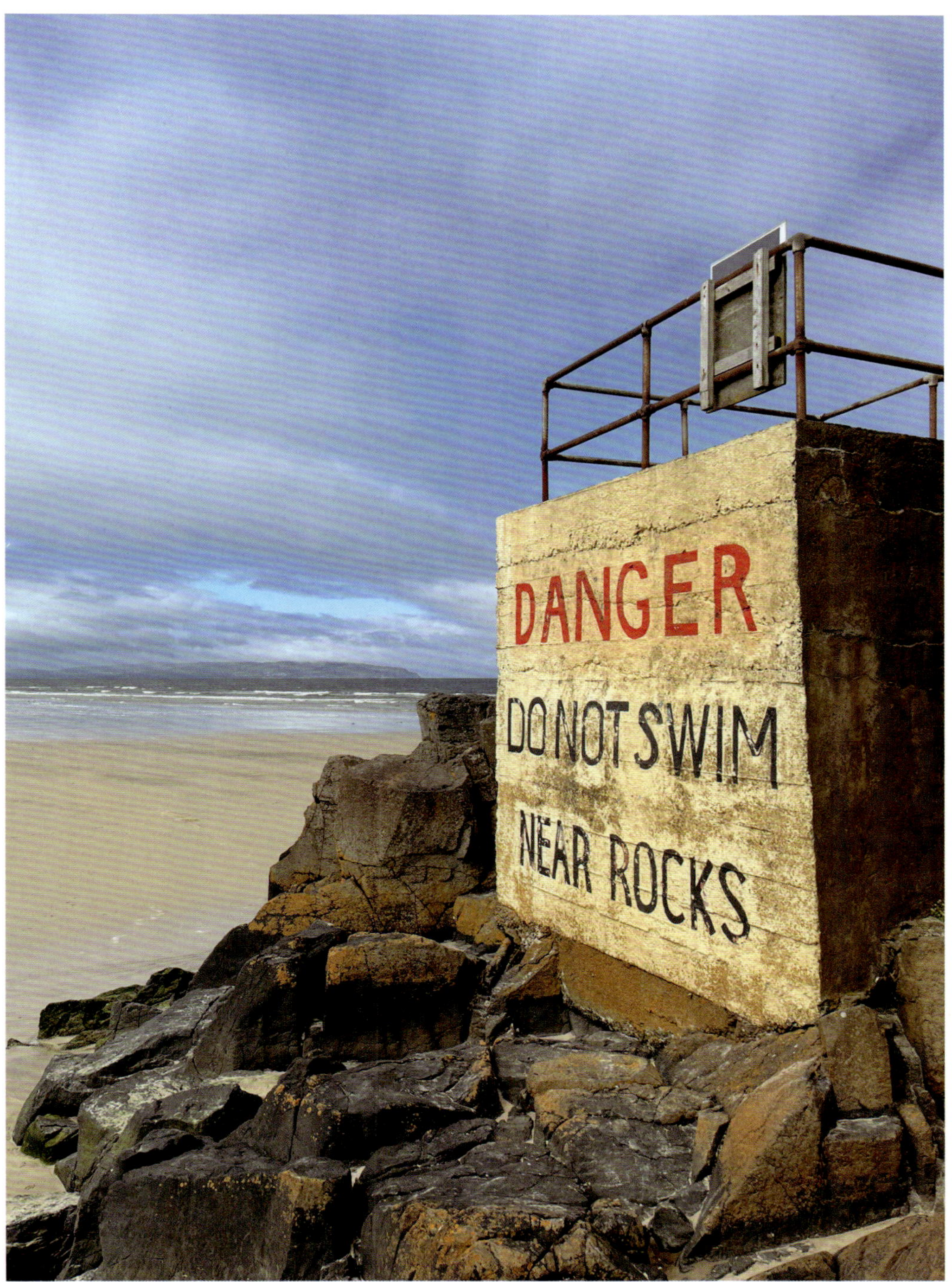
DANGER
DO NOT SWIM
NEAR ROCKS

131

Kishtey Çheh

PORT ERIN ❦ ISLE OF MAN

Liam Wiltshire has surfed on the Isle of Man's many beaches since he was a teen, yet it was on a surfing trip to Ireland in 2021 that he discovered sauna – at Bosca Beatha mobile sauna. Founded by Shirley Fitzpatrick 13 years ago, this mobile sauna and its nomadic owner pioneered the thriving Irish sauna scene, and Shirley has been crowned the 'Irish Sauna Queen'. Liam was hooked.

Liam bought a Lithuanian sauna and opened Kishtey Çheh ('Hot Box' in Manx) on his hometown beach in Port Erin in 2023. Of the 200 inhabited British Isles, the Isle of Man ranks in the top four alongside Ireland, Jersey, and the Isle of Skye, and is celebrated for its natural beauty, adventure, and heritage. It's also the world's only UNESCO Biosphere nation.

Kishtey Çheh has a strong base of regulars and has become a beach hub of its own. It has two cold plunge pools, a wood-fired hot tub, and two showers. In summer, Foraging Vintners pops up next door, selling non-grape-based varieties of sparkling wines, rums, ginger beer, and ciders produced in their winery on the other side of the bay. Noa Bake House serves food all year round and in the winter a catering van offers tea and coffee and snacks. Easy parking and public toilets complete the set of first-rate amenities.

➔ kishteycheh.im
❄ Sea/cold plunge 📍 54.0870, -4.7593

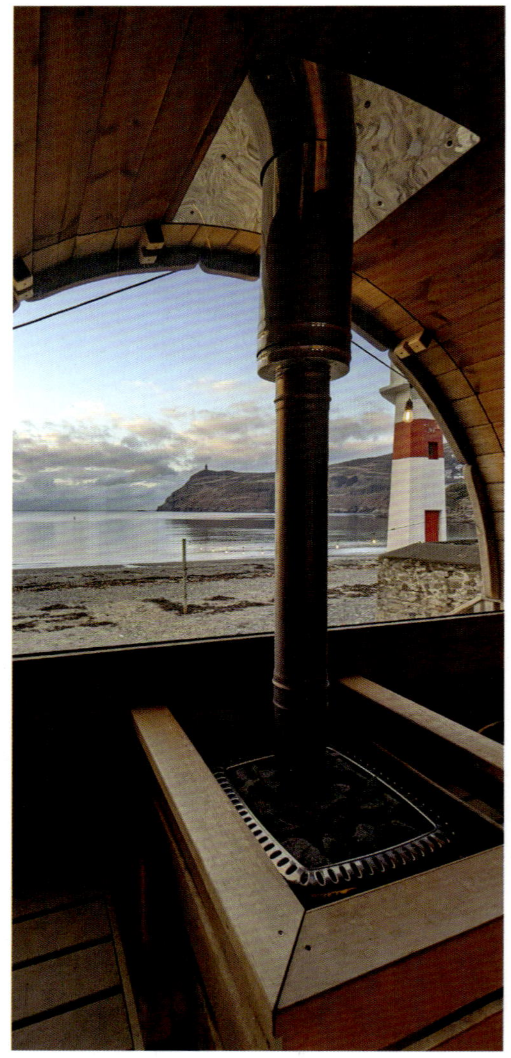

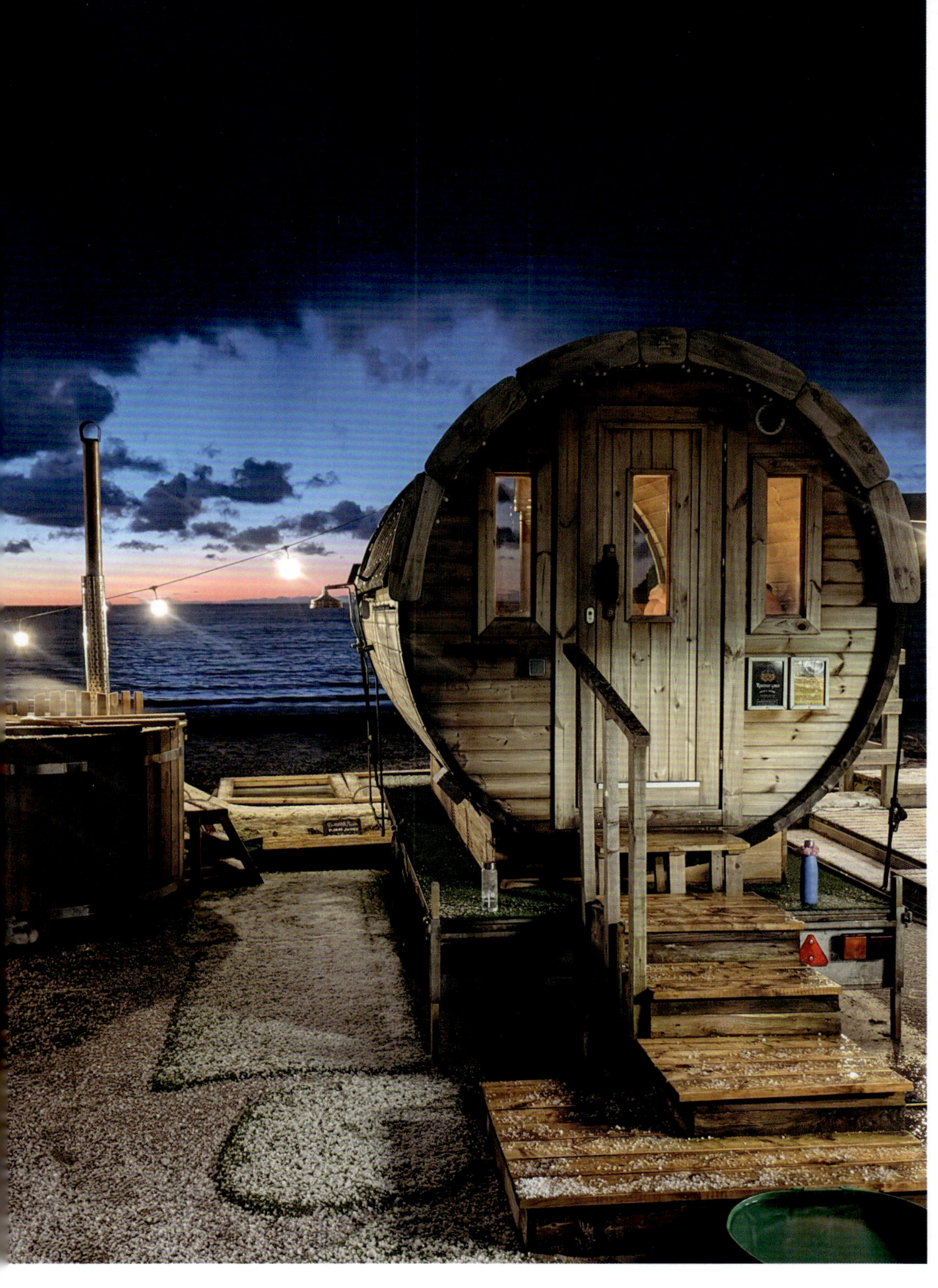

132

Sauna by Green Creek Hut Company

FENELLA BEACH & LAXEY BEACH ❁ ISLE OF MAN

During the Covid-19 pandemic, commercial airline pilot-turned sauna builder, Nick Davies, shifted his focus to creating and renting quirky huts that maximise the experience of being outdoors. Using his recycling and upcycling skills he crafted this bespoke sauna, in which a piece of driftwood guards the stove, an old dustbin on the roof holds water for the shower, and a solar panel powers a battery to light the sauna during nighttime sessions. These are worth a visit, as the Isle of Man is a stargazer's paradise with 26 registered dark sky sites.

This sauna is one of several bespoke huts that Green Creek Hut Company operate, and it moves between Fenella Beach in Peel and Laxey Beach. In the past, Nick had been the caretaker of a private Swedish-owned sauna, used by a local swimming group. At Fenella Beach the sauna is overlooked by Peel Castle, also known as the Fortress of the Black Dog, and originally constructed by the invading Viking king Magnus Barefoot in the 11th century. Nick also runs storytelling sessions based on Manx myths and legends. There is ample car parking, good access to the sea, and catering on offer.

greencreek.im Sea
54.2251, -4.6987 (Fenella Beach)
54.2245, -4.3922 (Laxey Beach)

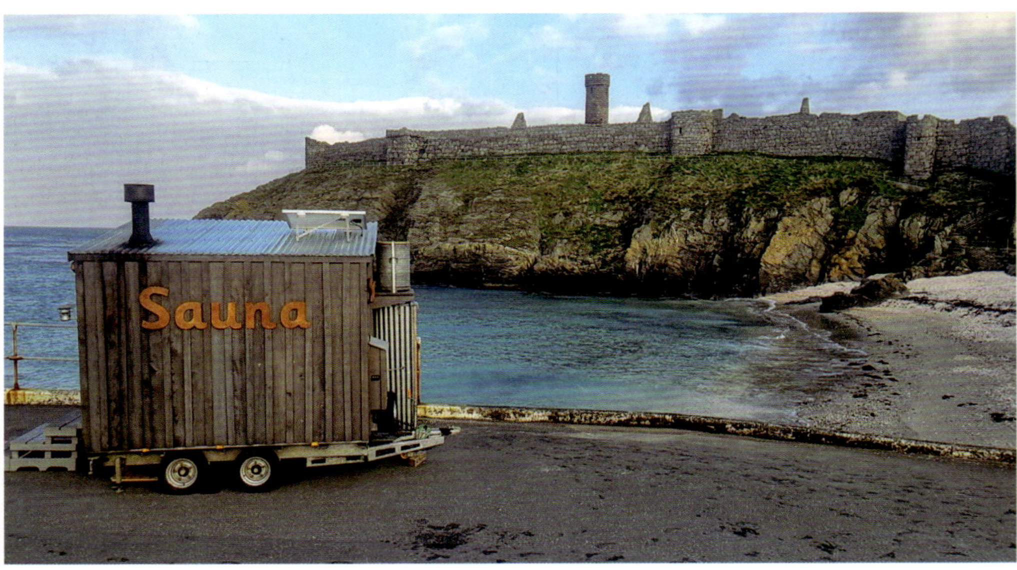

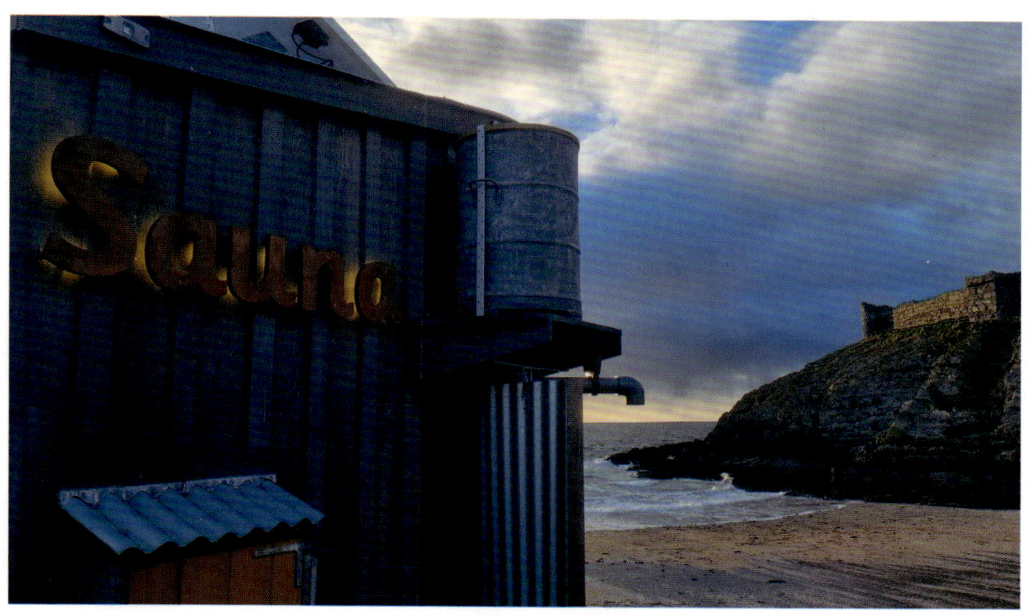
Sauna

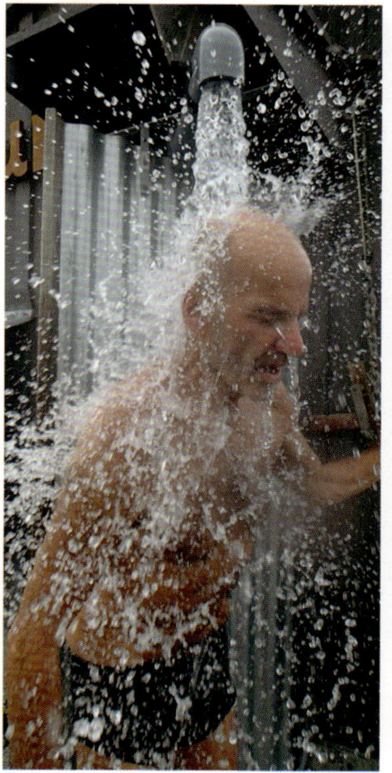

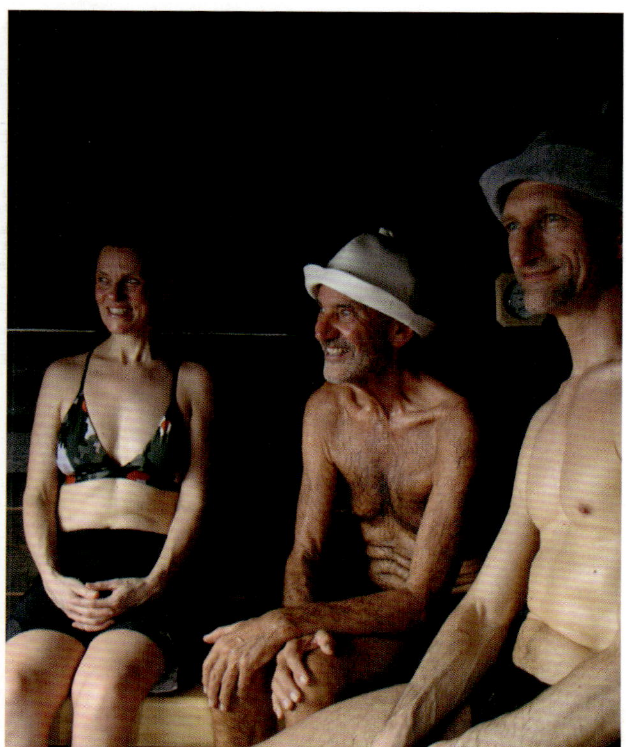

133

Wyld

LIVERPOOL ❦ MERSEYSIDE

For many years, British sauna fans have looked longingly to the waterfronts of Scandinavian cities with their floating saunas. Why, oh why, with our long dark winters, don't we have such spaces to warm the heart and lift the soul? Well, now we do, thanks to Wyld at Princes Dock in Liverpool. This Finnish-style floating sauna opened in 2024 with space for 24, access to the sea, two ice baths, cold barrels, and heated and unheated outdoor showers. Views from a giant picture window take in shiny skyscrapers and clean waterways, which have been granted an 'excellent' rating by the Environment Agency, thanks to four oxygen pumps and regular testing.

Wyld's exterior features Japanese *shou sugi ban* charred wood, and interiors are clad in thermally treated alder and spruce. Lockers, swimsuit dryers, underfloor heating, mirrors, basins, hairdryers, and eco-friendly salt scrubs give it a luxury feel and an aesthetic that fits within the dock's historic, modernised character. This vast network of waterways is UNESCO-recognised and fundamental to Liverpool's identity.

Everything is automated; access is gained via a code sent to your phone, and an hour before a booking, the sauna turns on, and it goes off when it's empty. 'We want to democratise sauna and cold-water therapy in the urban environment,' say Wyld founders Jon Miller and Tom Berendsen. 'It shouldn't be a luxury, but part of everyday life, at reasonable prices.' Wyld is just the sort of inclusive floating bathhouse that other British cities are crying out for.

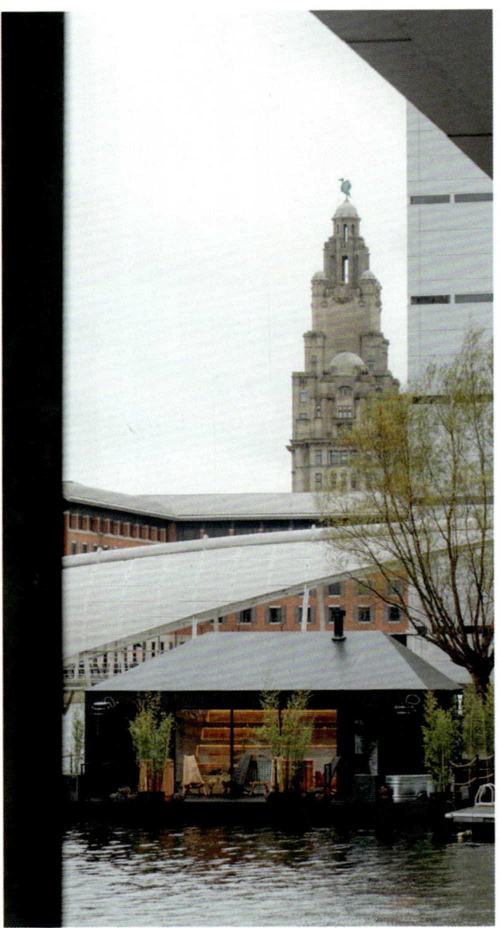

wyldsauna.com

Sea/ice baths/barrels/cold showers

53.4091, -2.9994

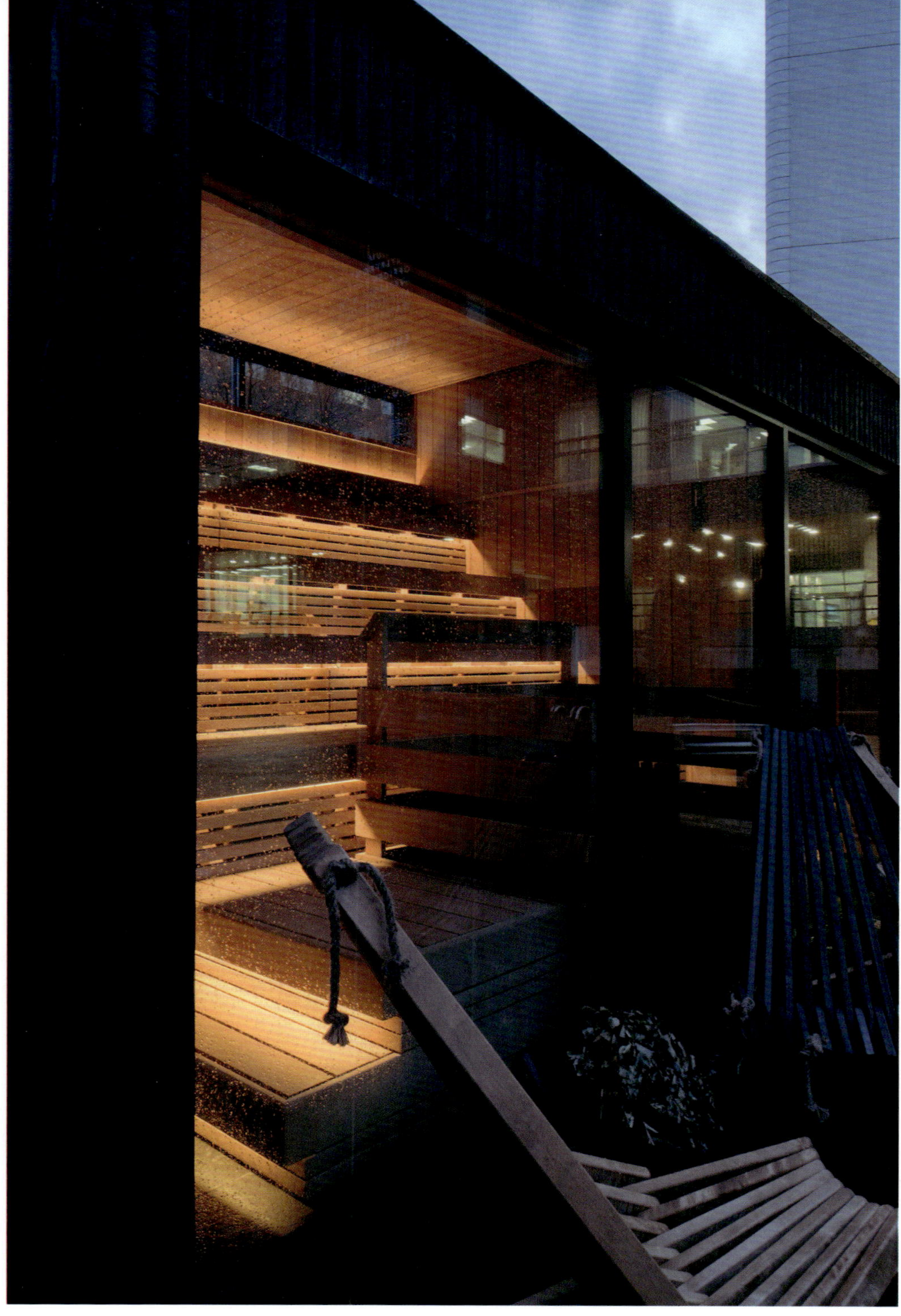

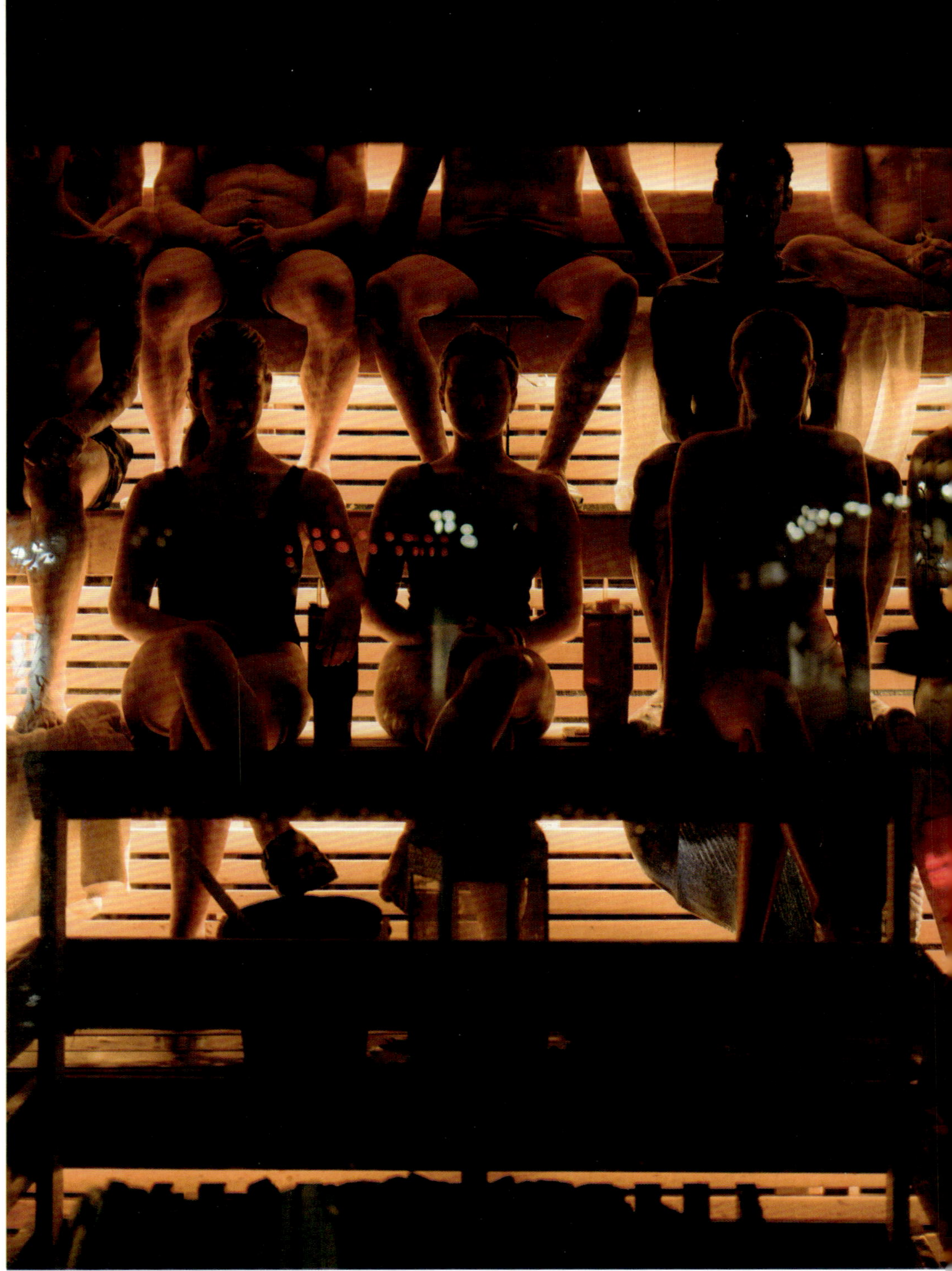

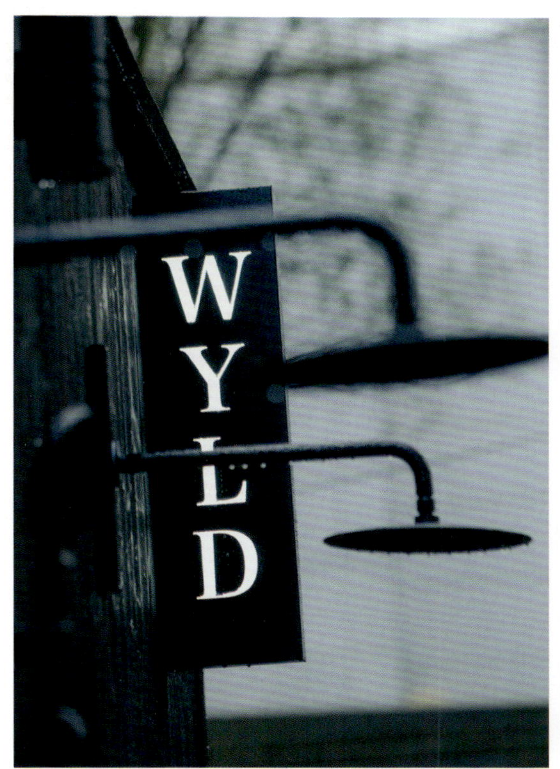
WYLD

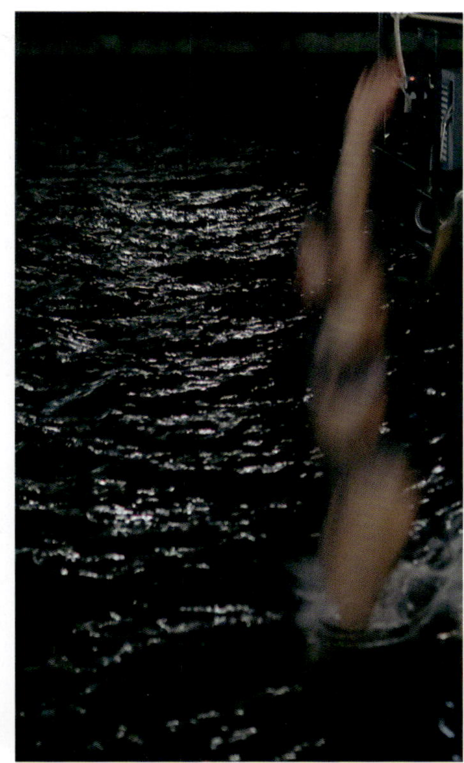

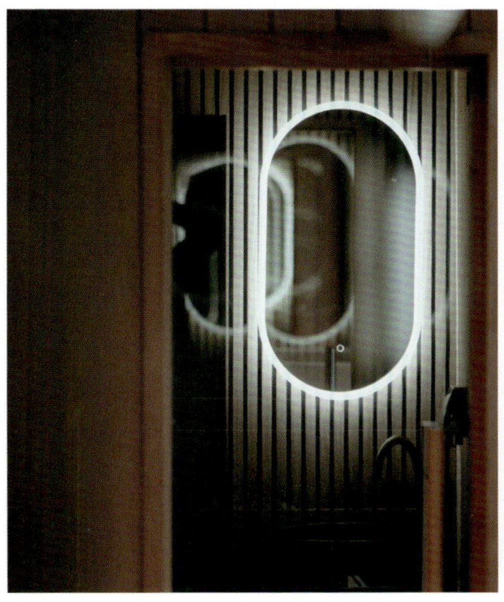

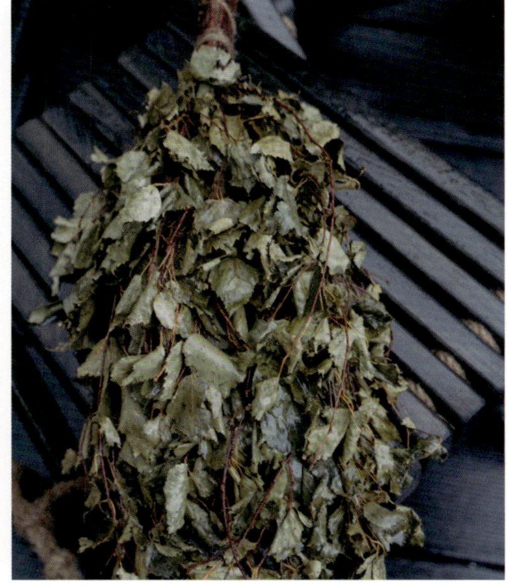

More

134 Watersedge

BISHAMPTON ❦ WORCESTERSHIRE

Watersedge is a family-run wellness lake with paddle-boarding, cold-water swimming, yoga, pilates, tai chi and two saunas. Organised activities include sound baths, breathwork and fire walking.

watersedge.club

Lake/ice bath 52.1563, -2.0000

135 Detox Wirral

LEASOWE BAY ❦ MERSEYSIDE

Detox Wirral runs two sauna tents at the end of the Gunsite car park, which is very popular with walkers, sea swimmers, paddle-boarders and kayakers getting down onto the beach at Leasowe Bay. Generally it's open from Friday to Sunday, but it's worth checking the tide.

detoxwirral.co.uk

Sea/bucket 53.4241, -3.0949

136 Mersea Sauna

CROSBY ❦ MERSEYSIDE

Louise Gallagher runs Mersea Sauna at Crosby Marine Lake next to the Crosby Lakeside Adventure Centre. Sauna sessions tie in with organised swimming on the lake through the summer, and there are changing rooms, showers and an ice bath.

merseasauna.com

Ice bath 53.4701, -3.0292

137 Whitmore Lakes

WHITMORE ❦ STAFFORDHSIRE

There are multiple lakes at Whitmore Lakes which have been used for fishing over the years. Since early 2024, the Swan Lake has been converted into a swimming lake, and a mobile sauna was added to the bank a few months later. To use the sauna you have to first purchase a two-hour swimming slot, and then add a one-hour sauna session.

whitmorelakes.co.uk

Lake 52.9768, -2.2851

138 Wild Sauna Club

STONEY STANTON ❦ LEICESTERSHIRE

Open-water swimmer Laura Mayfield felt most wild saunas were on the coast, so she made it her mission to provide mobile community sauna sessions to the Midlands. She has a large horsebox conversion and operates across a number of open-water swimming venues, one of which is beside the crystal-clear waters of Stoney Cove.

wildsaunaclub.co.uk

Lake 52.5427, -1.2725

139 Roots and Rocks

MYTHOLMROYD ❦ YORKSHIRE

This horsebox sauna is close to a number of Hebden Bridge's cold-water swimming spots, including Gaddings Dam, the location of the award-winning documentary Wildwater. Catherine Lennox is a dedicated and knowledgeable sauna host. The community centre next to the sauna offers changing facilities, showers and toilets for sauna users, and there's a catering van outside.

rootsandrocks.co.uk

Barrel/bath 53.7301, -1.9840

140 Hearth Space Sauna

LITTLE STAINFORTH ❦ YORKSHIRE

Hearth Space moves between two nature-soaked sites. The first, at Capernwray Diving Centre, is next to the clear waters of Jackdaw Quarry, popular with scuba divers and open-water swimmers. At the second site at Little Stainforth, the sauna sits on the riverbank.

hearthspace.co.uk

Quarry/river 54.1003, -2.2808

141 Hewn Yorkshire

FORCETT ❦ YORKSHIRE

Hewn consists of 12 glamping cabins with individual wood-fired hot tubs and a sauna located 250 metres up a track out of the quarry. Guests and locals can book it on a private, hourly basis and use it as they wish, making up their own routines as they go. A copper shower is fixed to the side of the sauna.

➡ hewnyorkshire.co.uk
❄ Shower 📍 54.4926, -1.7480

142 Sauna Hetta

MORPETH ❦ NORTHUMBERLAND

Sauna Hetta sits tucked in the dunes on Druridge Bay near Morpeth. The coastline is owned by the National Trust and the Crown, except for a mile-long stretch where Hetta sits. This belongs to Hemscott Hill Farm, a family home offering beachside glamping pods, barns and cottages. A private gate leads to the beach and the sauna, which draws local swimmers who come to enjoy the peace (the nearest village on either side is a mile away) and spot the odd pod of dolphins.

➡ saunahetta.com
❄ Sea/bucket 📍 55.2574, -1.5651

143 Northumbrian Sauna

HARLE ❦ NORTHUMBERLAND

GB ice swimmer and sauna master Fenwick Ridley has three sauna tents and can accommodate up to 20 people in guided sessions. Retreats and communal sessions run on the shore of Sweethope Loughs, a perfect place for cold-water immersion. His night sessions are popular as this is one of the darkest places in Europe.

➡ northumbriansauna.co.uk
❄ Lake 📍 55.1351, -2.0859

144 Salty Saunas

TYNEMOUTH ❦ TYNE AND WEAR

Louise Tupling and Mary Riley have been swimming in the sea for more than 20 years, and their tent sauna was originally just for their own use. These days they have two tent saunas and offer regular sessions in beach locations on England's north-east coast, and on request.

➡ saltysaunas.com
❄ Sea 📍 55.0236, -1.4247

145 Drumagosker Rural Sauna

LIMAVADY ❦ N IRELAND

Drumagosker Rural Sauna is 20 minutes inland from HotBox Sea Sauna on Benone Strand, and it's home to Nemo, the original HotBox sauna. The land is owned by Anna Isaksson's aunt and uncle, who run five-star accommodation on site. The rural spa features a cold plunge and can be hired for wellness retreats in the lush Irish countryside.

➡ hotboxruralsauna.com
❄ Cold plunge/shower/bath 📍 55.0167, -6.885

146 The Wee Sauna

BALLYGALLY ❦ COUNTY ANTRIM

Ballygally Beach is one of many award-winning beaches on the scenic Causeway Coastal Route, with white sands, dramatic boulders and gentle tides. At the eastern end, in the Coast Road car park is The Wee Sauna. There are no toilets or facilities at this wilder spot, but the slipway offers a route into the sea and bathers can jump off its wall.

➡ facebook.com/theweesaunani
❄ Sea 📍 54.8988, -5.8586

147 A Scenic Sauna

BALLYGALLY ❦ COUNTY ANTRIM

On the western end of Ballygally Beach, in the main car park, sits A Scenic Sauna, a six-seater, right in the heart of the action. Car park toilets offer a place to change.

➡ facebook.com/people/A-Scenic-Sauna/61554134446296/
❄ Sea 📍 54.8994, -5.8605

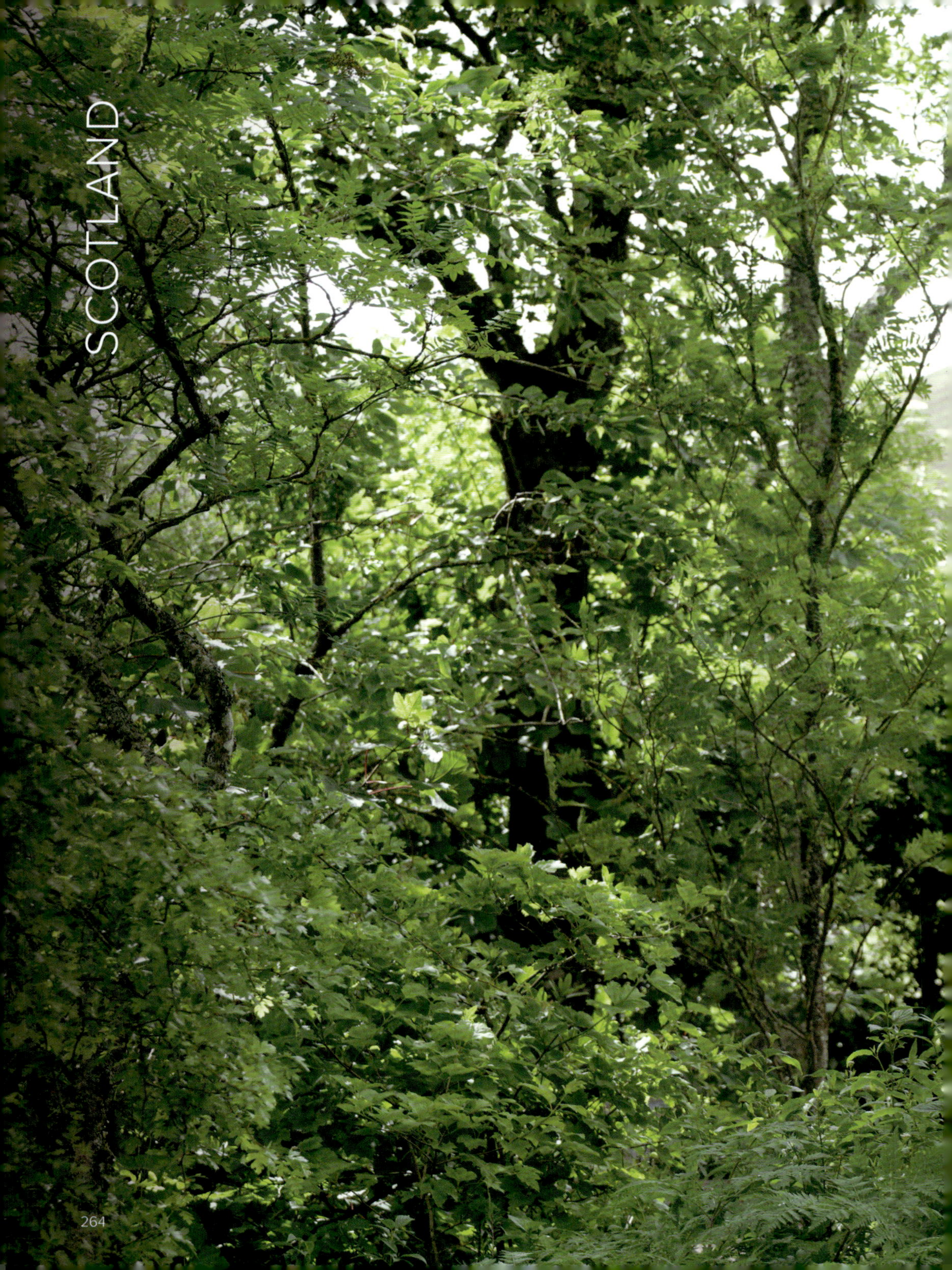
SCOTLAND

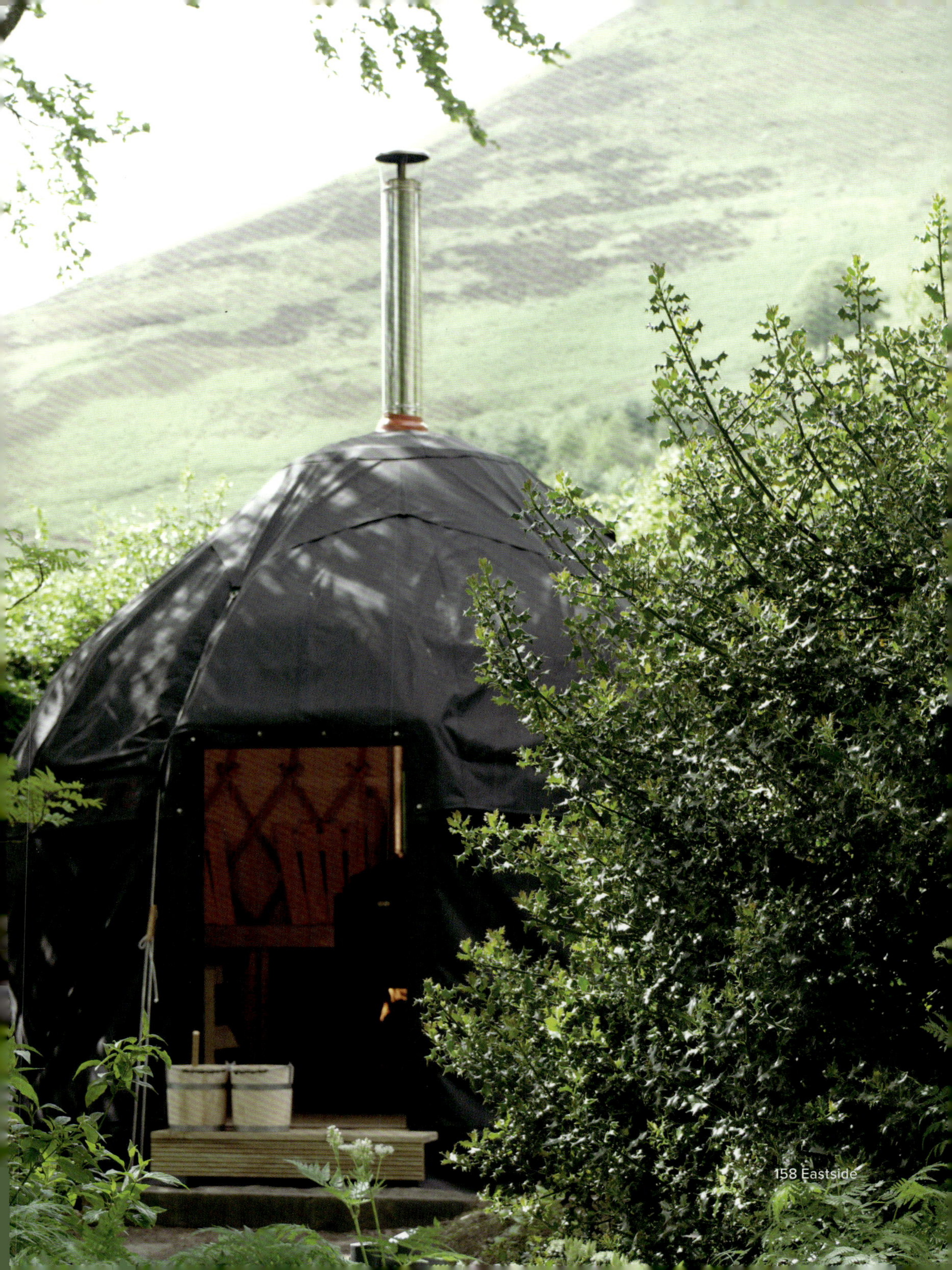

148

The Green Goddess Wild Sauna

ISLE OF ARRAN ❦ NORTH AYRSHIRE

What better way to enjoy the Isle of Arran than through the steamy windows of a vintage truck converted into a sauna, especially when beaches, streams and natural pools offer cold dips in such abundance? One such location, Blackwaterfoot Beach, has direct access to the clean waters of Drumadoon Bay, and both the bay and the sauna truck belong to the 640-acre Drumadoon Farm Estate.

The Isle of Arran is covered in rare Scottish temperate rainforest, rich in threatened biodiversity. Part of the estate's mission is to rebuild this fragile ecosystem, and tree planting, between November and April is also offered, along with archaeological programmes in conjunction with Archaeology Scotland, and artist-in-residence programmes.

The sauna truck is part of Drumadoon's travelling spa, a new concept that includes whiskey barrel cold plunges and Swedish Hikki hot tubs (filled with local spring water), a chill-out tipi with a fire pit, changing tents, outdoor showers and a composting loo.

The sauna moves around the estate, in rhythm with the seasons and in tune with its fauna and flora, enjoying each location at its best. Guided sessions include making sauna hats and whisks from locally foraged birch and kelp, and storytelling -recounting myths and legends of this ancient landscape; Arran was famous for its death rituals and is packed with 10,000 years of human history.

Coastal and beach stopovers include warm saltwater seaweed baths, and 'Celtic Rainforest' sessions which take people into the rainforest restoration project.

And the sauna truck is not just for the estate; around 4,500 people live on Arran, and the truck, which seats 14 people, is open to everyone. It can be hired for private full-day bookings, and travels around the island, pitching up wherever a beautiful burn, a fossil-studded beach or a moment of peace demands it.

→ wildsauna.scot

Sea 55.5057, -5.3459

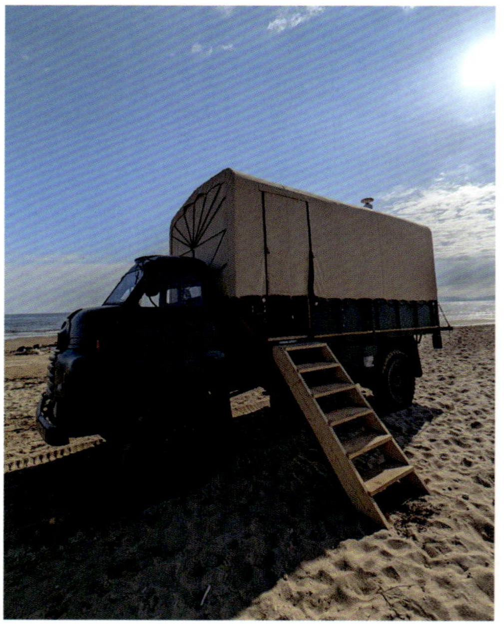

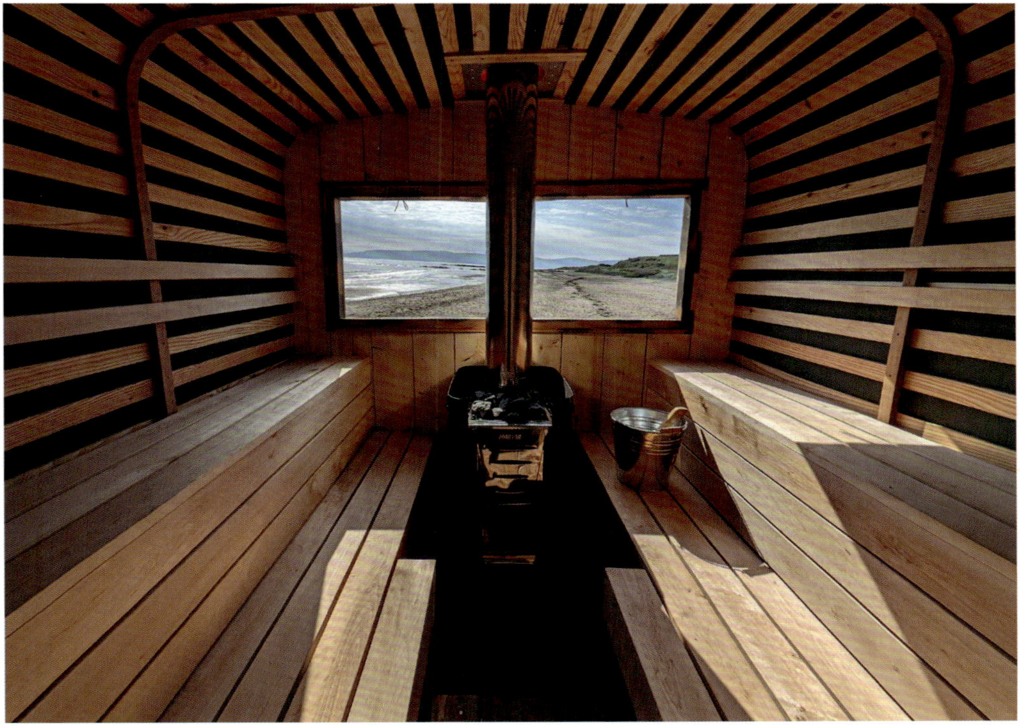

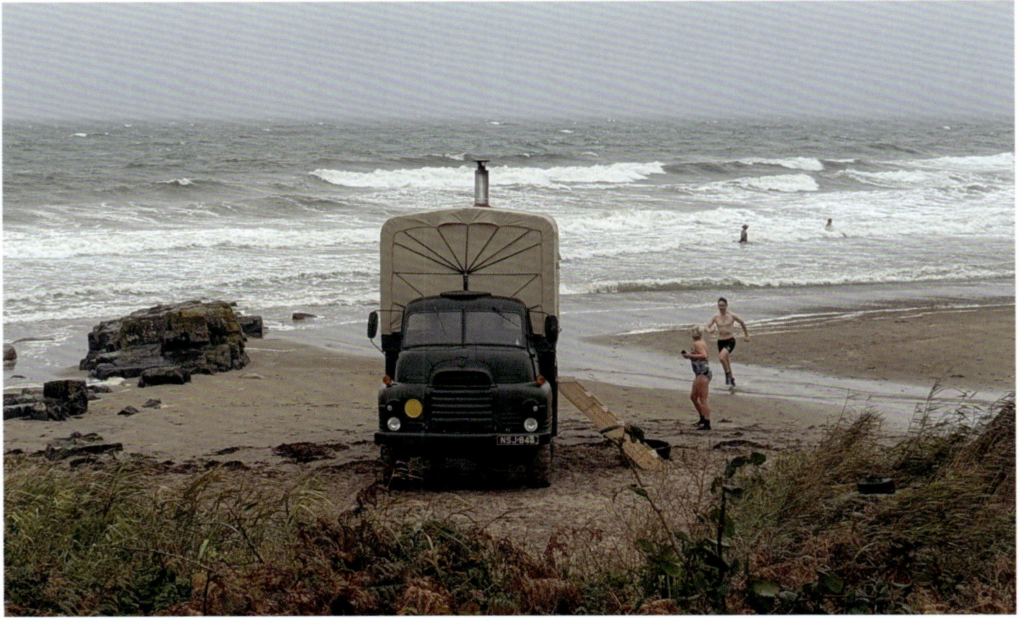

149

West Coast Wellness

OTTER FERRY ❦ ARGYLL AND BUTE

The renaissance of Evanachan Farm reads like a fairy tale. When all four Barge siblings came back to the family home on Loch Fyne during the Covid-19 pandemic, they swam in the loch, spotting otters and seals and dreamed of how they could move back to Scotland and make successful lives on a much-downsized sheep and dairy farm. Together, they pooled their family skills – among them a doctor, an architect, a caterer, a brewer, a boat builder, a fish farmer, a yoga teacher and a nonagenarian grandmother. From this impressive collective West Coast Wellness was born.

Yoga classes are held in geodesic domes with views over the loch, and there's wild swimming, hill walking, nourishing food and community too. The Lochside Sauna was a natural addition, built from reclaimed timber (mainly aspen) found on the 350-acre estate. Loch Fyne is a sea loch, and there are cold showers to rinse off the salt and a river-fed freshwater plunge pool. The sauna slots neatly into most of the retreat offerings and is open for drop-in sessions and private bookings for up to 16 people. Lochside Sauna is only part of the plan – saunas at different temperatures, a mix of natural elements, and a variety of settings (among them a bijou horsebox sauna next to the river) are all on the drawing board.

➔ westcoastwellnessuk.com
❄ Loch/shower/cold plunge ⊙ 56.0278, -5.2926

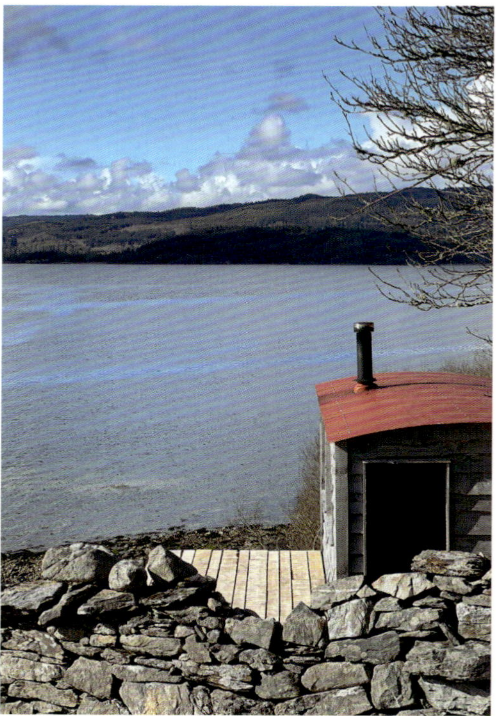

150

Saltbox Sauna

LEWIS ❦ OUTER HEBRIDES

Travelling between Lewis, Harris and Uig, Saltbox is the only wood-fired sauna in the Outer Hebrides. It's the brainchild of Norma MacLeod, an STA Open Water Coach and ex-competitive swimmer based in Stornoway. In 2019, Norma co-founded Immerse Hebrides, which runs retreats, swim tours and boat trips around the islands, and she knows all the beauty spots. Servicing them with a mobile sauna was a natural next step.

Saltbox is the very definition of a wild sauna – often there are no toilets or running water, but that doesn't stop bathers who like their nature raw.

A permanent sauna with space for ten, offering rituals and ceremonies, sits at Bayble Beach on Lewis, with plans for saltboxes on other islands too.

saltboxsauna.co.uk

Sea 58.1974, -6.2089 & many more

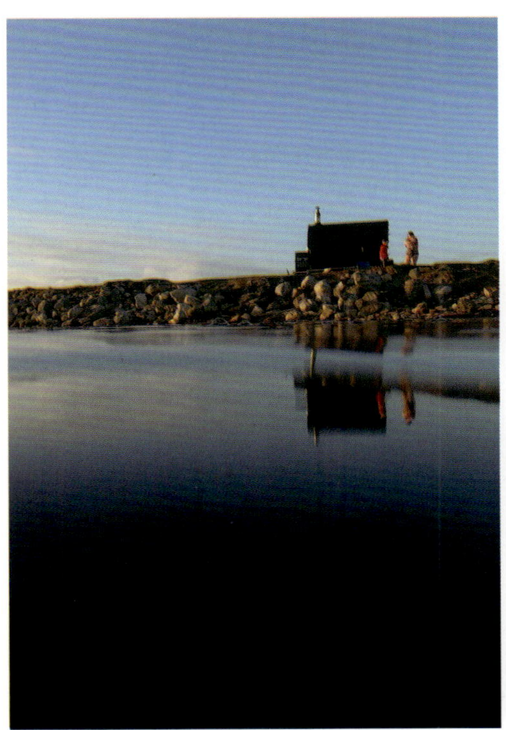

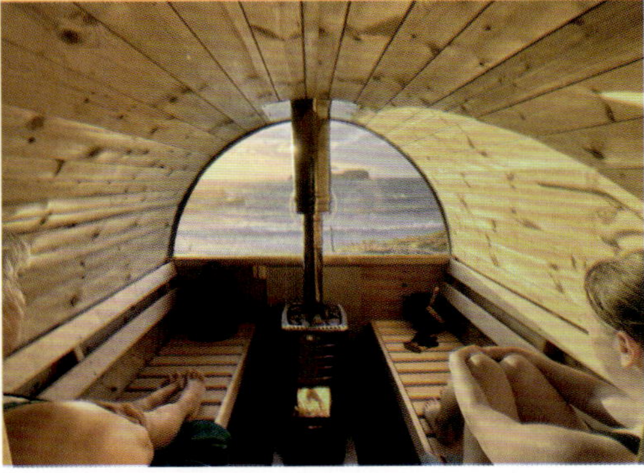

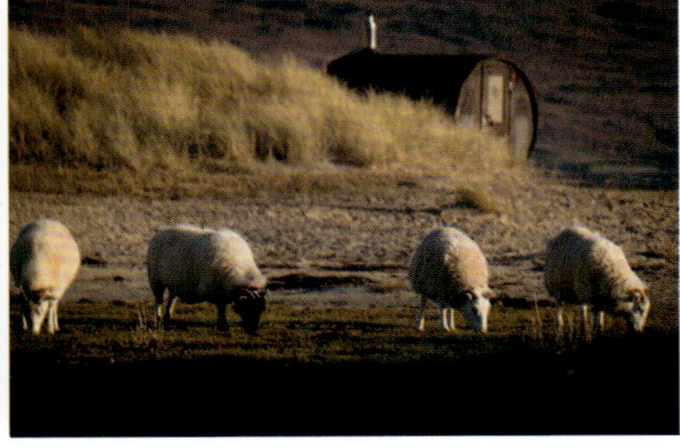

151

Braw

INVERKIP ❦ RENFREWSHIRE

Tommy Ryan-Roche got into sauna when he started training for an ultra-marathon three years ago. It was 42 miles through the Scottish Highlands, 6,500 feet of elevation, and in the winter. 'It was horrendous; my body was beaten up,' Tommy laughs, 'but my mind and my cardio were fine. I think that was down to how you regulate temperature in your body, which is the benefit of sauna.' But for Tommy, there's something deeper, beyond muscle recovery. 'I found that it went beyond the rehab part. I used to love going in and sitting for half an hour by myself with no phone. My mind would just stop, and I'd be forced to sit.' It was, he says, an awakening moment. 'Because your mind never gets to shut off. Between work, your goals, exercise and the family, it just never stops. And it's so good to just sit down, and it all stops, you know?'

He bought a barrel sauna from Latvia and christened it Braw, meaning 'fantastic' in Scottish slang. Tommy and Braw are now a firm weekend fixture at Lunderston Bay – the closest sandy beach to Glasgow and a popular spot for families.

➔ brawsaunas.com
❄ Sea/barrel/shower 📍 55.9219, -4.8712

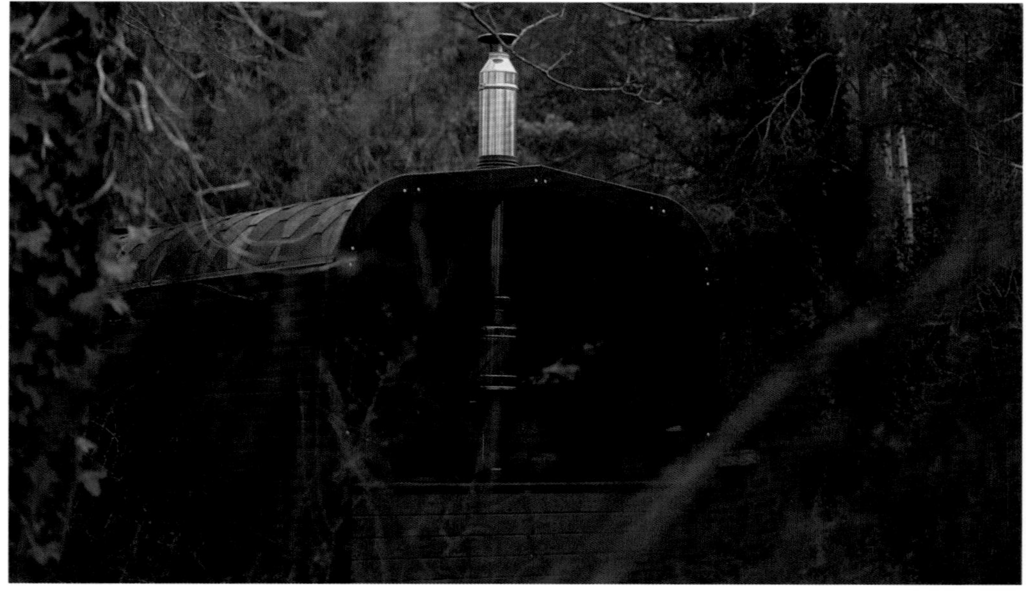

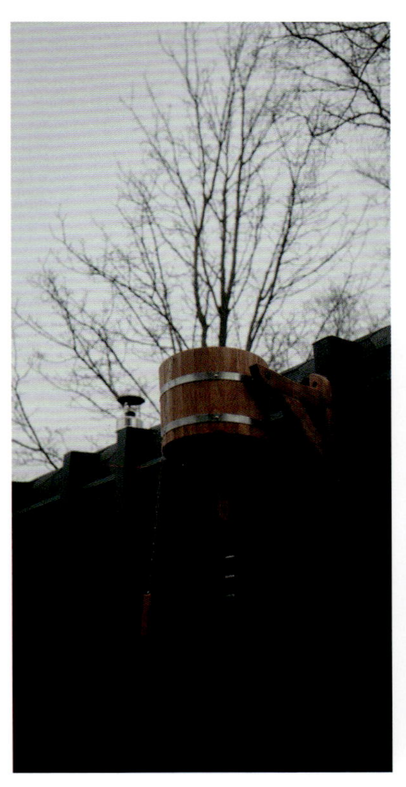
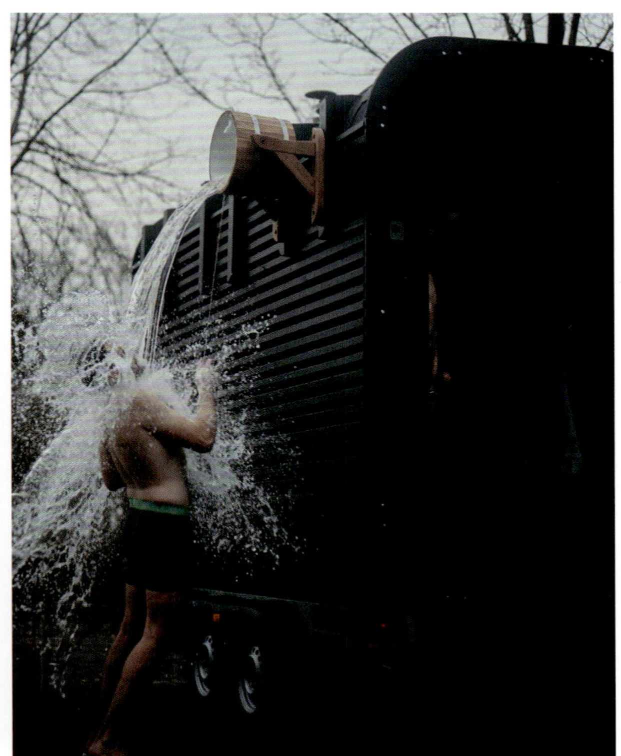
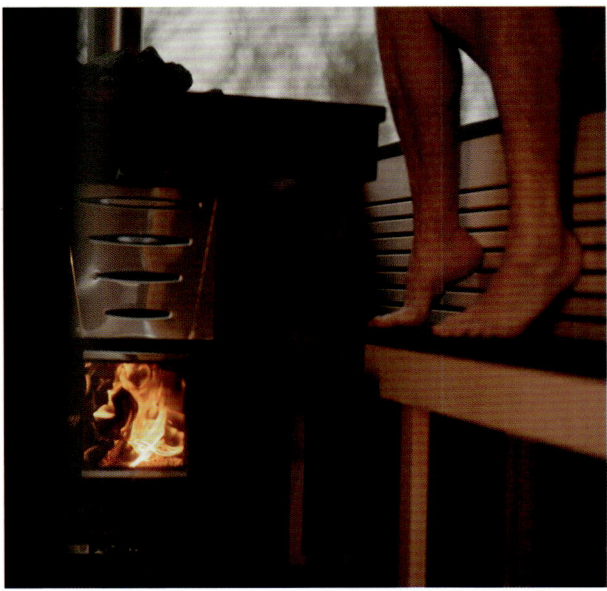
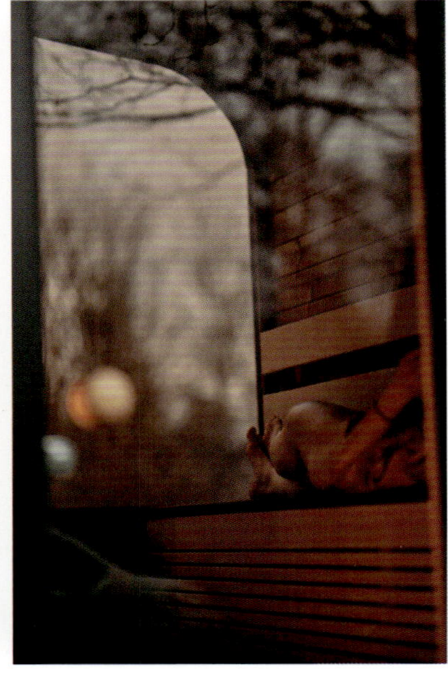

152

Arisaig Sauna

ARISAIG ❦ INVERNESS-SHIRE

James and Rebecca opened Arisaig Sauna in 2024 and it has quickly become known among seasoned sauna-goers for its intense heat, regularly reaching 90-100°C. Guests enjoy stunning views of the Skerries, Eigg, and Rum, along with a signature coffee scrub made with locally sourced grinds, the by-product of the collaboration with founding company Glenfinnan Coffee Co, started by James and his brother Iain. This is not unusual; other sauna cultures also mix coffee grounds with oil as they are packed with chlorogenic acids, which have anti-ageing properties and reduce fine lines, sun spots and redness.

A tarp hanging from two trees constitutes a changing area, there's a suspended watering can shower and a saltwater and seaweed bath. And the sea. It's tricky getting in at low tide (rock shoes are a must), but at high tide it's perfect for an exhilarating 'dook'.

Surrounded by trees and crystal-clear waters, Arisaig Sauna is also a favourite of local mermaid Jill, who swims around the bay from her house at high tide, often accompanied by curious seals. With an extra-large burner at the heart of it all, Arisaig Sauna is able to deliver a sauna experience as intense as the wild beauty of the landscape. The suggestion is that visitors park in Arisaig and walk 10 minutes to the sauna. There's a great pub and seafood shack in the village to create the perfect day out.

arisaigsauna.com

Sea/seaweed bath | 56.9055, -5.8468

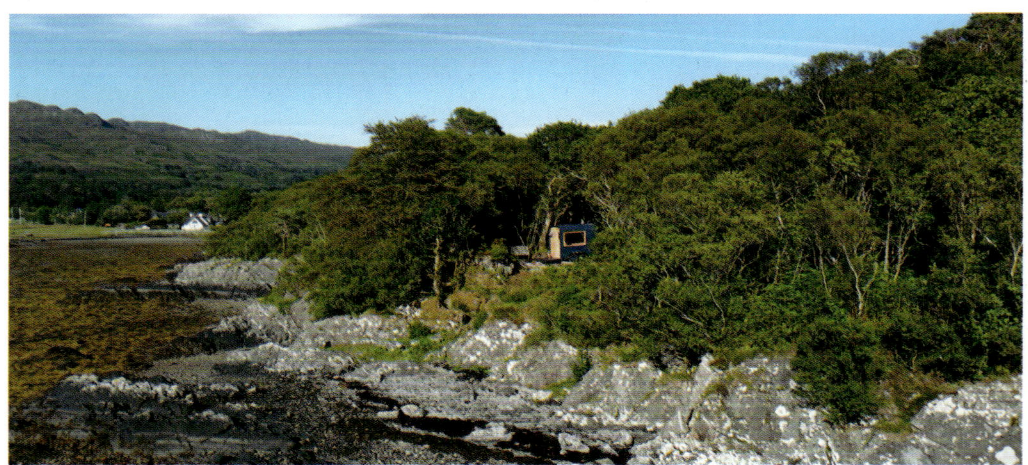

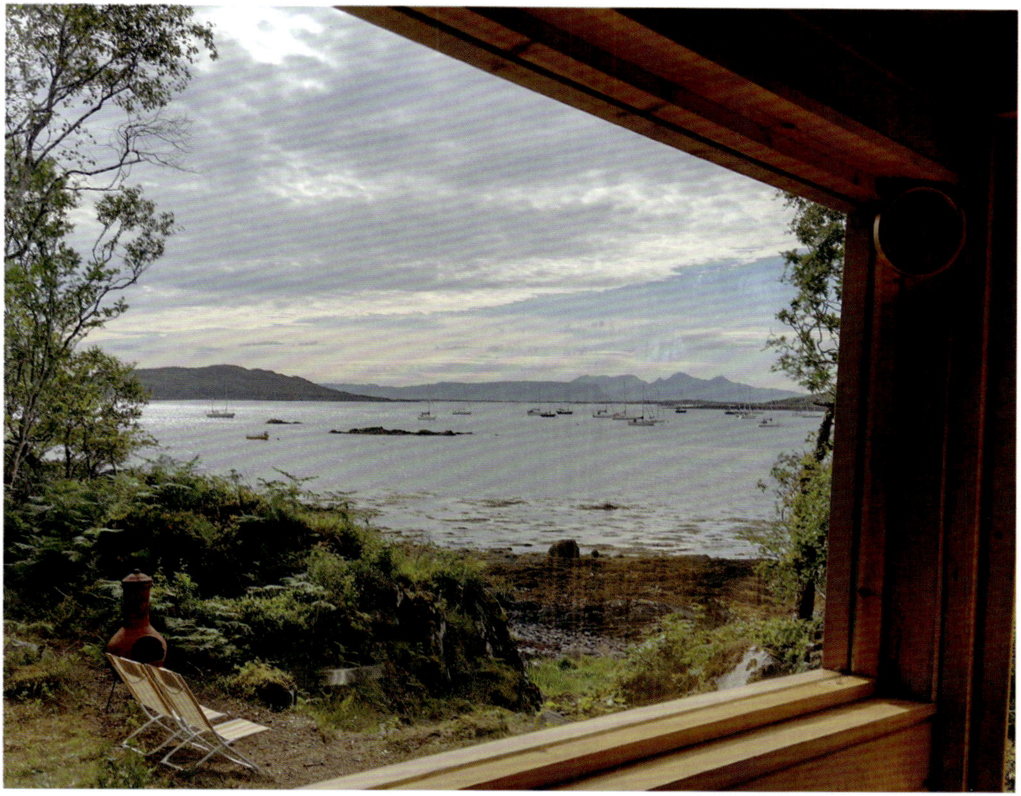

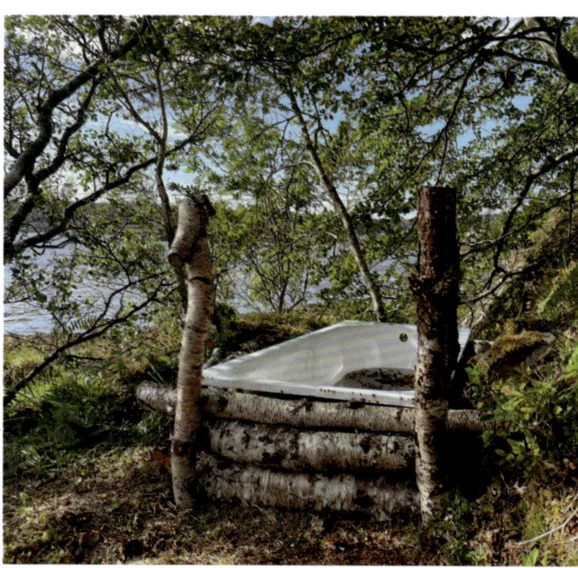

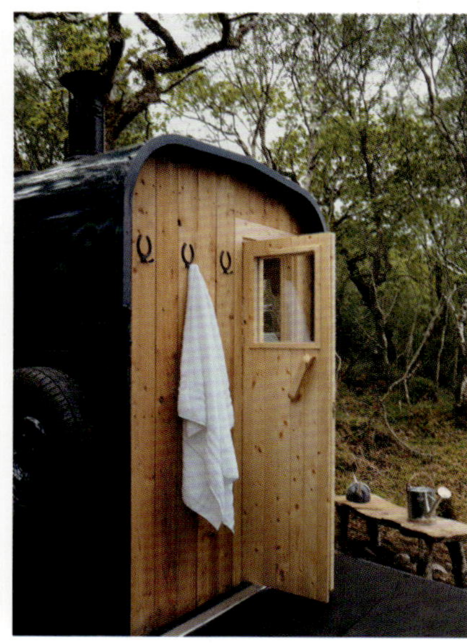

153

Bracken Hide

PORTREE ❦ SKYE

The Scottish/Estonian sauna connection is strong in Scotland, not least on the Isle of Skye. Here, the four-star 'wilderness hotel' Bracken Hide offers 27 'hides', or peaked wooden cabins, and two 'iglu' saunas set around a stream-fed pool. Iglu saunas feature wooden shingling, typical of Estonian rustic saunas, and their style has been popularised by the likes of David Beckham and film director Guy Ritchie.

Guests at Bracken Hide are entitled to a free 30-minute sauna session, and more sessions can be booked. The hotel also features a high-end restaurant and a whisky bar.

➔ brackenhide.co.uk

❄ Natural pool 📍 57.4142, -6.2165

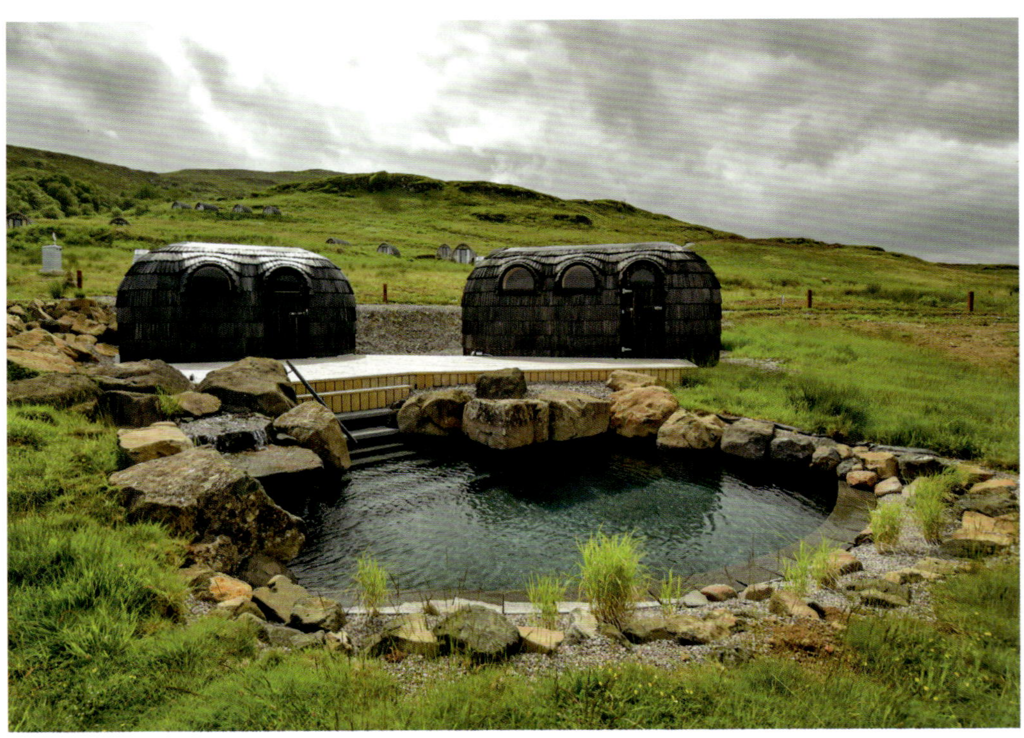

154

Eastwood Forest Sauna

LOGANSWELL ❦ GLASGOW

Eastwood Forest sauna draws athletic types who know that sauna is good for tired muscles. Triathlon-loving founder Johnny McBeth knows this too, and when his late father bought a plot on a former golf course, they talked about building a sauna on it. After his father passed, Johnny set to work, creating a 12-seater space in thermo pine from Aviemore. A large picture window and generous benches ensure the sauna doesn't feel cramped; four ice barrels and outdoor showers allow for cooling off; and a 'summer house' offers drinks, snacks and a place to relax.

➔ instagram.com/eastwoodforestsauna
❄ Barrel/shower 📍 55.7424, -4.3591

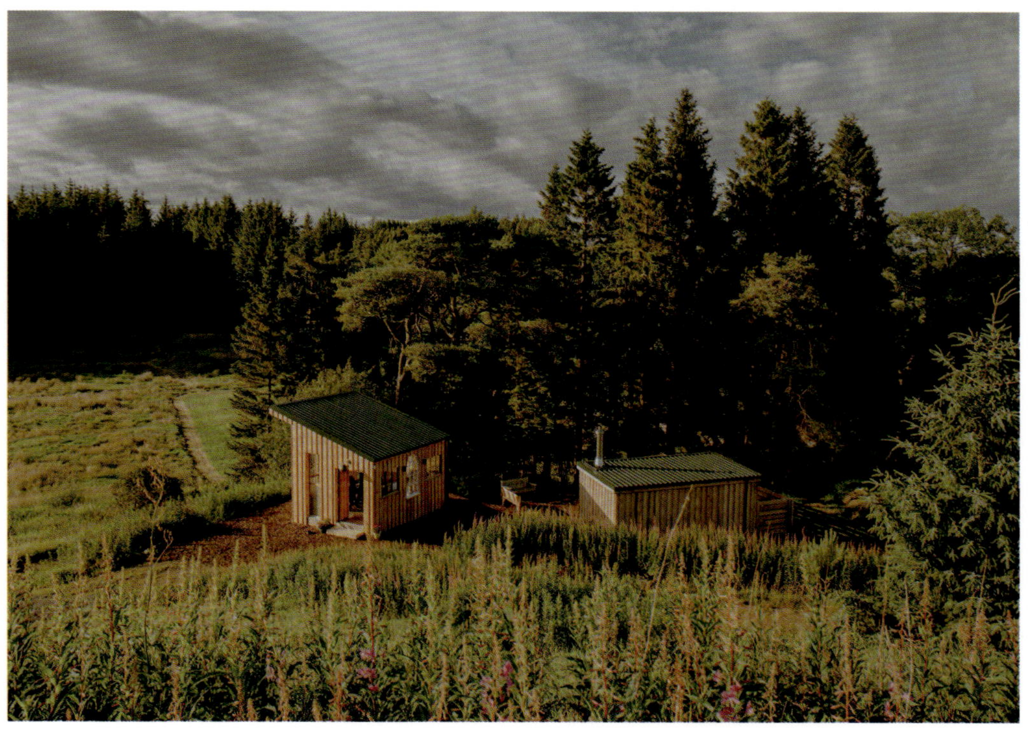

155

Hot Tottie Sauna

LUSS ❦ ARGYLL AND BUTE

Full disclosure: a 'hot tottie' in Glaswegian is a hot jacket potato, and there's nothing untoward about Kieran Izzett and Conlan Nimmo's sauna on the shore of Loch Lomond. Located at Luss on a private estate, it offers spectacular views across the loch to Ben Lomond, and there is a river running into the loch right by the sauna which is great for a cold 'dook'. The boys are cold-water swimmers, and they get plenty of Glaswegians stopping by along with locals and swimming groups from Luss. Their idea? To replicate the old bath-house tradition where people meet up, but this time in a beautiful location.

➔ hot-tottie.com
❄ River/loch 📍 56.1005, -4.6351

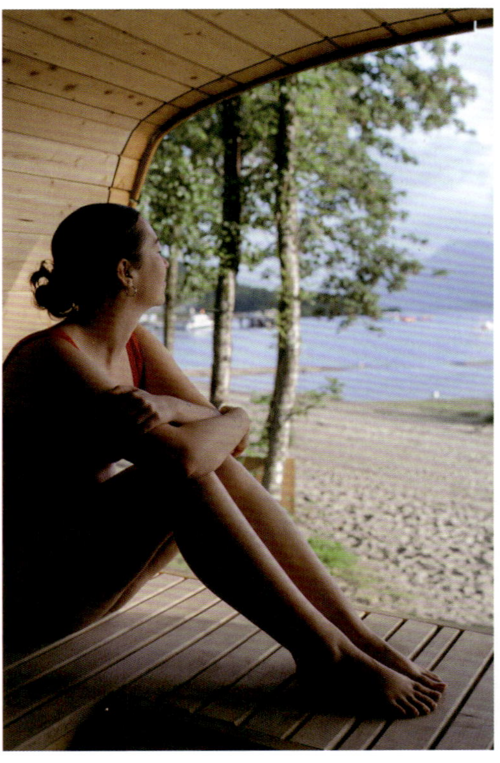

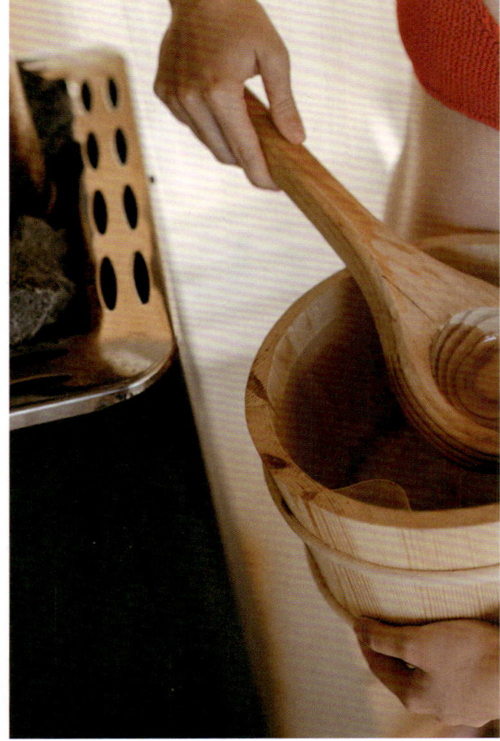

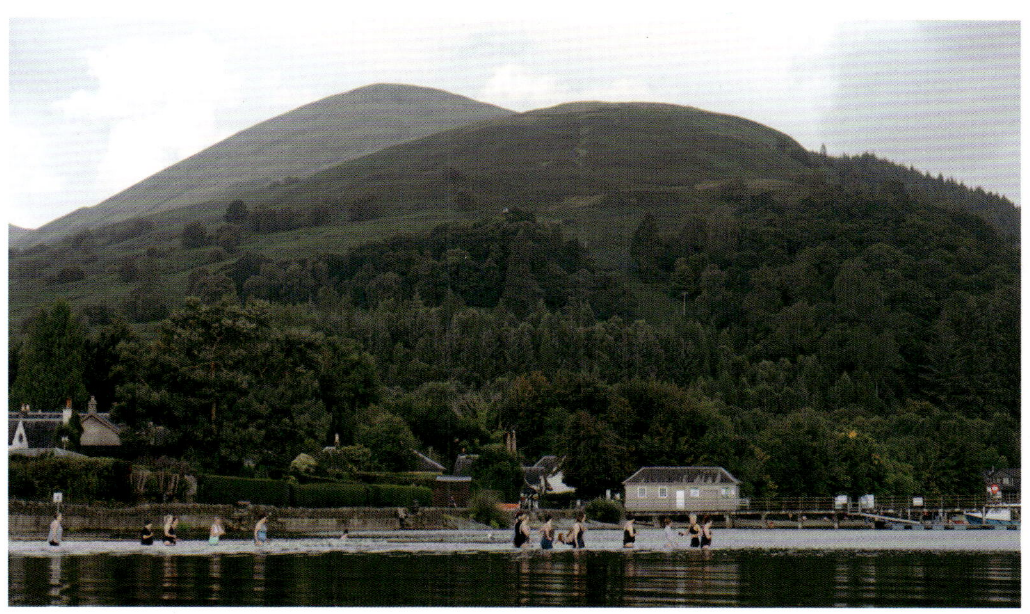

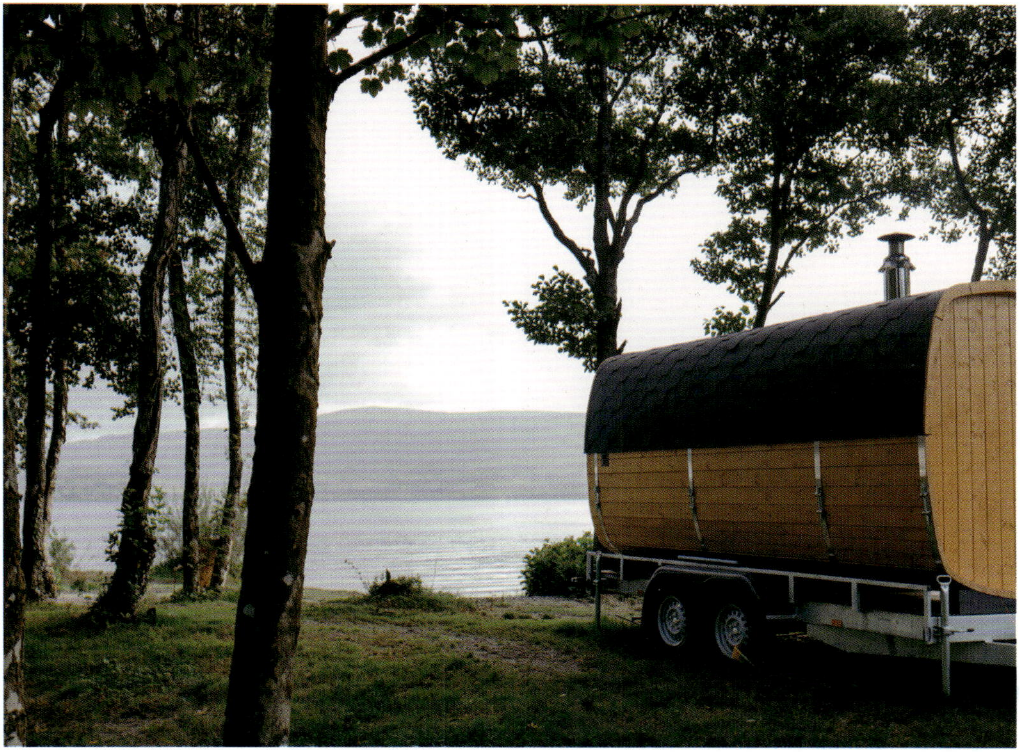

156

The Treehouses at Lanrick

LANRICK ❦ PERTHSHIRE

All you see when you approach the sauna on the Lanrick Estate is a metal door carved into the landscape and a Hobbit-like hillock of a roof that echoes traditional Nordic designs. Fifth-generation estate owner Simon Dickson worked with BAS architects and made the sauna with wood salvaged from the land, mostly larch, which was diseased and in abundance. The roof looks like an extension of the forest floor – and that's because it is an extension of the forest floor; instead of having a sedum roof, it's decked with bluebells, snowdrops, ferns, and grasses.

Guests can stay at Lanrick in any of the five treehouses, which come with a log-burning stove, a tree-top terrace, and an outdoor heated copper bath. The sauna is theirs to use for free, and it's open every day from 1.30–7.30 pm. It holds up to five at a time, but even when Lanrick is full, there are only ever 15 people staying there. The River Teith is 150 metres away, but it's full and fast-flowing; safer swim spots within a ten-minute drive can be found at Lochs Lubnaig and Venachar in the Trossachs National Park.

➔ lanricktreehouses.co.uk
❄ Cold plunge 📍 56.2030, -4.1242

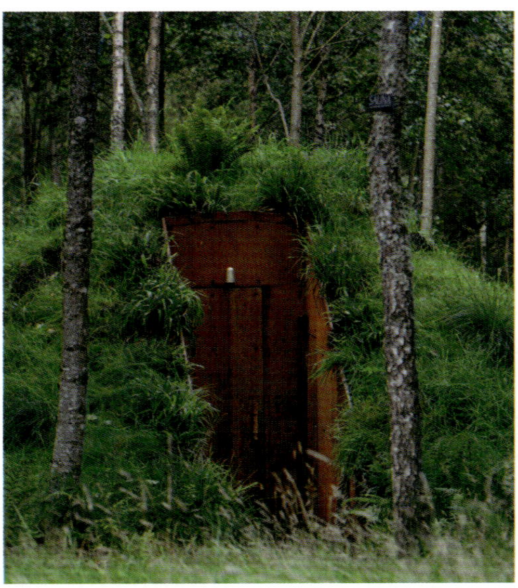

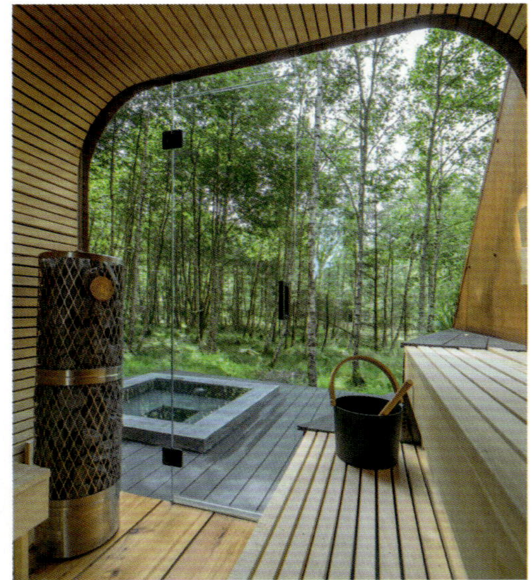

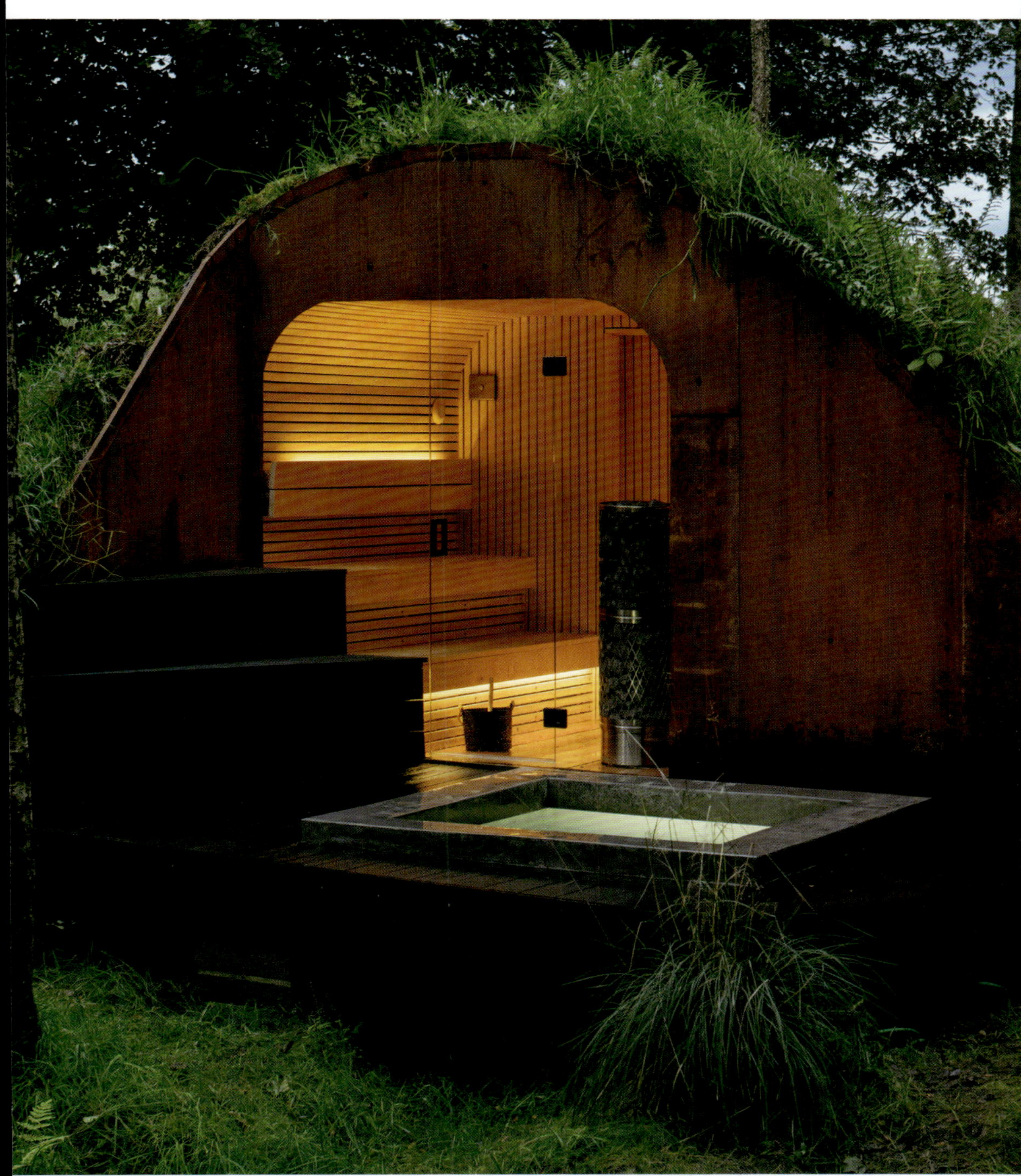

157

Nowhere Sauna

CRIEFF ❦ PERTHSHIRE

There's a secret activism in the sauna community against the go, go, go mentality – and Lauren Gentry and Susanna Macintyre, founders of Nowhere Sauna, encourage it. 'There's a pressure point in society, and the awareness of wellness is a response to where we are at,' says Susanna. 'There's a need to stop, a need for space for a different flow.' With their partners, they built a six-seater horsebox sauna and placed it beside the Mill Pond at Comrie Croft. This 231-acre farm near Crieff is home to 12 nature-based enterprises and offers accommodation, home-grown food and drink, and activities and relaxation in the great outdoors. The bath tub and waterfall bucket are fed by the burn, and Nowhere Sauna draws a creative crowd of parents, artists, musicians and freelance workers who all want to connect with something bigger than themselves.

nowheresauna.com
Bath/bucket 56.3863, -3.9408

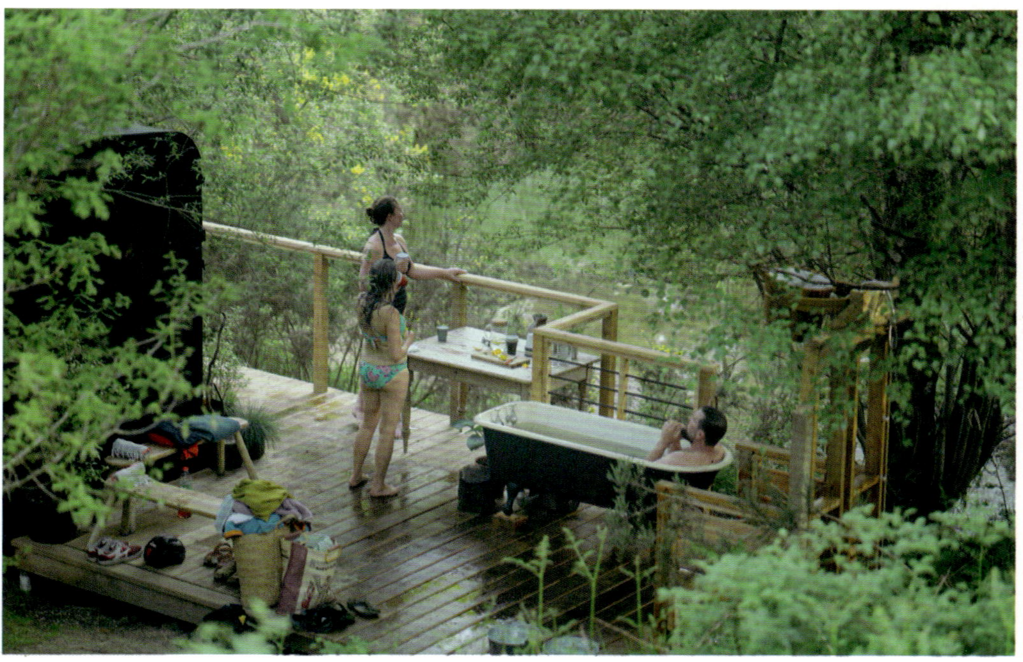

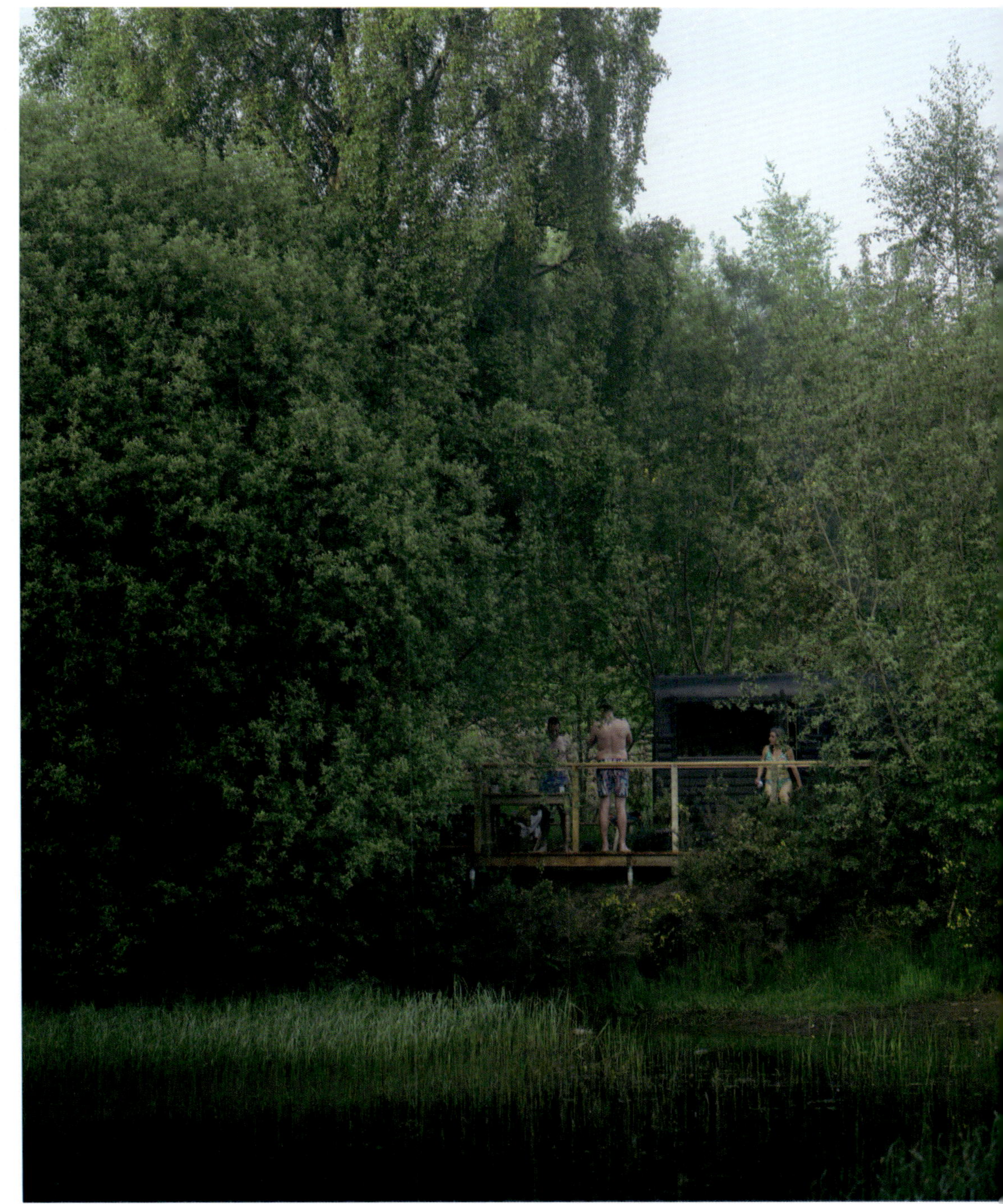

158

Eastside

PENTLAND HILLS ❦ MIDLOTHIAN

Eastside is part of an 18th-century farmstead and consists of five elegantly modernised holiday cottages, as well as a sauna yurt. This is the latest addition, an alternative to a hot tub, and guests are entitled to a free two-hour session (additional sessions can be booked). The yurt holds up to seven people; Finnish sauna robes, towels and drinking water are provided.

Next to the yurt sauna is a stream-fed cattle trough that has been fashioned into a cold plunge. There's fantastic hill walking from the doorstep within the heather-clad Pentland Hills Regional Park, and the sauna is a most welcome end to a day of hiking. Eastside owner Michael Rummey says, 'Two-thirds of people who stay want to use the yurt sauna. It's one of the reasons people book to stay here. It has wide appeal as it doesn't get too hot (it's typically around 50-60°C). It's not necessarily for aficionados, it's more relaxed. Take a drink and enjoy it. No egg timers needed.'

➜ eastsidecottages.co.uk/journal/eastside-sauna
❄ Cold plunge 📍 55.8290, -3.3033

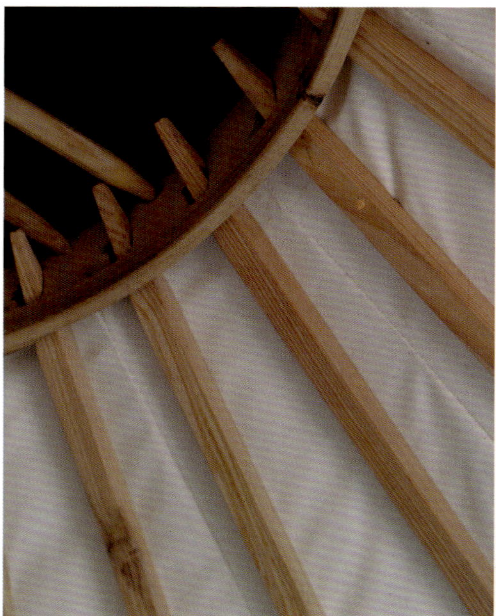

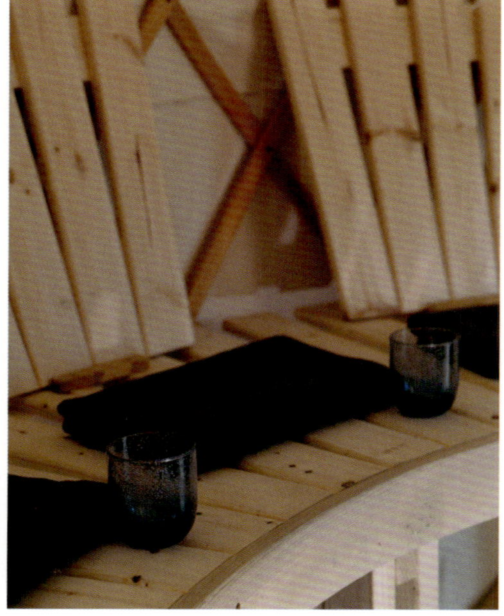

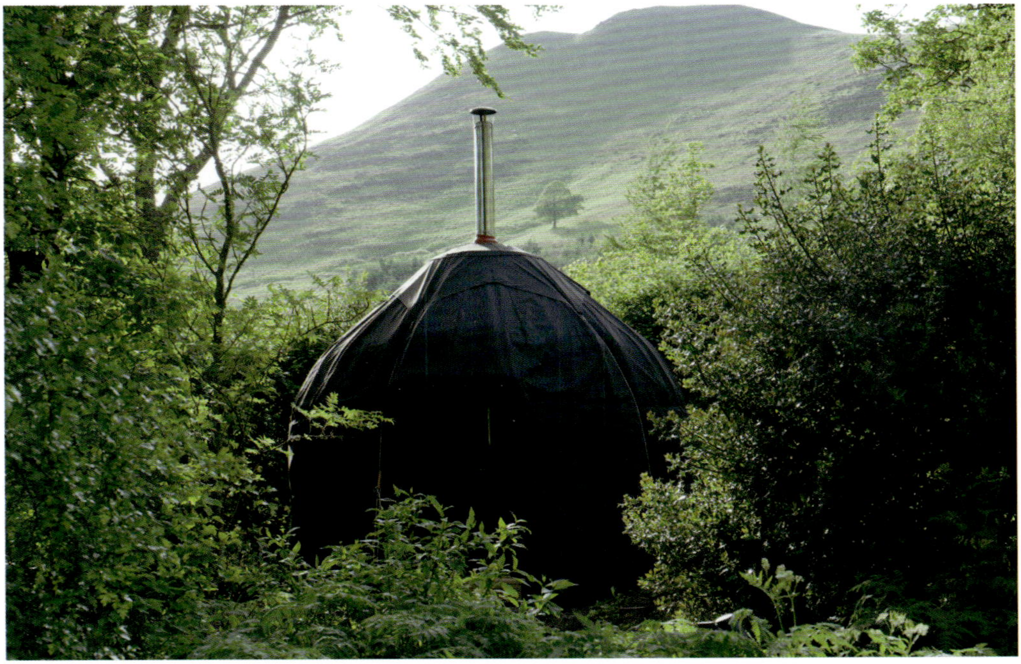

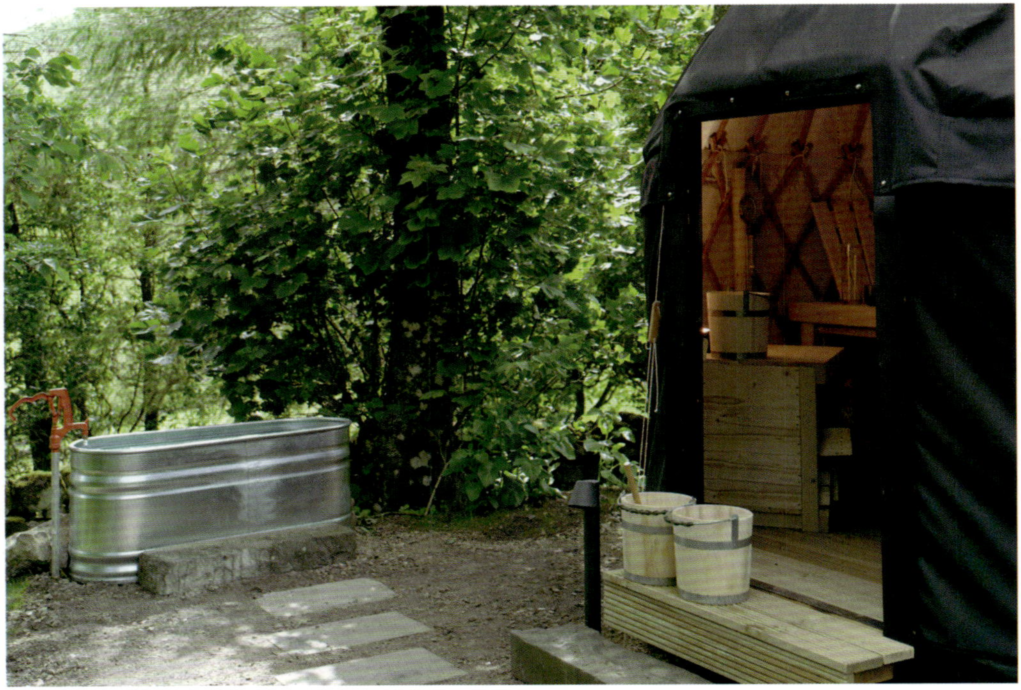

159

Soul Water Sauna

PORTOBELLO & GRANTON ❦ EDINBURGH

When she moved to Edinburgh from England, Kirsty Carver launched a 'time bank' and built a community that would exchange time and skills instead of money. Many of this community came with her when she opened Soul Water Sauna on Edinburgh's Portobello Beach in 2022. It's still there, and such is its popularity that Kirsty opened a second, bigger Soul Water Wild Spa at the other end of Edinburgh, in Granton in 2024. Set in a post-industrial landscape, this spa feels wild – but not deserted; one sauna named Big Bear holds up to 18 people and its sibling Little Bear holds up to eight, there are showers, changing rooms, cold plunges made from beer stills, a beach and windswept views of the Firth of Forth. Next to Soul Water Wild Spa is The Pitt, a not-for-profit community-facing outfit that brings together a food market, coffee shops, bars and a music and events space.

Kirsty offers a range of sessions, often based on traditional sauna rituals, although she emphasises that 'it doesn't have to be serious; you can have a lot of fun in the sauna. With the sauna floors often strewn with birch leaves and body scrub, we're reminded that a sauna that looks like it has given birth to a tree is a good sauna'

soulwatersauna.com · Sea/cold plunges
55.9511, -3.1013 Portabello
55.9833, -3.2419 Granton

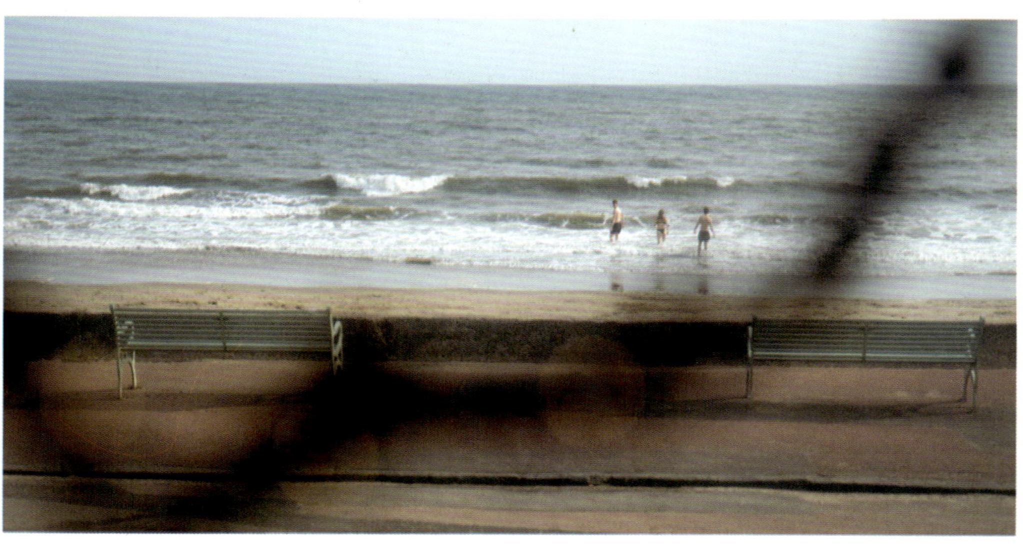

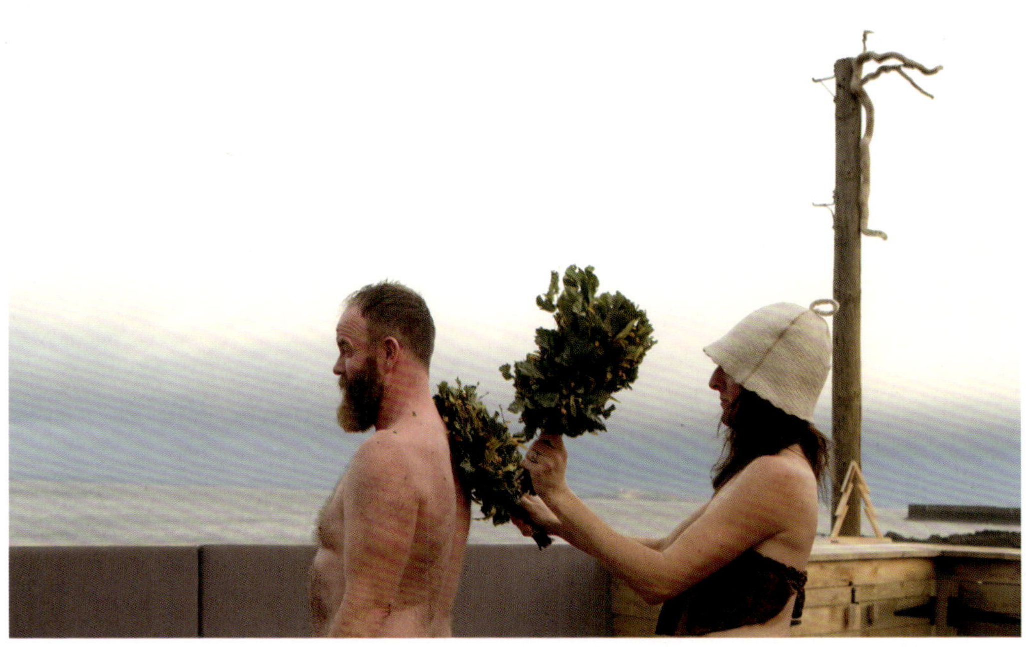

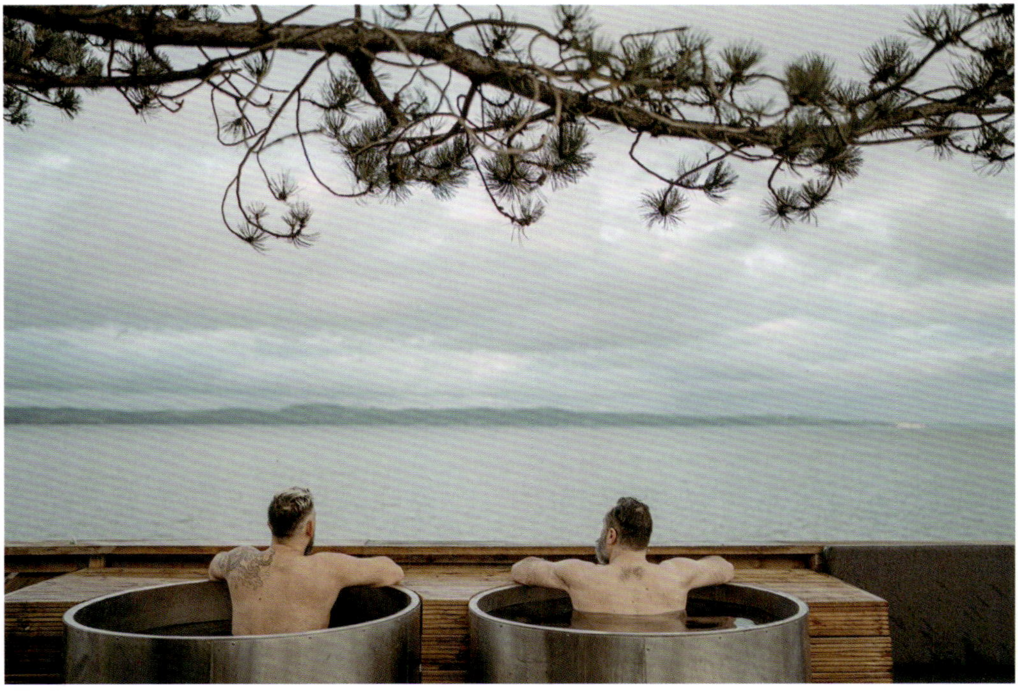

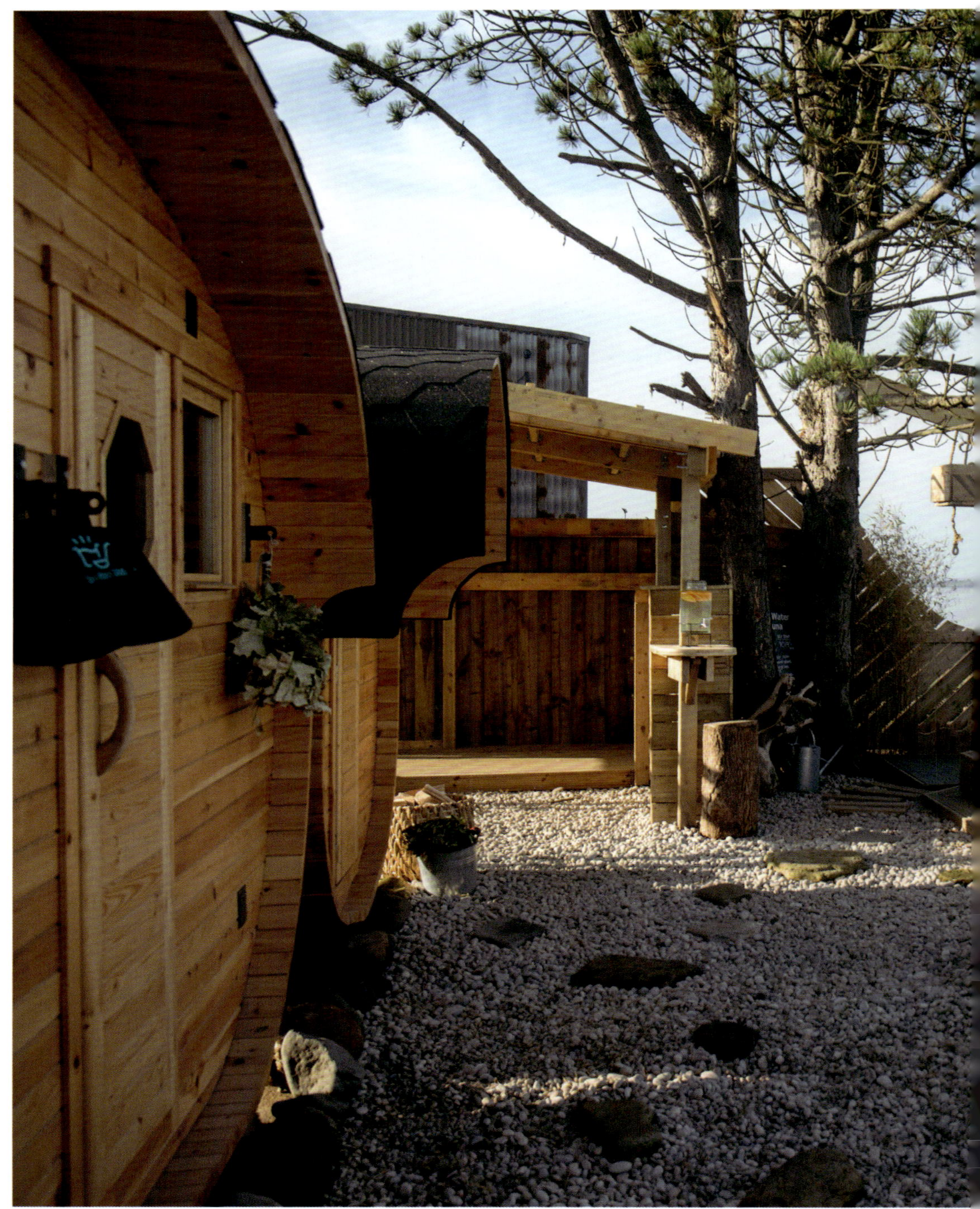

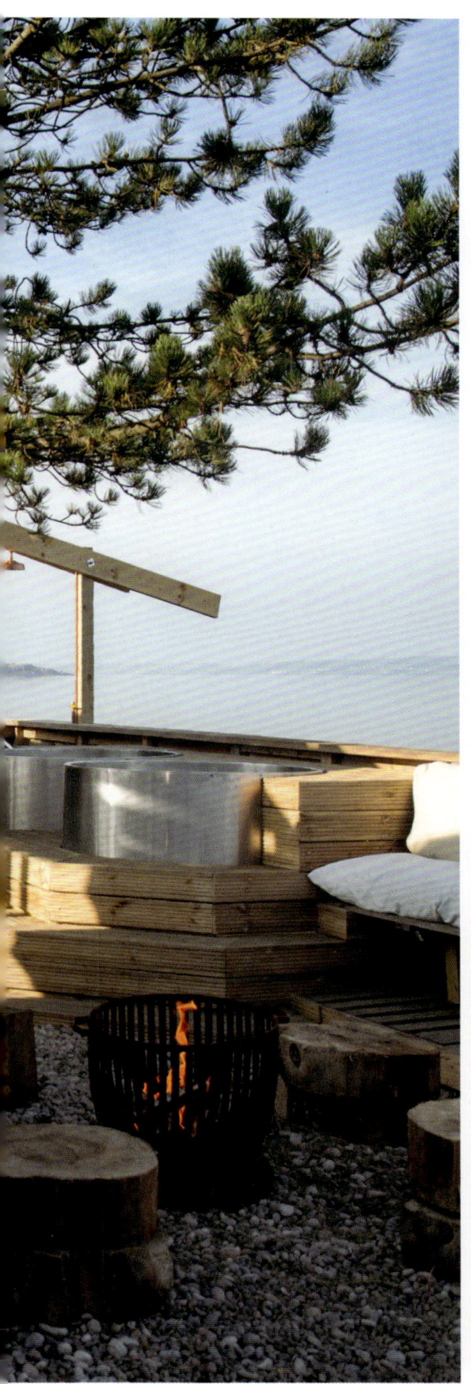

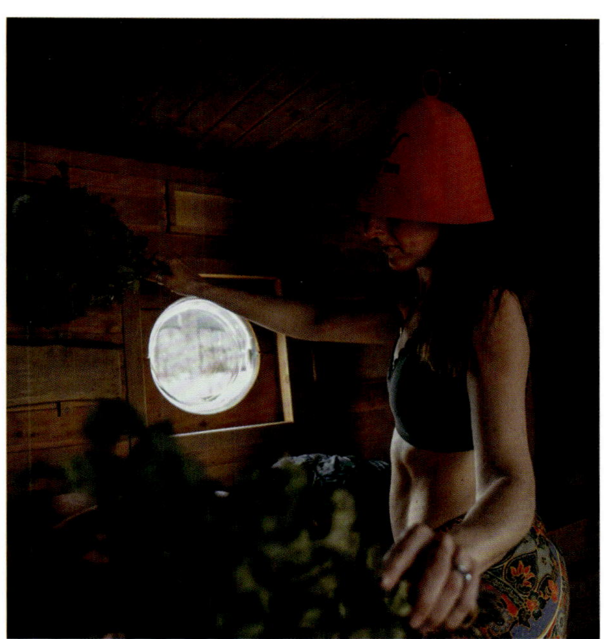

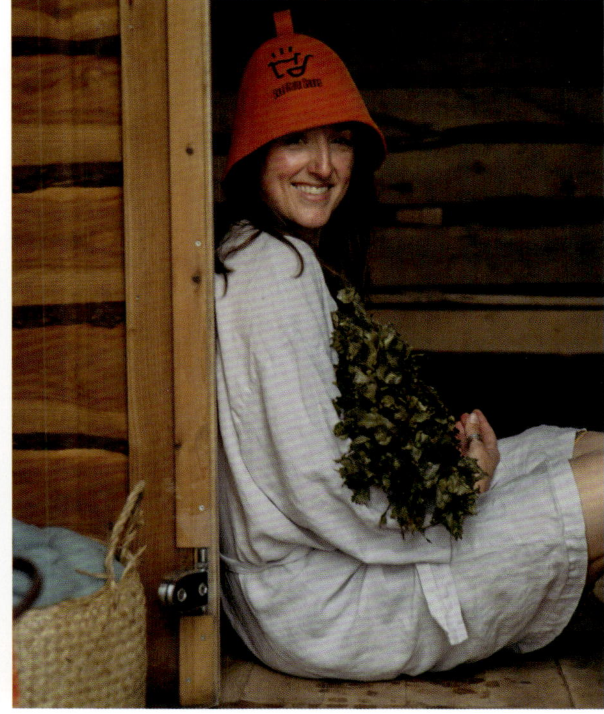

160

Braan Sauna

DUNKELD ❦ PERTHSHIRE

Fraser Potter owns The Taybank and has transformed it into a destination hotel in Dunkeld, a picture-postcard town on the River Tay. His partner Kim is a keen cold-water wild swimmer who runs a sauna on the grounds. She started by renting her first sauna from Haar (now in Shetland). It had no access to the fast-flowing River Tay, but a large metal cold plunge with great views over the river and the famous Dunkeld Bridge. However, Fraser is always building something, so it was only natural that they would build their own. They christened it 'Braan', after the Braan tributary that feeds into the River Tay, and it sits on the riverbank from October to March. It's available to guests at The Taybank and locals, where community sessions every week cost an eighth of the price of the normal session. Kim's mission, during the long, dark Scottish winters, is to get people outside and socialising in the steam.

→ thetaybank.co.uk/sauna
❄ Cold plunge/shower 📍 56.5646, -3.5840

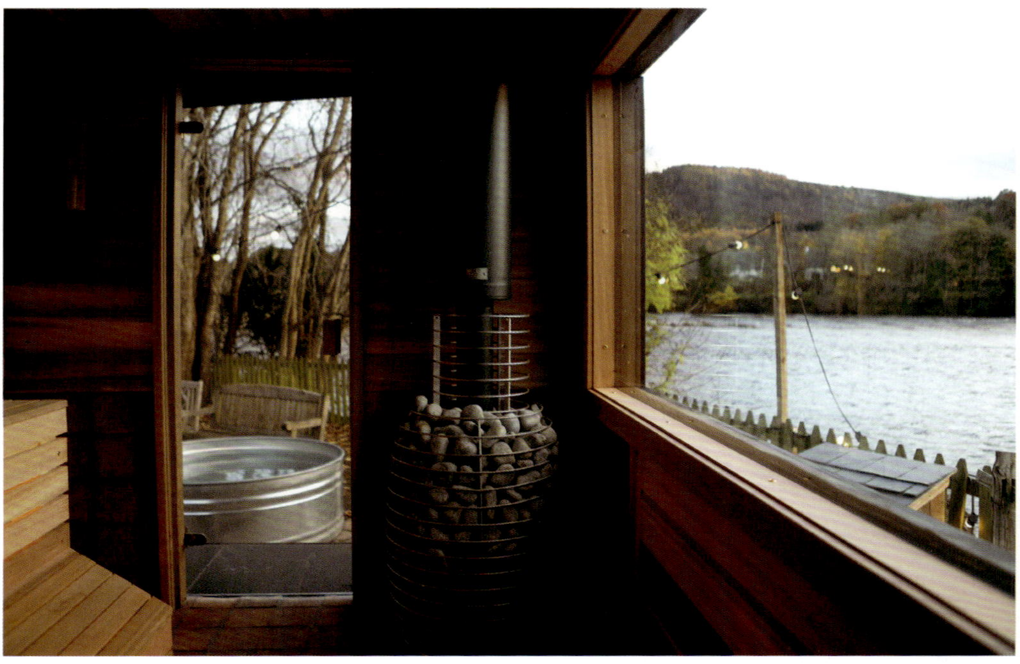

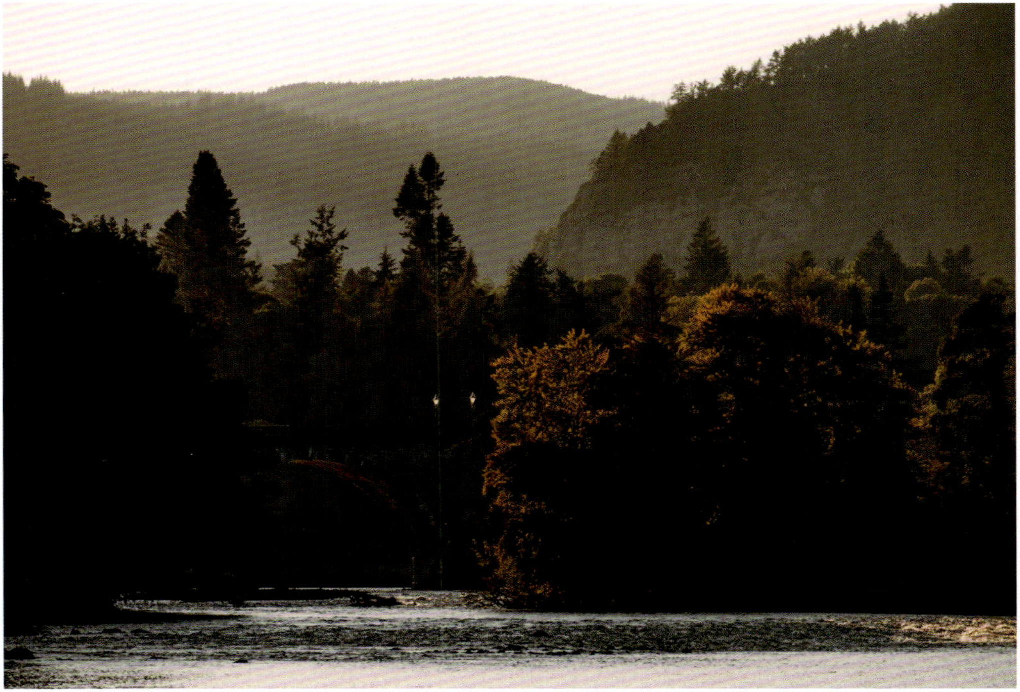

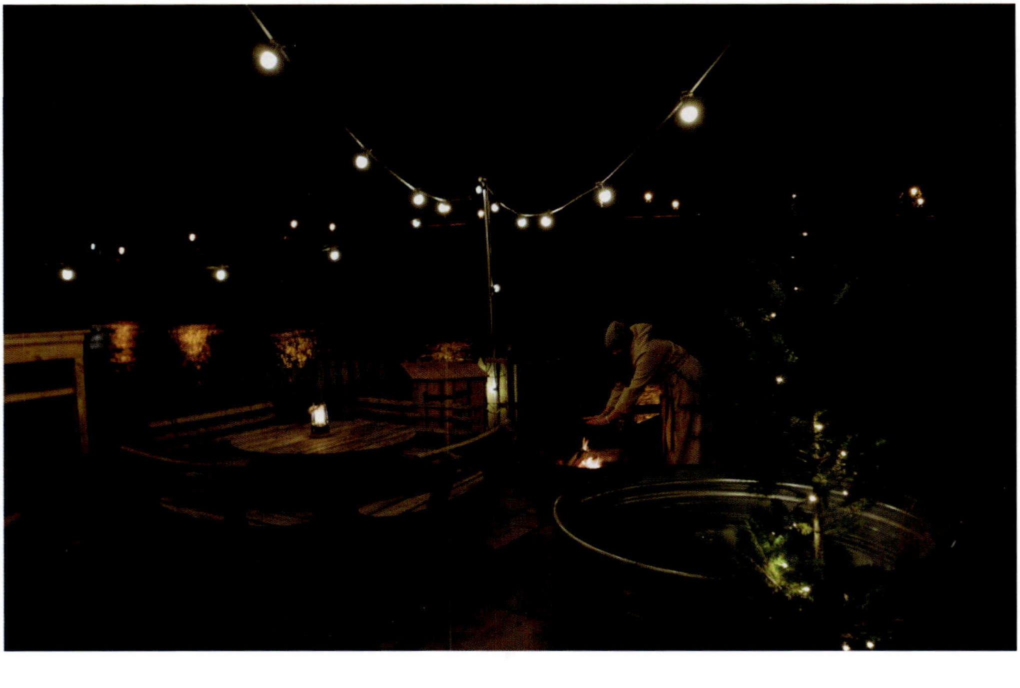

161

Lindor Curative Forest

NORMAN'S LAW ❦ FIFE

Rory MacPhee founded Lindor Curative Forest in Fife in 2020. A curative forest promotes *shinrin yoku*, or 'forest bathing' – mental and physical relaxation in nature. In Germany and Japan, it's prescribed by GPs as a successful treatment for good health and well-being. Lindor, which stretches across five acres of mixed woodland, supports addiction, recovery and grief, with nature as its core guide.

Rory, who has had previous careers as a maritime lawyer, boat builder and seaweed harvester, built the sauna himself with materials from the land. Inspired by earth structures, particularly those from Japan from the Jōmon era, he created a wooden frame and backfilled it with earth for maximum acoustic and thermal insulation.

Sometimes, instead of a sauna, Rory will light a fire under the cast iron bathtub filled with rainwater. He adds several handfuls of wrack (Fucus) seaweed and feels his skin soak it up. He offers this to visitors, especially those with certain medical conditions.

With eco-therapy at its core, groups can sit around the fire, lie in hammocks, engage in communal activities (such as Qi Gong) and learn green wood crafts. And other facilitators are invited to deliver their own wellness programmes at Lindor.

Rory distils leaves and pine needles to create water for the sauna, and bathers can rinse in water taken from a sacred well near Loch Leven. The well has been in use since pre-Christian times and has an ancient place of worship close by. Ten minutes from the forest by bike is a small loch for a plunge and swim.

'I invite people to walk slowly around the forest,' Rory says. 'This is not a place for mountain bikers and fell walkers, but for those who may struggle with anxiety, or have mental health issues, or who are going through end-of-life care.'

→ instagram.com/rory.macphee_crafts
❄ Well water ⊙ 56.3671, -3.1315 Exact location revealed on booking

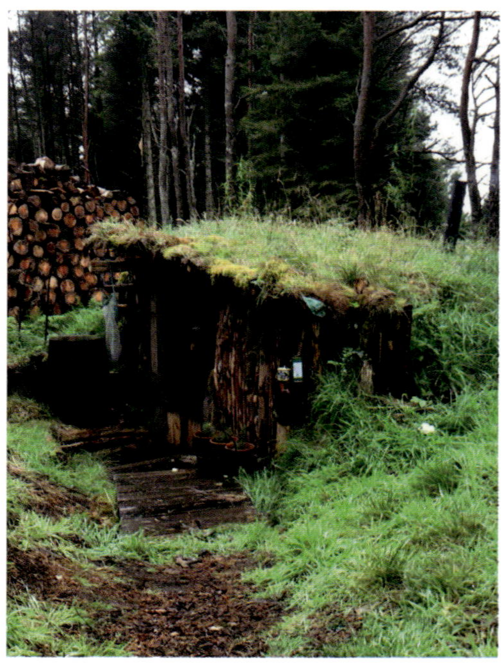

162

Smugglers Sauna

LOCH AN EILEIN ❦ ROTHIEMURCHUS

In the 18th and 19th centuries, crofters survived by making and selling illegal moonshine, which was smuggled out to towns and cities by middlemen. Smugglers Sauna is a nod to their shenanigans. It sits in the forest on the Rothiemurchus estate near Aviemore. Sir David Attenborough has called Rothiemurchus 'one of the glories of wild Scotland'.

This 10,000-hectare family-run, forward-thinking estate has been cared for by 18 generations of the Grant family and offers eight luxury self-catering properties, a camping and caravan park, and tons of activities. The sauna, which is only available for private hire, sits close to the northern end of Loch an Eilein and to the river that has two pools, perfect for a post-sauna dook.

It seats four comfortably and was built by Zeki Basan, a tree surgeon who used timber that he had felled and milled himself to line the interior. The boards are charred in a technique Zeki learned from his grandfather to preserve wood from the wild Highland weather and to stop 'beasties', such as woodworm, getting in. Zeki was born and raised in the Braes of Glenlivet and used the wood from old whisky barrels to clad the exterior. You can still smell the whisky.

➔ rothiemurchus.net/outdoor-activities-at-aviemore/activity/smugglers-sauna
❄ Loch/river 📍 57.1529, -3.8227

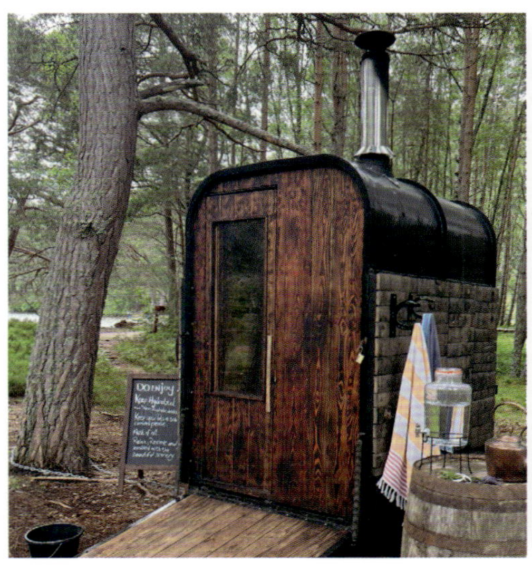

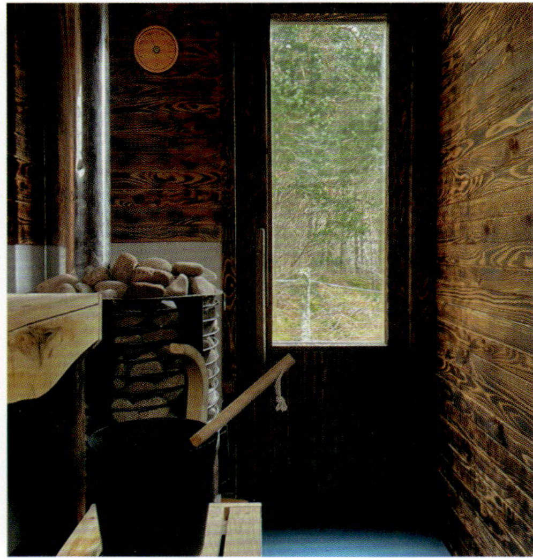

163

Elie Seaside Sauna

ELIE ❦ FIFE

Elie has always been one of Fife's starriest resorts: golf champion Tiger Woods is regularly spotted wandering its 17th-century streets, and Prince William and Kate Middleton would hide away at weekends here when they were students at the nearby University of St Andrews.

Its golden sands and sheltered harbour have long drawn huge groups of wild swimmers, whose numbers only swelled further during the Covid-19 lockdowns. At this time, local girl Judith Dunlop returned home to Elie and taught yoga on the beach, before setting up one of Scotland's first wild saunas – Elie Seaside Sauna. Dune Sauna occupies an elevated spot next to the beach at the far end of the harbour, while Shore Sauna is level with the shoreline; together, they have become symbols of the booming Scottish sauna movement.

Epic sunsets, showers and public toilets are on hand, and many rituals too, among them whisking with birch leaves grown in a local forest. Judith also runs a sister saunas at Cellardyke Tidal Pool, and East Sands in St Andrews, where she also performs sauna rituals and sauna yoga events.

➔ elieseasidesauna.com
Sea 56.1874, -2.8175

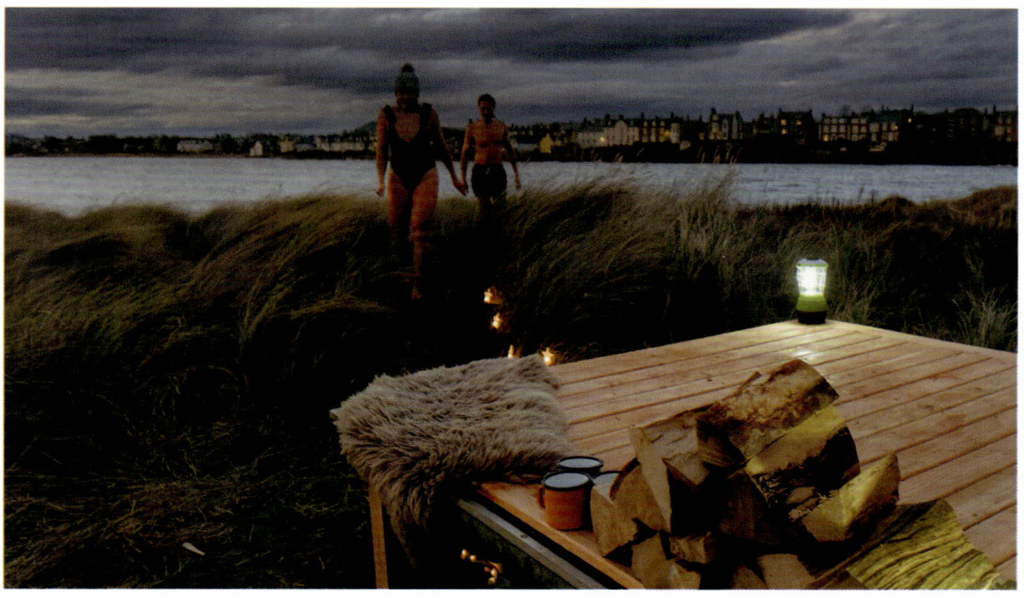

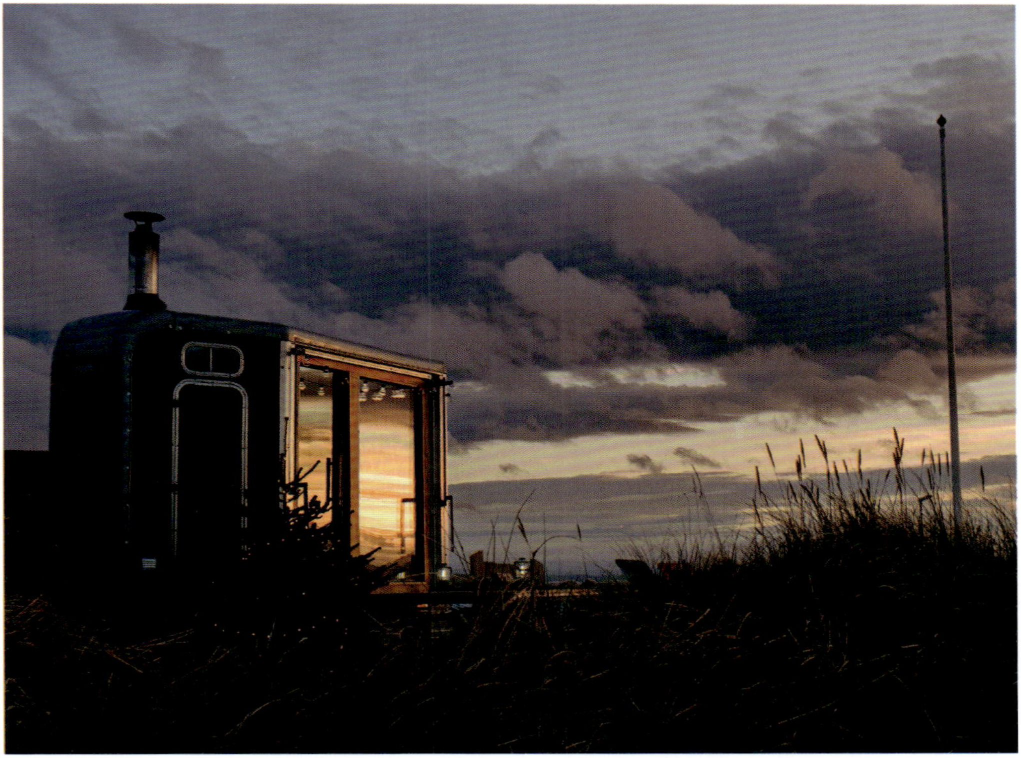

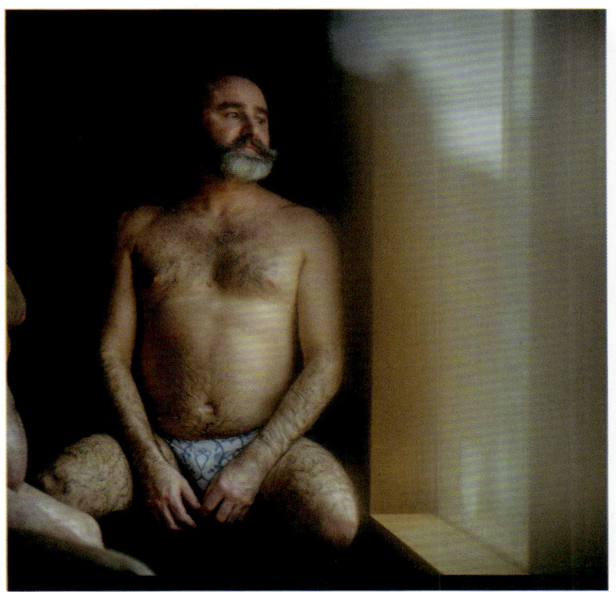

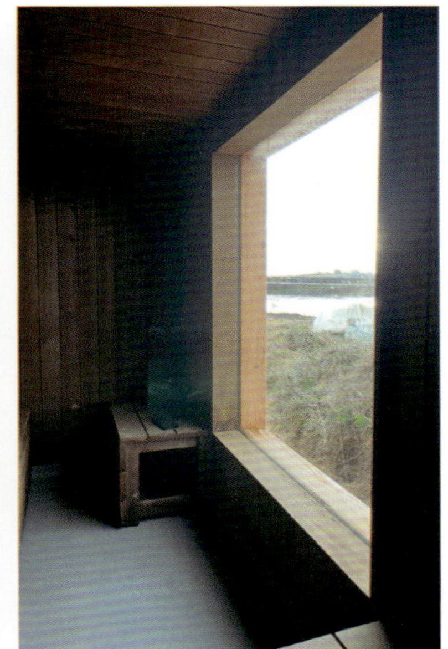

164

Wild Scottish Sauna

CUPAR & ST ANDREWS ❦ FIFE

In 2023, Jamie Craig Gentles and Jayne McGhie opened Wild Scottish Sauna on the stunning Kingsbarns Beach in St Andrews. This stunning two-mile stretch of coast is part of the Cambo Estate and features sand dunes, rocky outcrops and waves that are gentle (for the North Sea). Jamie and Jayne both run businesses in St Andrews and the idea was born after Jamie set up a cold-water swimming group called Bob & Blether that meets regularly on Castle Sands.

A second sauna with the same Scandi-influenced design followed at Eden Springs County Park in Cupar, where cold dips are serviced by a jetty and a loch. The fisheries consist of three lakes dedicated to fly fishing and are part of the Eden Springs Country Park. It's well serviced with facilities including a café that's open daily.

The newest addition is an 8-12 person sauna of the same design on West Sands, St Andrews. It sits next to Dook Cafe and the Blown Away Surf School. All three saunas ofrer private and community slots and special events from yoga to bootcamp and recovery.

wildscottishsauna.com Sea/Loch
56.3034,-2.6451 Kingsbarns
56.3073, -3.1133 Cupar
56.3468 , -2.8069 St Andrews

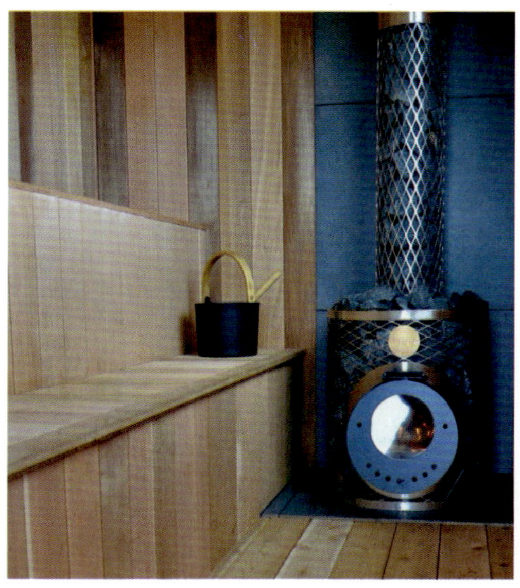

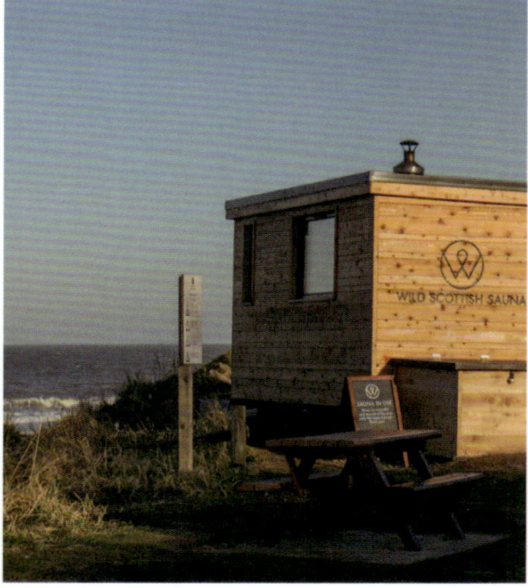

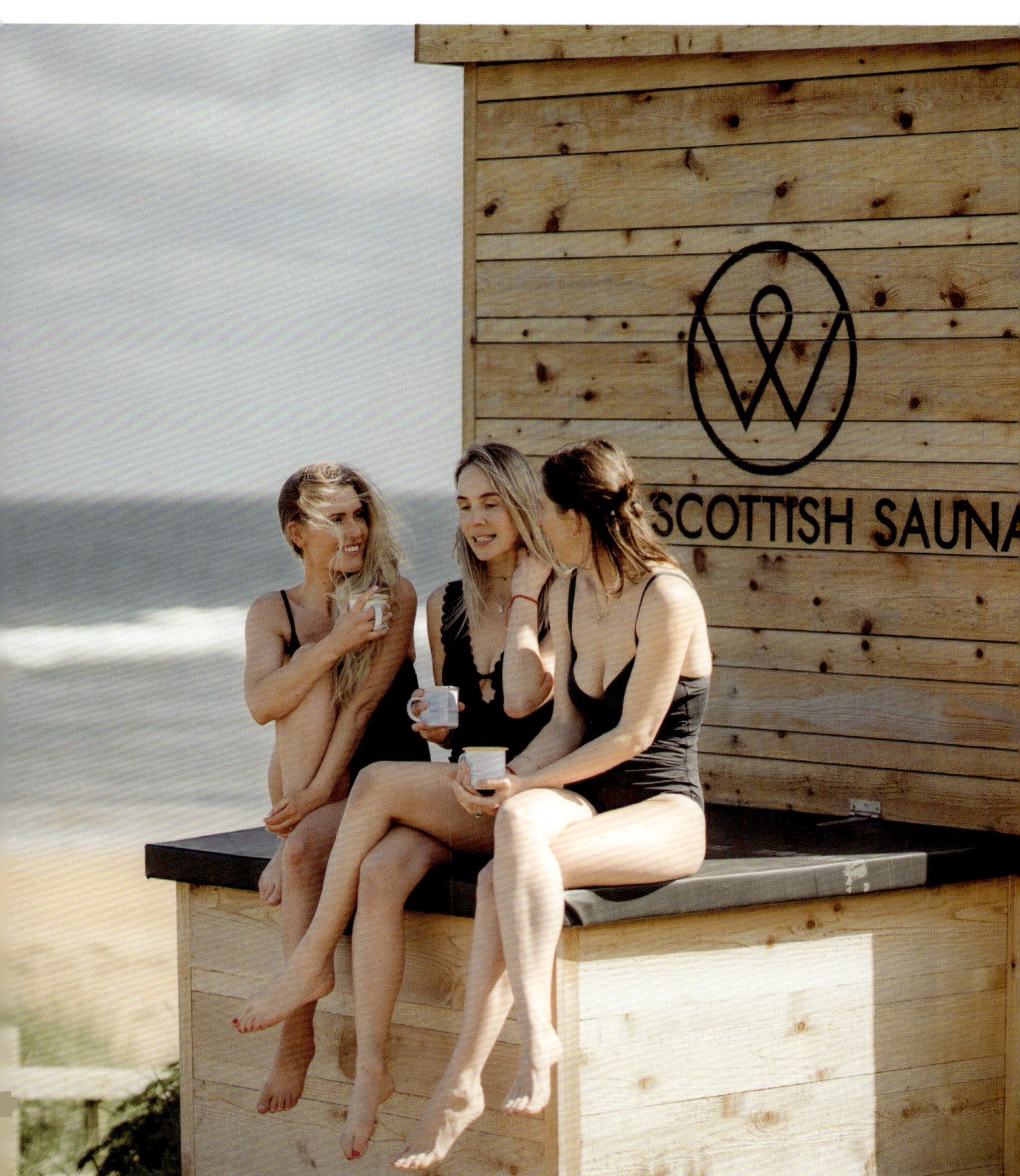
SCOTTISH SAUNA

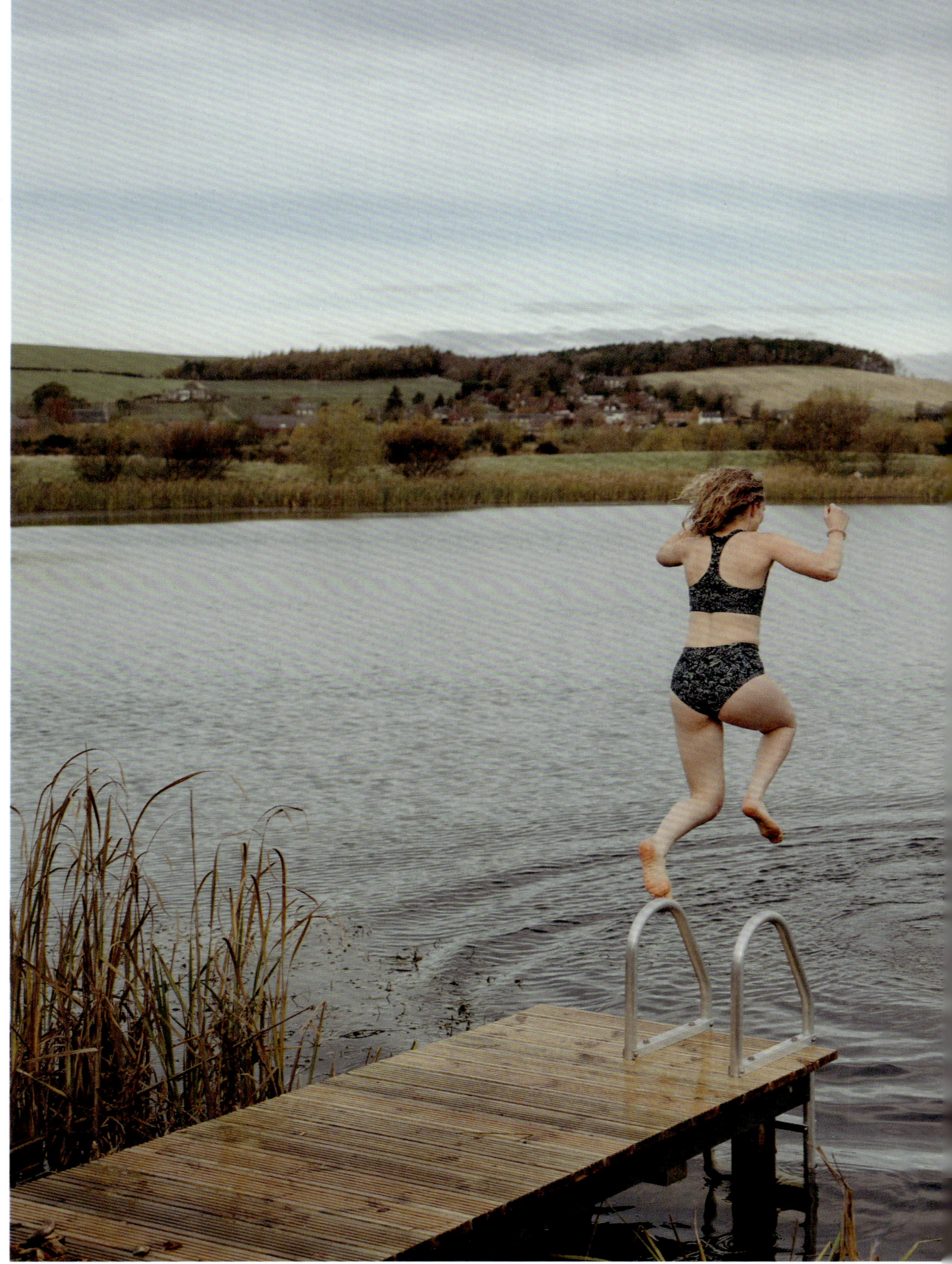

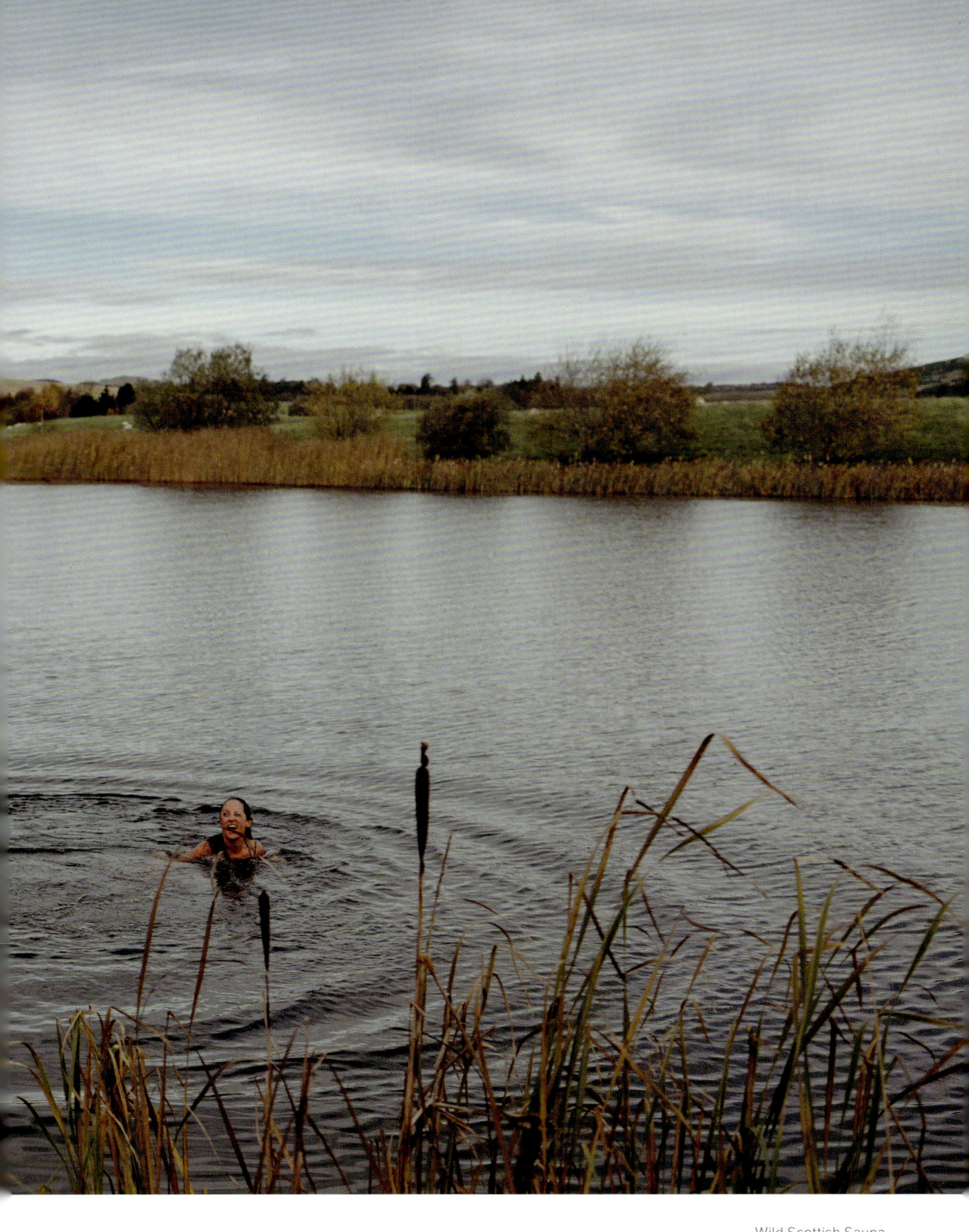

165

St Andrews Seaside Sauna

ST ANDREWS ❦ FIFE

The ancient city of St. Andrews has a long history of sea bathing and swimming around its coasts is a long standing tradition, so it was only a matter of time before it got a beach sauna. And now it has two. St Andrews Seaside Sauna sits in the car park of the East Sands Leisure Centre on the south end of the beach, and Wild Scottish Sauna sits at its northern end. Between the two is the legendary Cheesy Toast Shack. East Sands is a popular spot, and sauna bathers can watch surfers and kite surfers between dips. Both operators run sister sites and are well-versed in hosting leaf whisking, aufguss, yoga and more.

→ standrewsseasidesauna.com:
Sea 56.3328, -2.7787

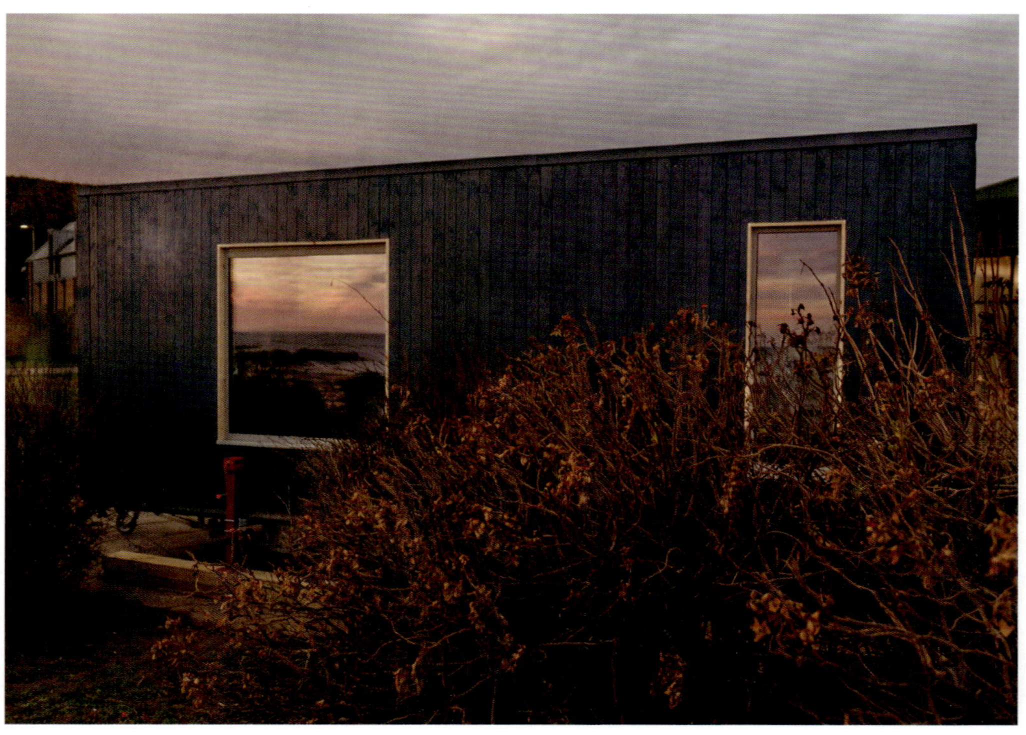

166

Cellardyke Seaside Sauna

CELLARDYKE ❦ FIFE

Tidal pool tourism is a popular pastime in Eastern Scotland, and the Cellardyke Tidal Pool has been a jewel on the Fife Coastal Path since the 1930s. In recent years, however, it had fallen into decline, so a band of locals formed the Tidal Pool Committee and raised £100,000 to restore it. Phase 1 consists of a newly renovated pool, an outdoor activity centre and a community-oriented sauna. This is owned by Judith Dunlop, a 'saunapreneur' who set up Scottish Seaside Saunas after lockdown and runs sister sites in Elie and St Andrews. Cellardyke has a tangible buzz: an Airstream sells coffees and snacks, there's a wood-fired pizza hut, and it's loved by locals and tourists alike.

cellardykeseasidesauna.com

Tidal pool 56.2286, -2.6797

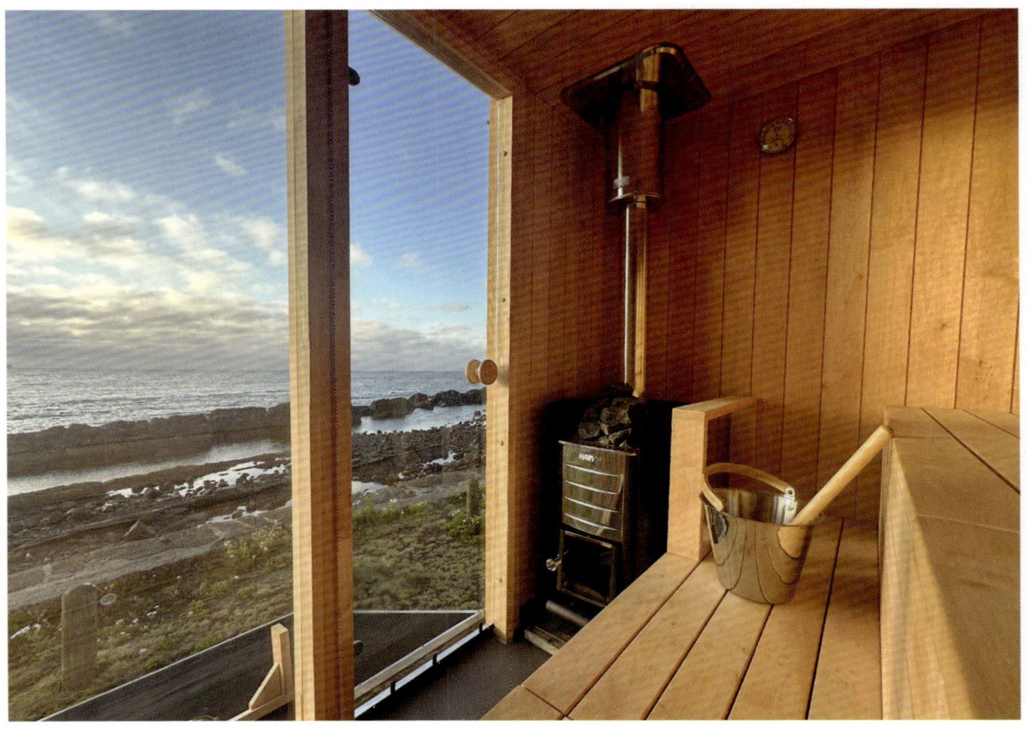

167

Wild Braemar Sauna

BRAEMAR ⚘ ABERDEENSHIRE

Perched on its own, 400 metres high, in the middle of the Cairngorms National Park, Wild Braemar Sauna certainly lives up to its name. There's nothing surrounding this six-seater horsebox sauna, which owner Annie Armstrong built and then towed to an isolated swim spot on the Mar Estate outside Braemar.

Annie is a local nature guide and outdoor educator who runs Wild Braemar, which offers bespoke day retreats in nature – think walking, foraging, sketching, forest bathing – and sauna. Most of her clients are guests at The Fife Arms, Braemar's full-blown, old-school Highlands hotel, which was reopened in 2018 by eminent art collectors Iwan and Manuela Wirth.

Clad in local Scottish larch, the sauna sits in a secluded spot at a confluence between two rivers, with majestic views of the Cairngorms. Inside, it's fitted out in local aspen, with a wood-burning stove and pink granite sauna rocks taken from local rivers.

Annie guides guests into the River Dee even when air temperatures are below freezing. After enjoying what, for many, is their first cold plunge, bathers can relax in a bell tent decked out with sheepskins, cushions and a stove, and celebrate their courage with local cheeses, meats, soups, and Fife Arms whisky.

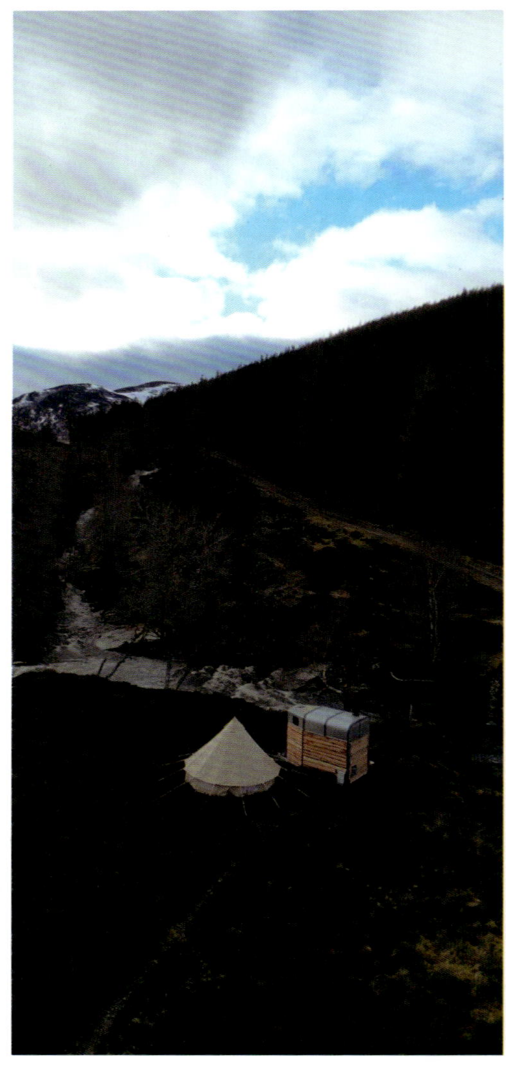

➔ wildbraemar.com/riverside-sauna
River 57.0061, -3.3993

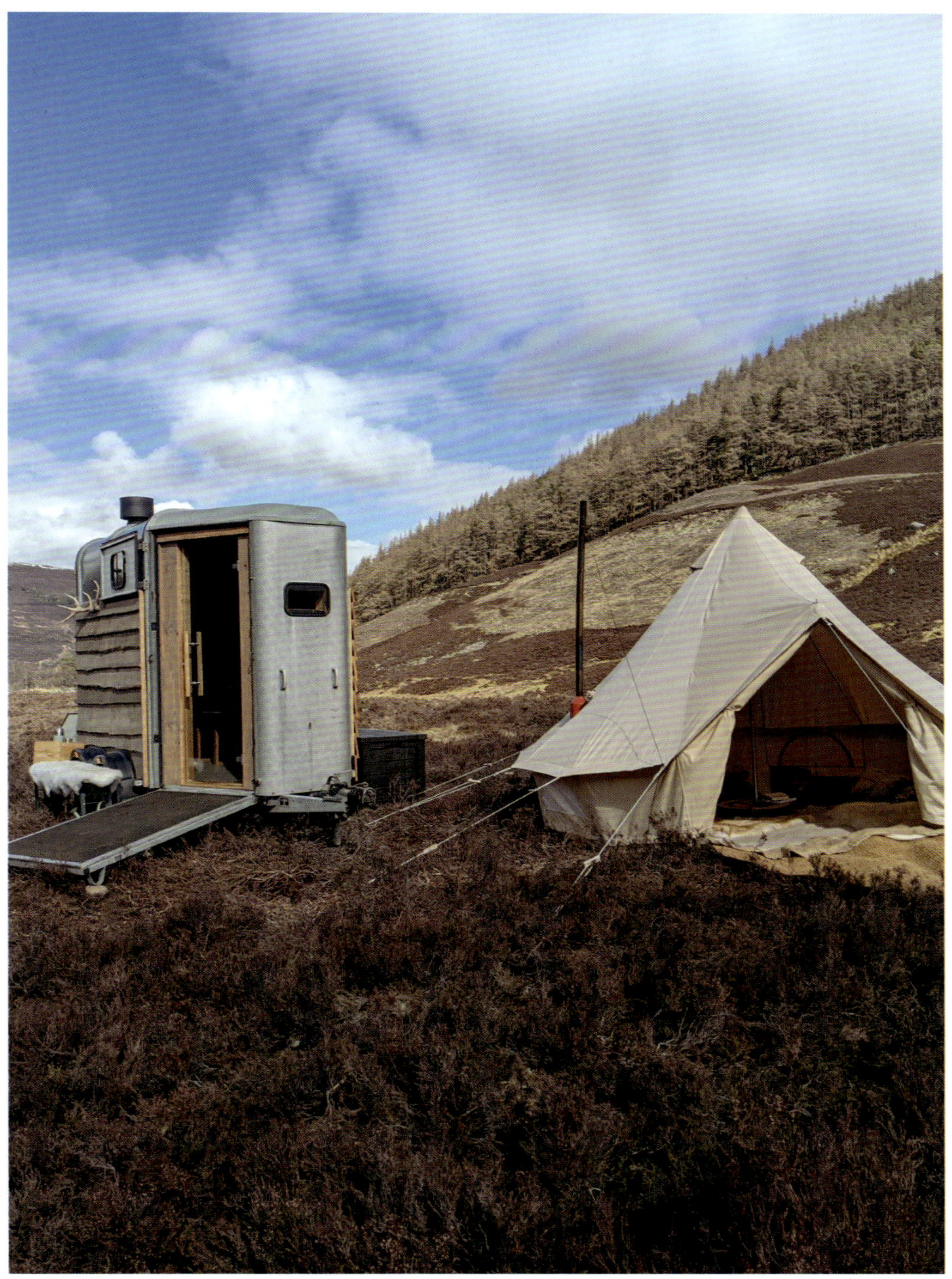

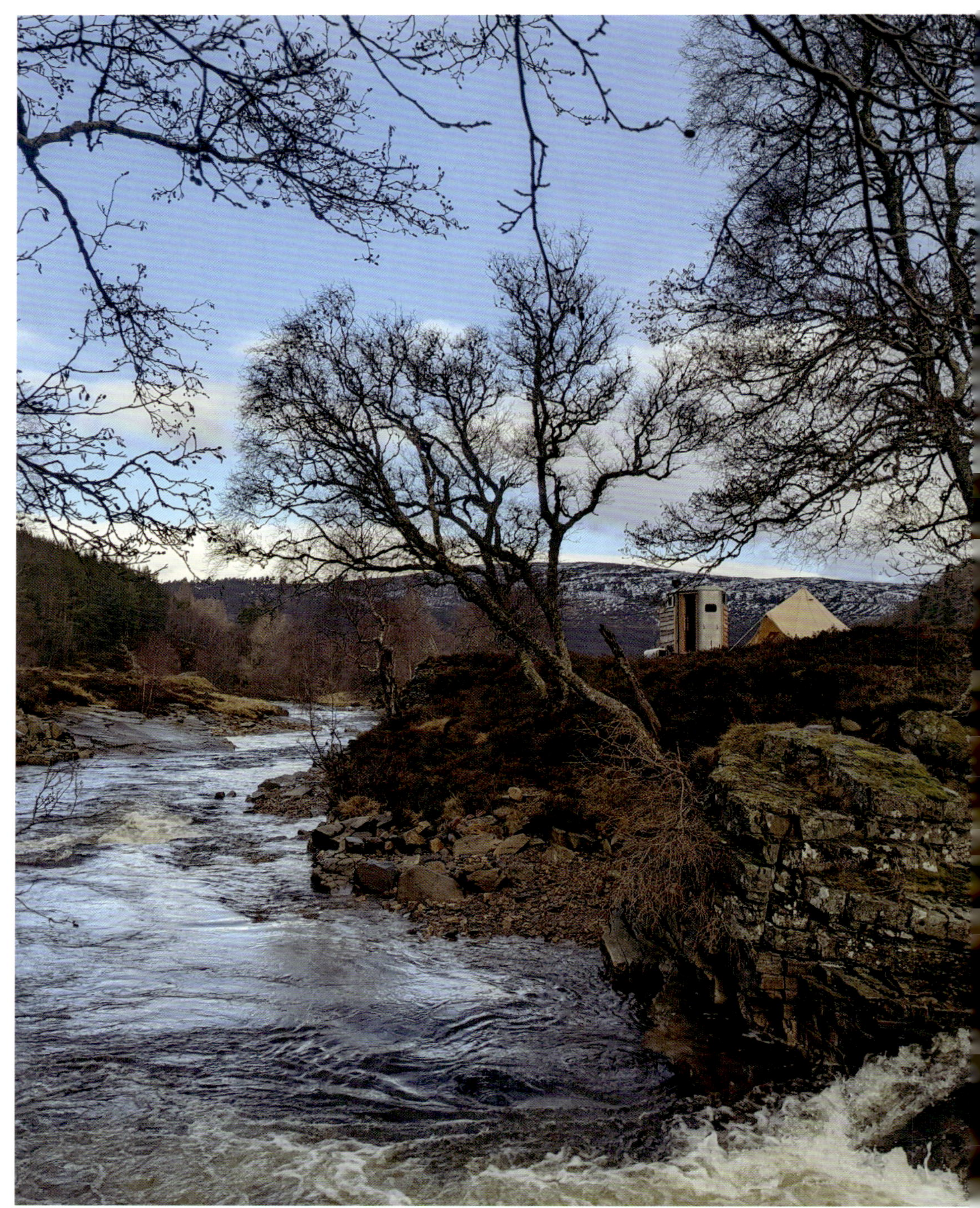

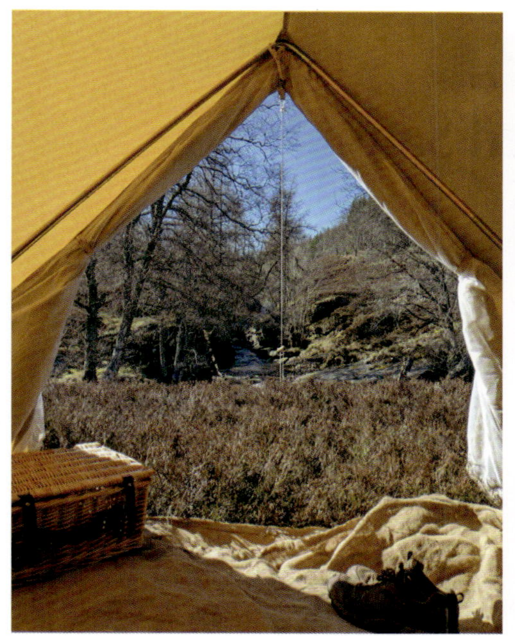

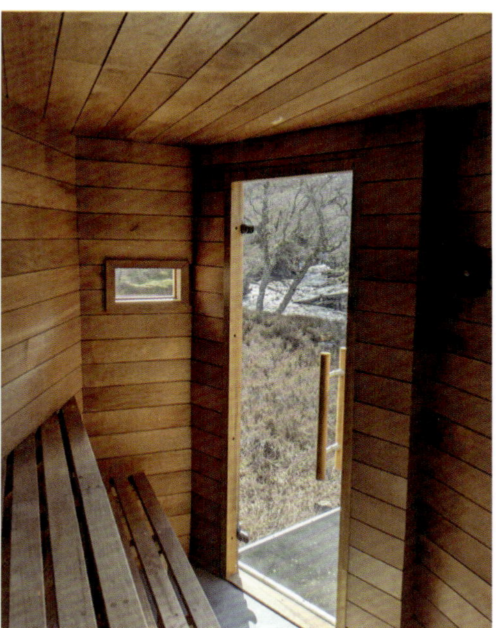

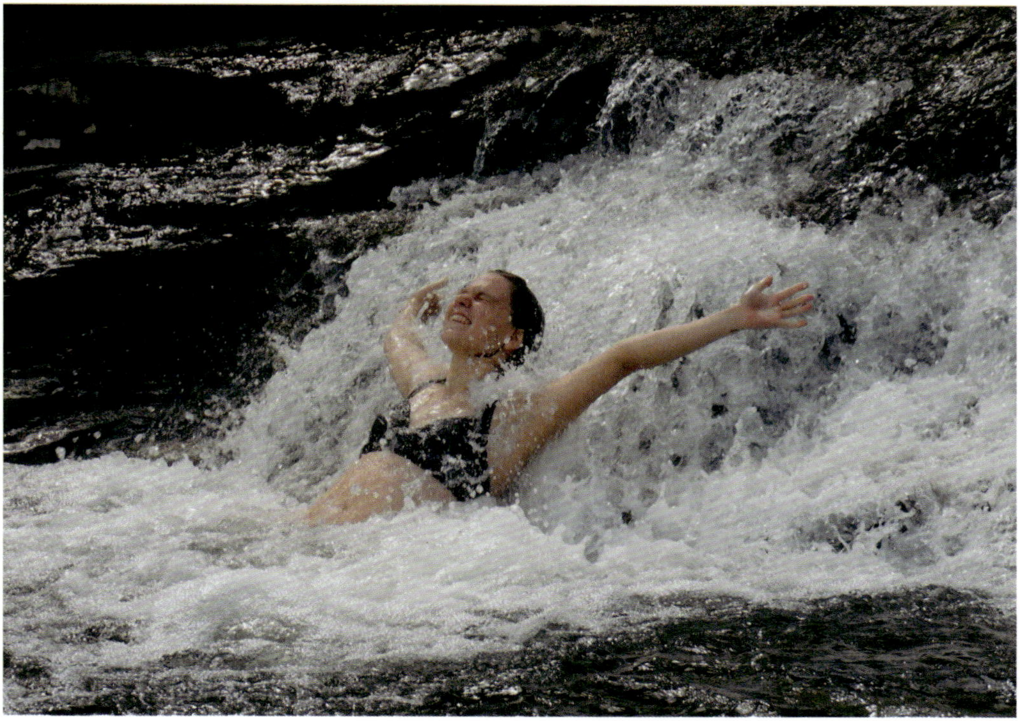

168

Watershed Sauna

FINDHORN ❦ MORAY

Elle Adams and Rupert Hutchinson were sitting in their freezing flat in Findhorn early in 2022, trying to work out a Scottish winter survival strategy. They saw a horsebox advertised on Gumtree and bought it – impulsively and in the dark. They parked it in a friend's garden and, with his help, converted it into a sauna. Elle charted their progress online, and her friends started asking if they could get warm too when it was finished.

In 2022, Watershed Sauna opened above the eight-mile-long Findhorn Beach. What started as a side hustle, set to run alongside the couple's sustainability consultancy Living Alive, has turned into a landmark project and an inspiration for many

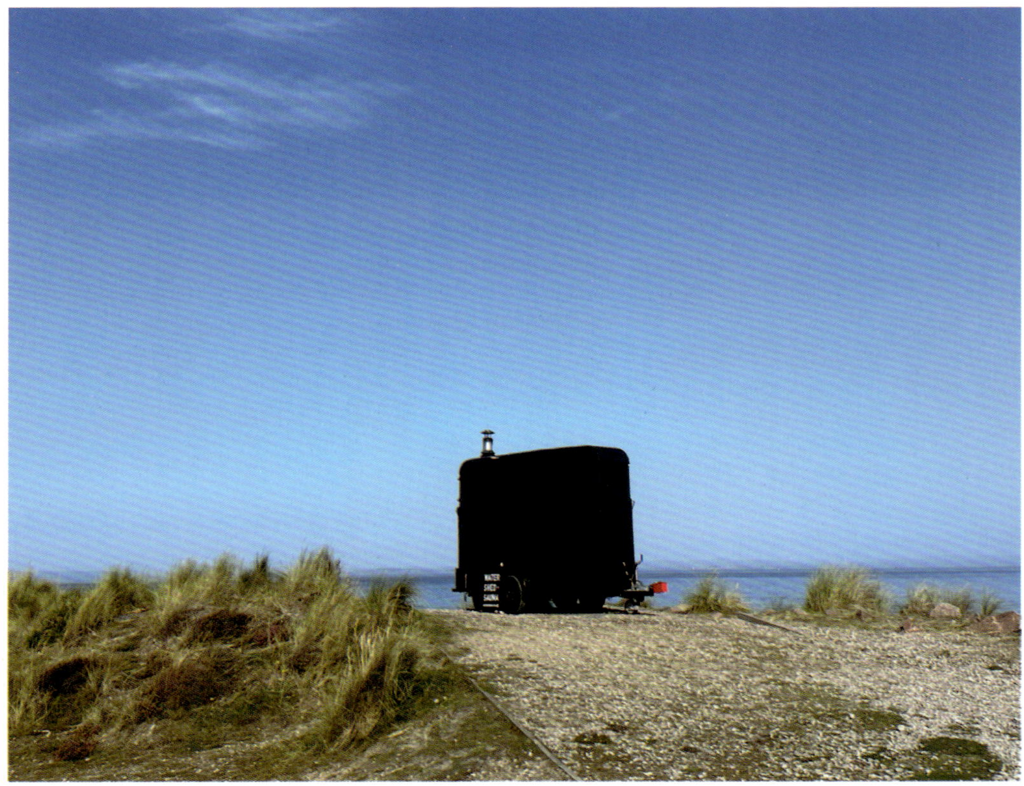

younger sauna operators. The sauna is made from local Douglas fir and painted black, with black water containers, buckets and dry bags to match. It both stands out and blends in with the grasses, gorse, sand and sea. Firewood is locally sourced, the granite stones for the stove were collected from the banks of the River Findhorn, and only locally produced pine or juniper berries are used in their essential oils.

Everything is thought out along the lines of: 'How are we serving the community? How are we looking after the environment? How are we making our living?' says Elle, 'Are we doing these things well?' A trip to Watershed Sauna suggests they are doing all things very well.

As well as fostering nature connections, Watershed nurtures social ones too. Elle is a director on the board of the Findhorn Village Conservation Company, which enabled locals to purchase the village from an absentee landlord in 2016; the village also owns the intertidal area. The hope is that other communities will follow Findhorn's lead and take ownership of the land.

When you book a session at Watershed, you can buy a seat for someone in need, and the Winter Wellness Programme provides subsidised spots for local residents. A fun addition is Sauna Bingo, where bathers can spot nine different sights and species – among them a basking shark, a dolphin and an osprey. With its microclimate and generous dose of sunshine, this is the 'Costa del Moray', and wildlife is abundant. Every completed bingo card wins a free sauna session.

➔ watershedsauna.com
❄ Sea/bucket 📍 57.6632, -3.6068

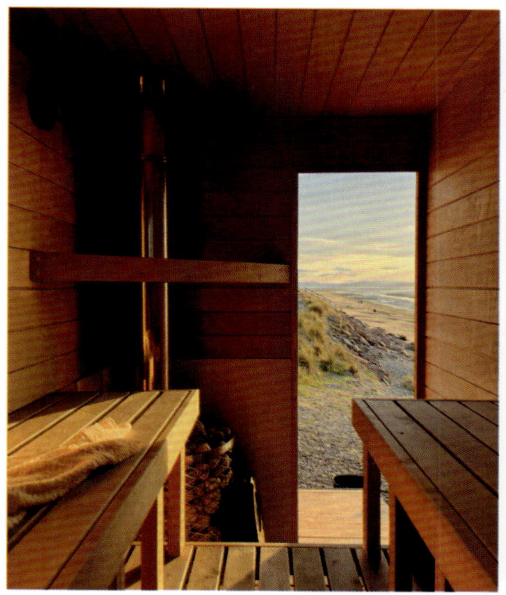

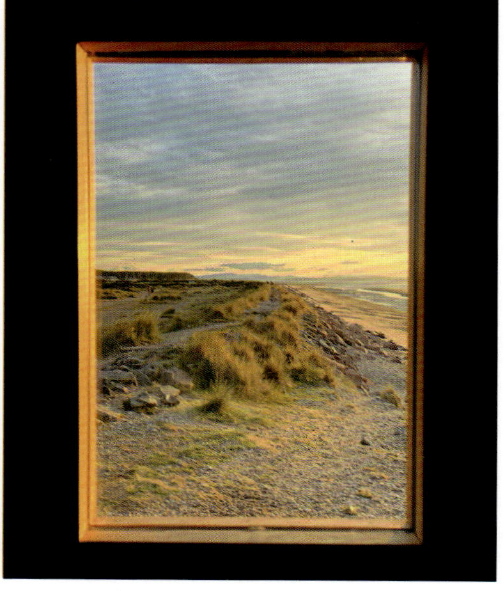

169

Sauna at the Kings

CULLEN ❦ MORAY

When Sauna at the Kings opened on Cullen Beach, it was the result of two years' planning by owner Becky Gorrara, whose partner Andrew runs Coffee at the Kings out of a converted vintage Airstream.

The black barrel sauna fits in with the shape of the arches of the viaduct that runs through Cullen, and, thanks to its elevated position on a piece of scrubland between the golf course and the sea wall, bathers get a great view of the famous Three Kings rock formation through the large panoramic window. The sauna seats eight, and there's fresh water for rinsing off and toilets on the beach.

Sauna at the Kings has its own essential oil, made in collaboration with a local aromatherapist, and Becky makes whisks with branches collected from local woodland. Cullen Beach is a busy spot. Blue Coast Surf and Paddle School is close by, and the Wild Dookers, a big group of swimmers, meet here. There are collaborations with yoga, Pilates and fitness groups, and great coffee and cakes.

saunaatthekings.co.uk
Sea/bucket 57.6939, -2.8347

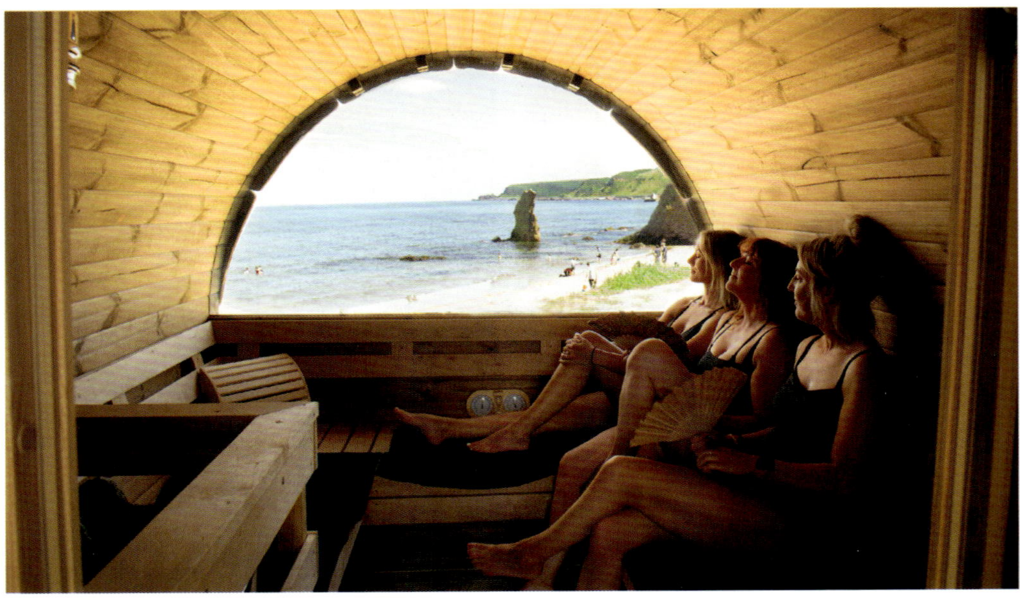

170

Sea Biscuit Sauna

ABERDEEN ❦ ABERDEENSHIRE

Debbie Thornton, a proud 'Aberdeen quine', opened Sea Biscuit sauna on Aberdeen's Esplanade in 2024. She had been a regular customer of Haar Sauna when it was on the Aberdeen Footdee beach (or Fittie, as it's pronounced locally) the year before. When it left, she missed it so much that she decided to build her own. The result is an intimate horsebox conversion for six, with two benches facing each other.

Debbie is now a sauna master trained in Lithuanian pirtis for multi-sensory sauna master sessions. She collaborates with many other wellness practitioners to organise events centred around sauna practice – silent discos on the beach, yoga sessions, ritual cleansing pirtis sessions, breathwork and reiki soul healing sessions, open-water swimming instruction days, cacao rituals and a lot of laughter.

A second sauna, Sea Biscuit 2.0, pops up at weekends in different North Aberdeenshire locations. Look out for her at Greenmyres Eco Bothy in Drumblade, Port Errol harbour at Cruden Bay and at Sandend Holidays, a campsite with access to a beautiful beach.

seabiscuitsauna.co.uk
Sea/shower 57.1451, -2.0732

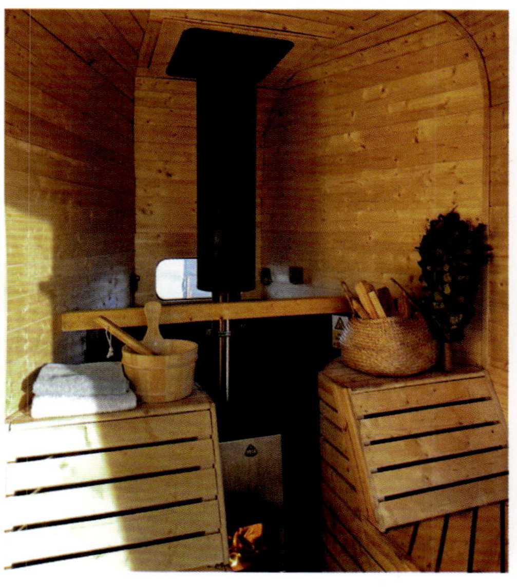

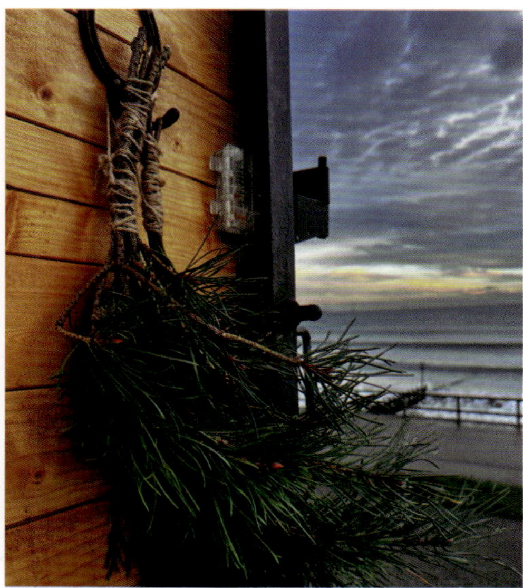

171

Haar Sauna

ST NINIAN'S BEACH ❦ SHETLAND

When it opened in 2020, Haar was the first horsebox sauna in Scotland; and everywhere it went – Aberdeen, the Cairngorms, the River Tay – it left an impression and a band of protégés who set up other saunas in its footsteps. It was the original firestarter. In 2023, its founders, Hannah Mary and her husband Callum, decided to take it home, back to Shetland, where Hannah Mary is from.

It now sits on the 750-metre-long St Ninian's Beach, a glittering horseshoe-shaped bay on St Ninian's Isle, which flanks a sand spit to mainland Shetland. The island houses the ruins of a Viking monastery, Neolithic graves and an abundance of puffins. It draws locals and tourists alike.

Haar is the Scottish word for the sea mist that frequently rolls off the North Sea. This can descend for days, and the sauna holds dedicated sessions for locals, among them men's mental health groups (suicide is the largest killer of men aged under 40 in Scotland). Haar is the only wild sauna operator on Shetland, and it's now setting its sights beyond 60 degrees North, to Scapa Beach on Orkney.

haarsauna.com
Sea 59.9706, -1.3310

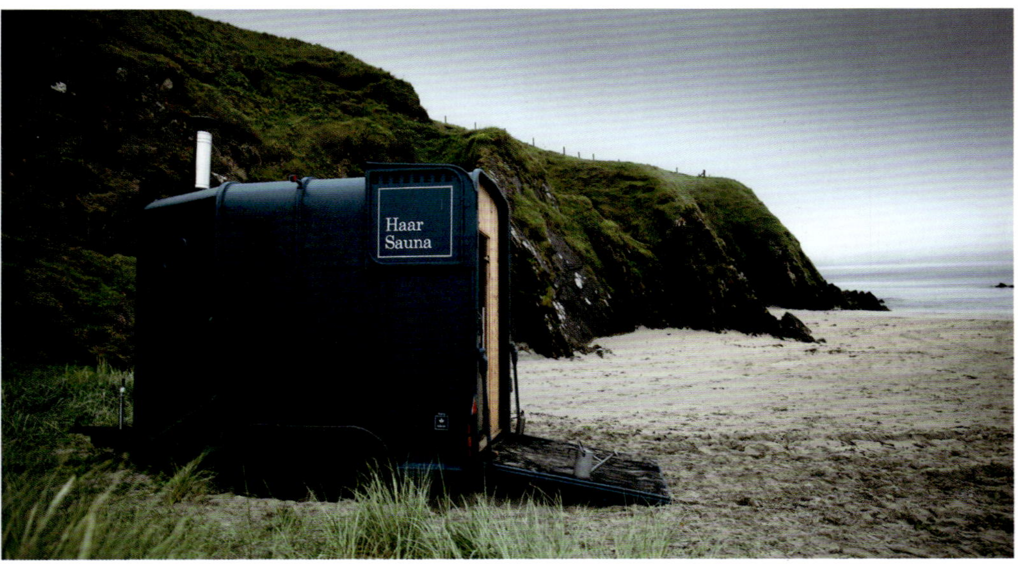

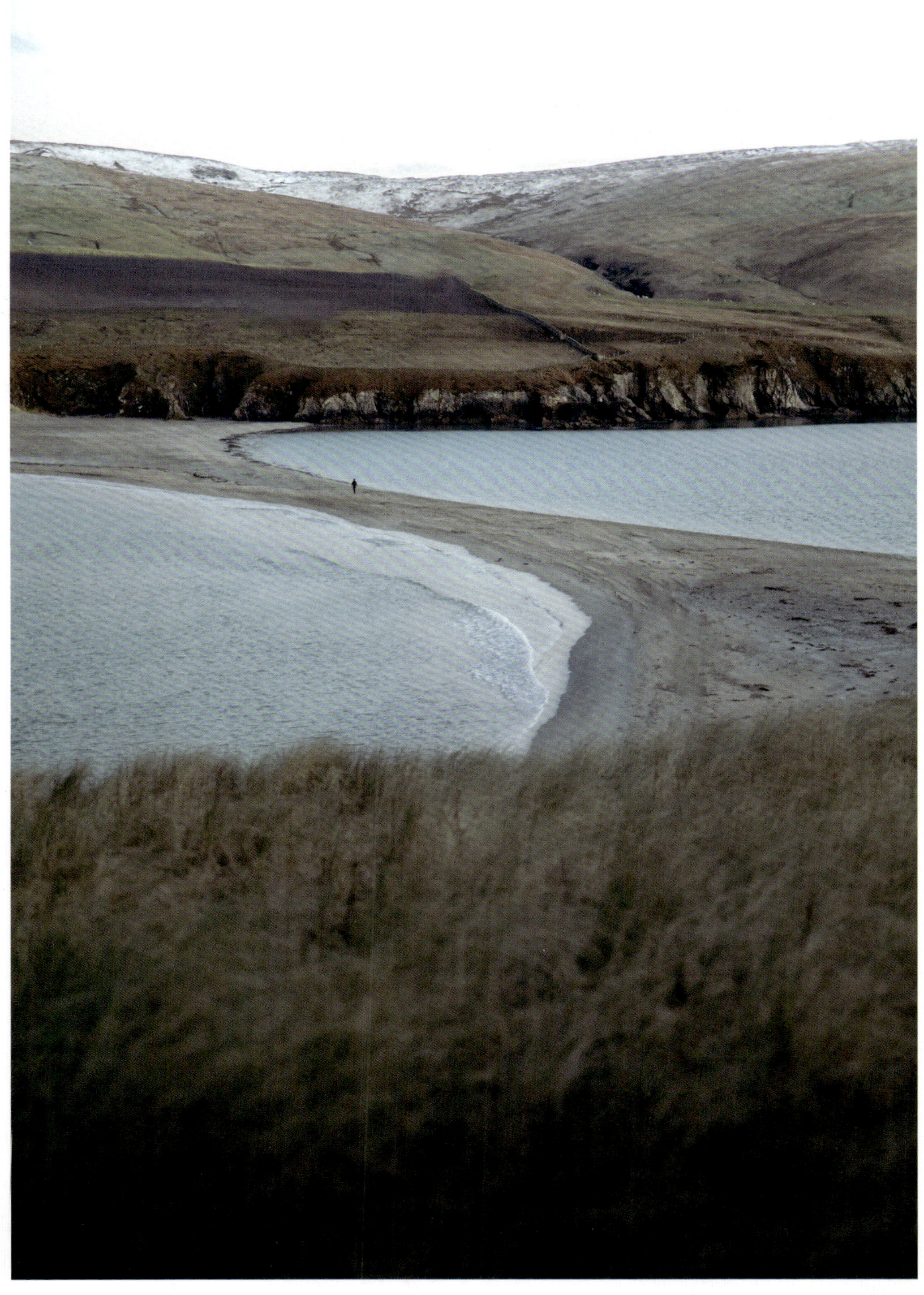

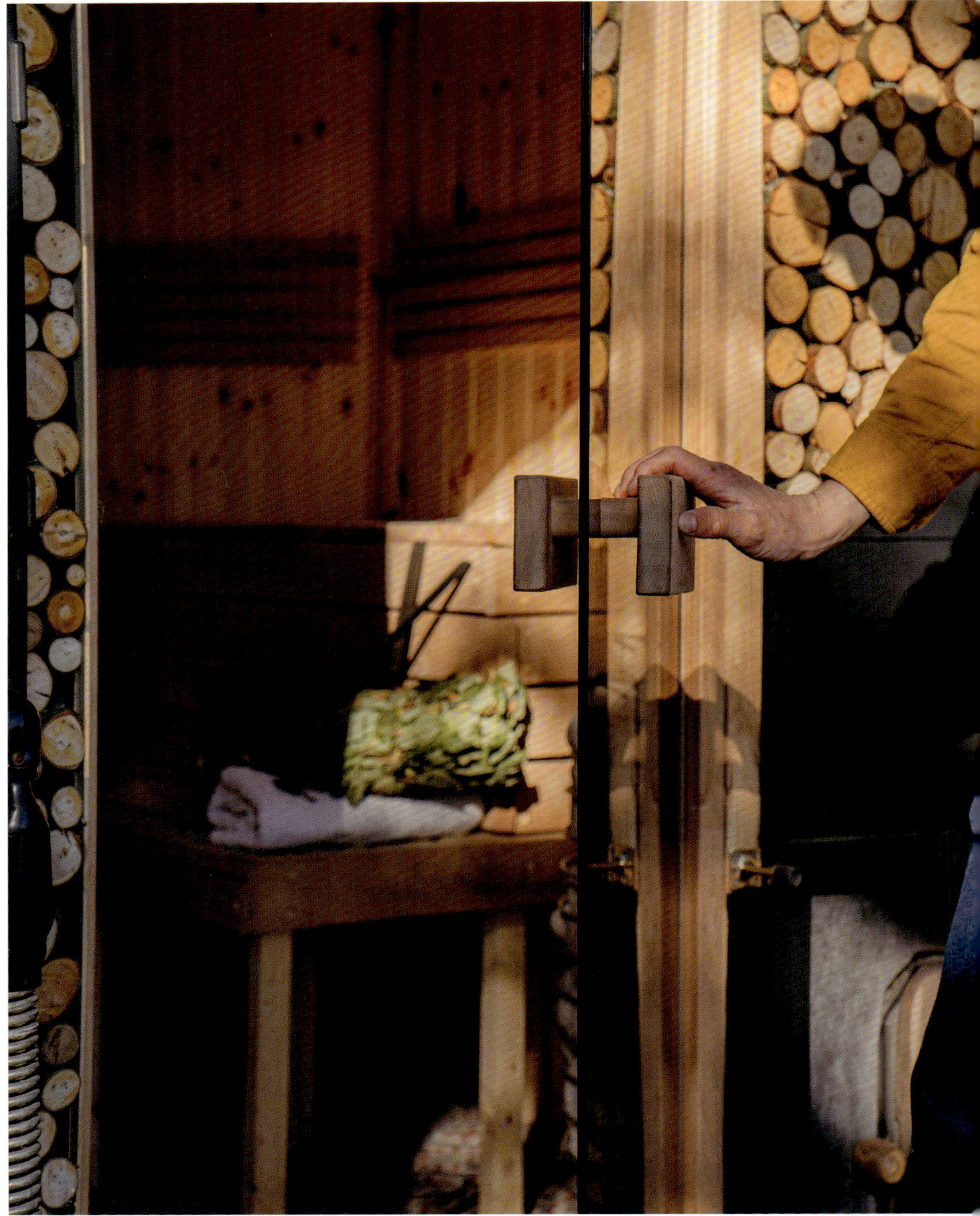

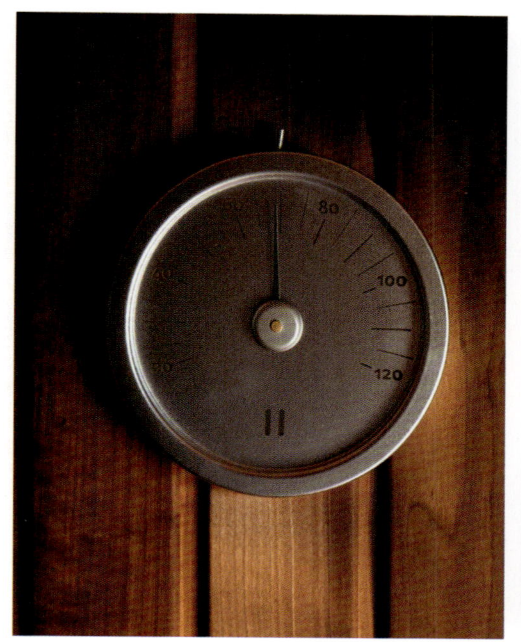

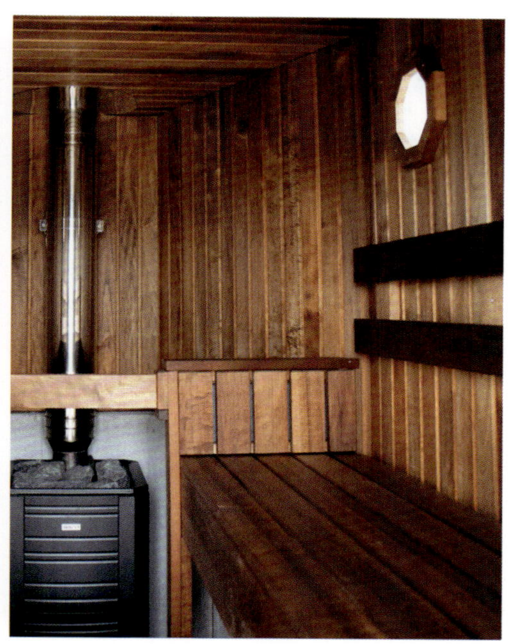

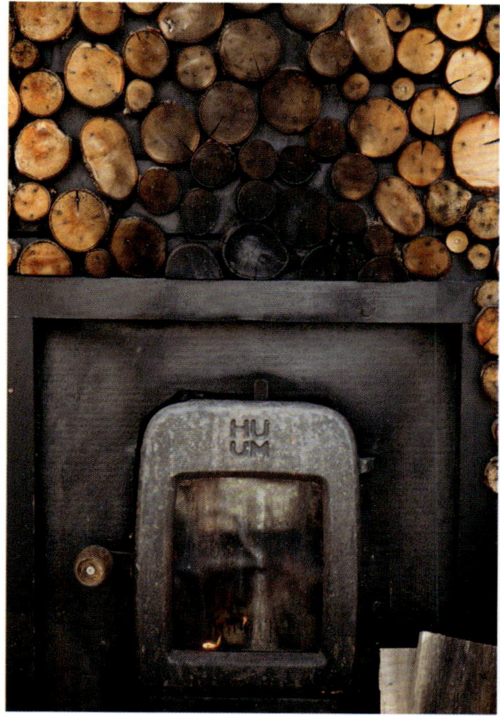

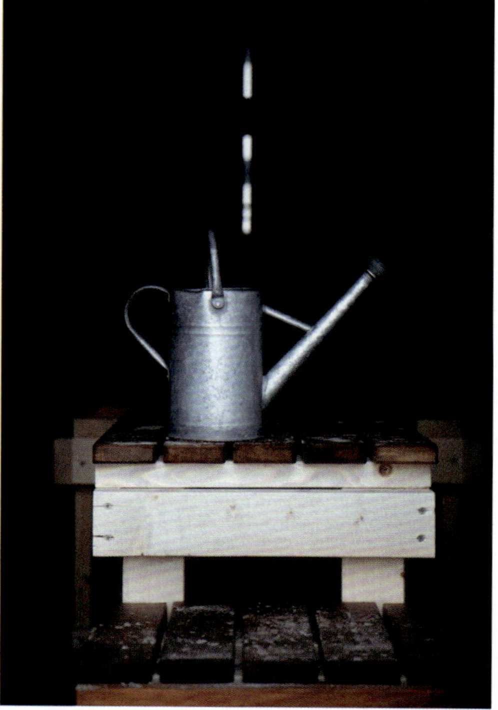

Haar Sauna

More

172 Stonesthrow Sauna

LAMLASH ✽ ISLE OF ARRAN

Stonesthrow Sauna's main site is at Lamlash Bay, a Marine Protected Area with great biodiversity and a wonderful view of the Holy Isle. This mobile sauna has a large picture window, and moves around the Isle of Arran offering sessions in other stunning seaside spots, among them Brodick and Whiting Bay.

stonesthrowsauna.co.uk
Sea 55.5304, -5.1290

173 Blackhouse Sauna

IRVINE BEACH ✽ NORTH AYRSHIRE

At Blackhouse, post-exercise muscle recovery and being outdoors whatever the weather are the focus. David Moore, one of Blackhouse's three founders got hooked on cold water therapy while preparing to hike up Mount Everest in 2019. The sauna is mostly parked at Ardossan's South Beach, on the coast south west of Glasgow

facebook.com/p/Blackhouse-Sauna-61555941230619/
Cold plunge/sea 55.6048, -4.6942

174 Happy & Wild

LUNDERSTON BAY ✽ INVERCLYDE

Lisa Boonsanong runs a pop-up tent sauna operation in various locations on the Firth of Clyde. She is a qualified open-water swim coach who has introduced loads of people to the joys of sauna and cold-water dipping since opening in 2021. Happy & Wild also provides sauna tents for private hire.

happyandwild.co.uk
Sea/loch 55.9306, -4.8762

175 Wild Bathing Sauna

TRALEE BAY ✽ ARGYLL AND BUTE

Jo MacLean, a cold-water swimming instructor, gives bathers a dose of the wilderness and open water around Oban. Her mobile barrel sauna holds six people, and she uses logs sourced from her own croft for the sauna fire.

wildbathing.co.uk
Sea 56.4956, -5.4223

176 Spear Sauna

NEWBRIDGE ✽ EDINBURGH

Adam Fisher and Rob Ng have provided converted horsebox and tent saunas for years. Their own magnificent 18-person permanent sauna is open to the public for optimal contrast therapy sessions at the Lost Shore Surf Resort near Edinburgh, the largest inland surf resort of its kind in Europe.

spearsauna.co.uk
Lake/drench buckets 55.9216, -3.4005

177 Sunnd Sauna

EDINBURGH/BRISTOL ✽ FESTIVALS & EVENTS

Olivia-Grace Smith and Luke Shields built their roaming sauna, *Sunnd* – meaning wellness, health, and joy in Gaelic – with hopes of reconnecting their guests to themselves, the environment and those around them. Based between Edinburgh and Bristol, you'll find them at festivals and events up and down the UK.

sunndsauna.com
Drench buckets 55.9788, -3.2888

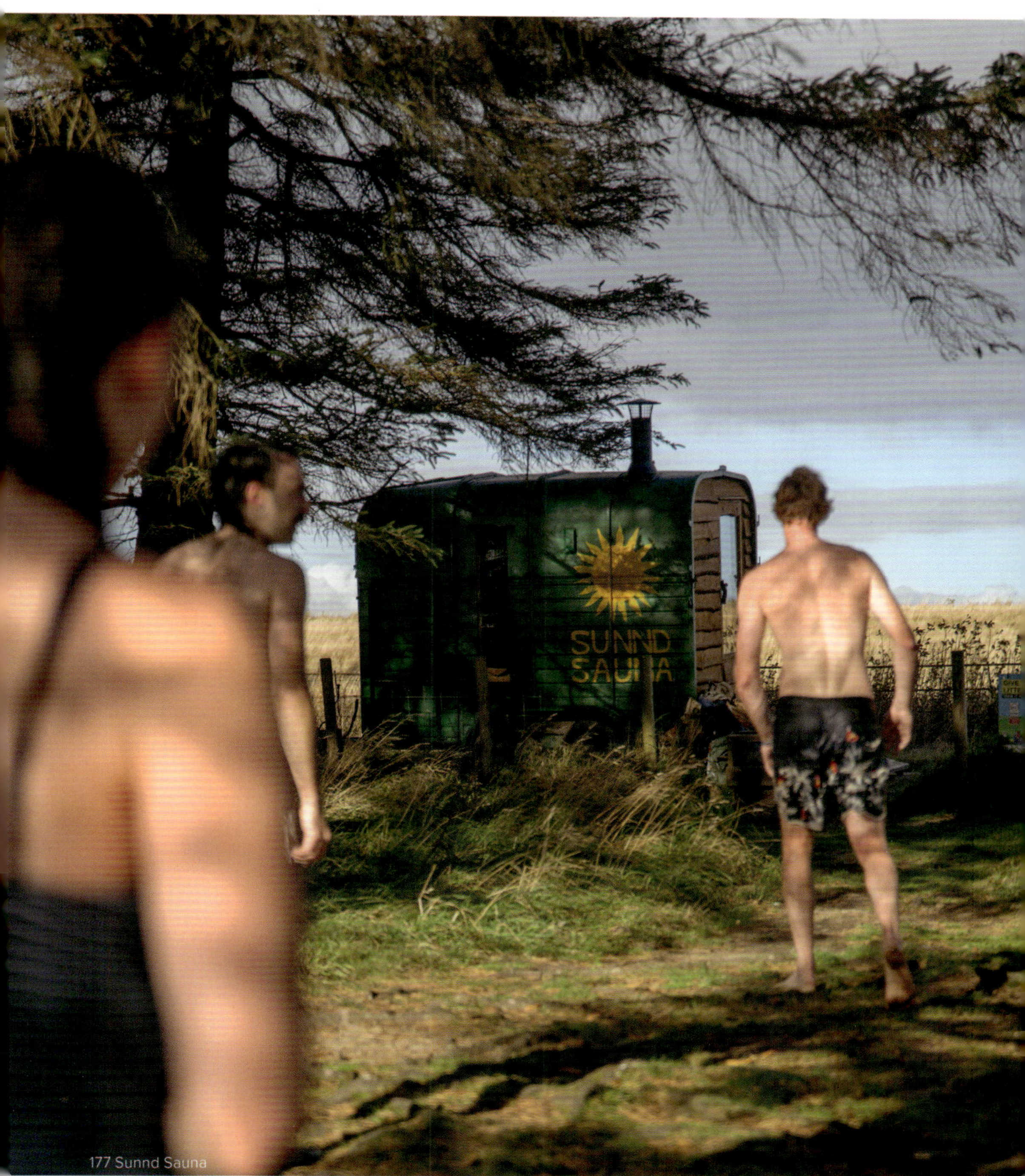

177 Sunnd Sauna

178 Cedar Hus

MELROSE ❁ ROXBURGHSHIRE

Cedar Hus's sauna is made from recycled Canadian cedar salvaged from an outbuilding on Laura and Willie Mitchell's farm. The mobile sauna moves around the Scottish Borders. Some sessions are offered in conjunction with high intensity cardio training or yoga. If they set up away from natural water, they have a shower and a bucket.

cedarhus.co.uk
Shower/bucket 55.5294, -2.6916

179 Viking Heat Retreat

BALMALCOLM ❁ FIFE

Tina Ronaldson's Viking Heat Retreat offers a barrel sauna with five recycled baths as cold plunges. The retreat offers discounted private sessions for local mental health charities and also welcomes teenagers.

instagram.com/viking_heat_retreat
Bath 56.2623, -3.0973

180 Taymouth Marina Hot Box

KENMORE ❁ PERTHSHIRE

The 'sauna with the slide' is a much-talked-about feature of the Wild Wellness lochside spa at Taymouth Marina. It's more than a gimmick, and you don't need to be staying at the marina resort to use it. Anyone can buy a two-hour pass, which includes use of the outdoor hot pool, spa bar, HotBox sauna, steam room, jetty – and slide, which swooshes you into the fresh waters of Loch Tay.

The resort consists of houseboats, apartments, and townhouses; guests in the latter two are entitled to a free spa session. Stately Munros and the surrounding countryside can be seen from the spa, and the marina itself is bustling with water sports, from kayaking and canoeing to paddleboarding and boat tours.

taymouthmarina.com
Loch 56.5791, -4.0042

181 Sauna Cairngorms

LOCH INSH, INVERNESS-SHIRE

Linda Thain runs sauna sesssions, both private and communal in conjunction with her yoga business. The sauna is set in the grounds of Loch Insh Outdoor Centre in Kincraig, right on the shores of the loch, ideal for a cold dip. Wild swimming is very popular here, but the site is also a destination for walkers, runners and cyclists.

yogacairngorms.com
Loch 57.1171, -3.9208

182 Hot Fox Sauna

DUNBAR ❁ EAST LOTHIAN

The Hot Fox Sauna sit on the banks of the lake at Foxlake Adventures in Dunbar. It is open to the public from Friday to Sunday all year round, and more frequently through the rest of the year. Access into the lake for a cold dip is easy, and many water-based activities can be booked separately.

foxlake.co.uk/sauna
Lake/barrel 55.9920, -2.5886

183 Highland Sauna

ROSEMARKIE ❁ INVERNESS-SHIRE

Highland Sauna has two mobile barrel saunas, one popping up every weekend on Rosemarkie Beach and the other available for gardens, events, festivals and parties.

highlandsauna.co.uk
Sea 57.5933, -4.1125

184 Stravaig Saunas

CRATHIE ❦ ABERDEENSHIRE

Louise and Stuart Thomson run a bespoke joinery business in rural Aberdeenshire. The couple were given a Harvia sauna fire as a 'random' wedding gift by Louise's sister, so they built a beautiful mobile sauna to house it. It can be booked for use on site, below their home and business, or for use in the surrounding area. There is a bath for plunging, plus a shower on the side of the sauna or buckets for rinsing.

deesidetimbercrafts.co.uk/stravaigsaunas

Shower/bath/bucket 57.0454, -3.1770

185 Arbikie Estate

LUNAN ❦ ANGUS

Arbikie is a 2,000-acre, family-run estate, with one of Scotland's most sustainable distilleries. Mirrored ÖÖD House cabins, complete with mirrored saunas and showers, provide a place to stay and relax.

arbikie.com

Cold plunge 56.6655, -2.5276

186 Glen Dye Estate

BANCHORY ❦ ABERDEENSHIRE

The Woodland Sauna on the Glen Dye Estate is only open to guests staying on the estate. Sessions are for three hours, with guests responsible for lighting the fire. There are plenty of distractions while the sauna hots up, among them two large plunge baths and a 'natural' waterfall-type shower.

glendyecabinsandcottages.com

Bath/shower 56.9653, -2.5735

187Stonehaven Paddleboarding

STONEHAVEN ❦ ABERDEENSHIRE

Dave Jacobs describes setting up Stonehaven Paddleboarding as his midlife crisis. He used driftwood to construct the horsebox sauna, which is a great addition to the water-based experiences that he offers in the harbour and beyond. Dave runs everything himself and only takes bookings and requests through personal messages. He suggests people visit at times that suit, like when the tide is in and it's only a short walk to the sea. Driftwood Sauna has no minimum age policy and families are actively encouraged to come and under-8s go free. Groups who want to try a 'clothing-optional' sauna can also come early, when the harbour is quiet.

shpb.co.uk/sauna

Sea/shower 56.9582, -2.2030

188 Barbossauna

ABERDEEN ❦ ABERDEENSHIRE

A native of Brazil, Fabio Barbosa has been in Aberdeen since 2008, where he's a keen surfer in the waters off Footdee beach. Horsebox conversion, Barbossauna is open seven days a week all year round for communal sessions or private hire. A second horsebox acts as a changing room and offers some privacy in this busy, touristy area. If there is room, walk-ins are always welcomed. Everyone is offered a loyalty card – have seven saunas and get one free. Local sports clubs and fitness centres started enquiring about a mobile sauna for when they host events, and to cope with such demand, Fabio has built another horsebox sauna.

barbossauna.co.uk

Sea/shower/watering can 57.1448, -2.0729

189 Largo Castaway

LARGO ❦ FIFE

Antonia and Steve Pettifer have long known how contrast therapy can be so beneficial for pain relief. They also know how much fun sauna is and wanted to share the experience with their local community. They opened Largo Castaway Sauna in 2025, running sessions at the weekend and on holidays. The sauna is right by sea, a perfect location.

largocastawaysauna.co.uk

Sea 56.2123, -2.9239

The Wild Sauna movement today

WHERE NEXT?

Trying to document the British sauna scene today literally means today, because by tomorrow it will have moved on – morphing, maturing, expanding. So where and when did it all begin and where does it go from here?

SAUNA FESTIVALS

In the 1980s and 1990s the birth of the Wild Sauna movement owed much to the festival scene – it's where many have their sauna epiphanies. At festivals people often become more open, free and adventurous – and willing to try new things, like a wood-fired sauna. During the summer months, many mobile operators hit the festival circuit, following in the footsteps of Lost Horizon and Sams Sauna (Magic Hat Sauna) that went 30 years before them. Since then, festivals have grown their wellness spaces, and mobile wild spas such as Slomo and The Wandering Wild Spa offer saunas, hot tubs, drench buckets and cold plunges away from the crowds.

Still, saunas at festivals are one thing, but an actual sauna festival? Popular in all the sweat bathing nations, a sauna festival brings people together to sweat in all sorts of set-ups, from home-grown truck conversions to floating saunas and traditional smoke saunas. It was only a matter of time before the UK caught on to this most original of wellness festival, and The Saunaverse debuted in Hackney's Community Sauna Baths in 2023. Here, around 300 bathers, from newcomers to sauna diehards, come together to enjoy a sweaty celebration in wood-fired saunas and cold plunges. Music, workshops, dance and rituals make up the mix, and include Baltic whisking, sound baths and wholly British inventions such as 'Laugh-guss' (a mix of laughter yoga and *aufguss*) and sauna life-drawing classes, the latter two both thanks to London artist Barry Sykes.

DIVERSITY AND INCLUSIVITY

What we know so far about the Wild Sauna scene is that, generally, women who swim are the first arrivals; they're followed by their male counterparts and by athletes who know how good sauna is for muscle recovery after exercise. Then come the younger bathers, drawn to the digital detox and the real-life encounters sauna offers. But what about everyone else? The sauna door may be open to all, but not everyone comes. For those with chronic anxiety, chronic pain, chronic fatigue, the idea of being in a swimsuit in a dark, hot box can be overwhelming and intimidating, and operators have to work hard to reach those communities who might benefit from sauna the most.

The Community Sauna Baths operates sites all over London, in some deprived areas of the city. It studies closely which communities are not coming to sauna, and collaborates with charities, practitioners and individuals to try and reach these groups. In conjunction with the charity Care4Calais, CSB runs sessions for refugees and asylum seekers who offer gardening in exchange for sauna and lunch. It also collaborates with Latin American Women's Aid, Age UK, English for Change and other charities, and offers free

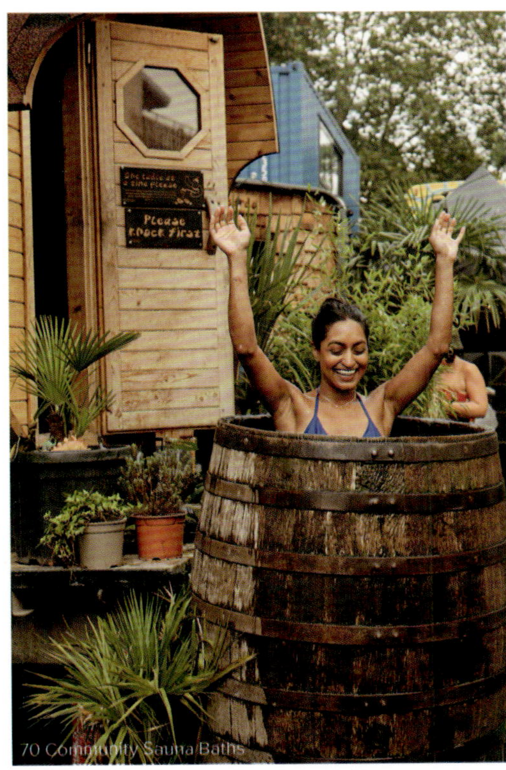

70 Community Sauna Baths

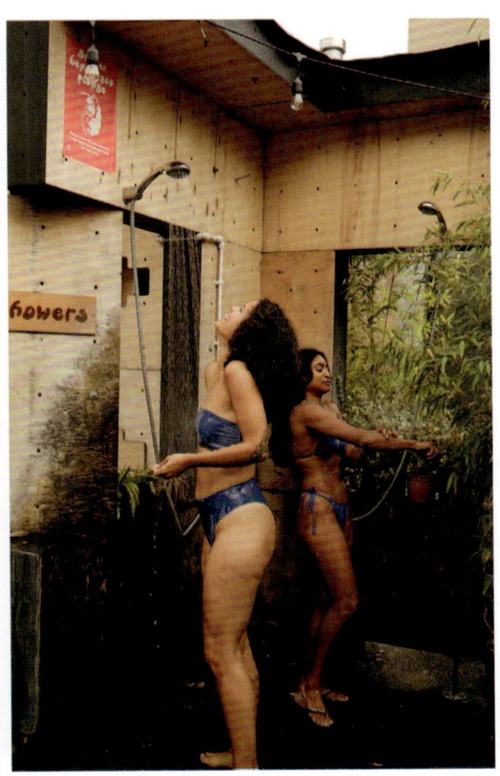

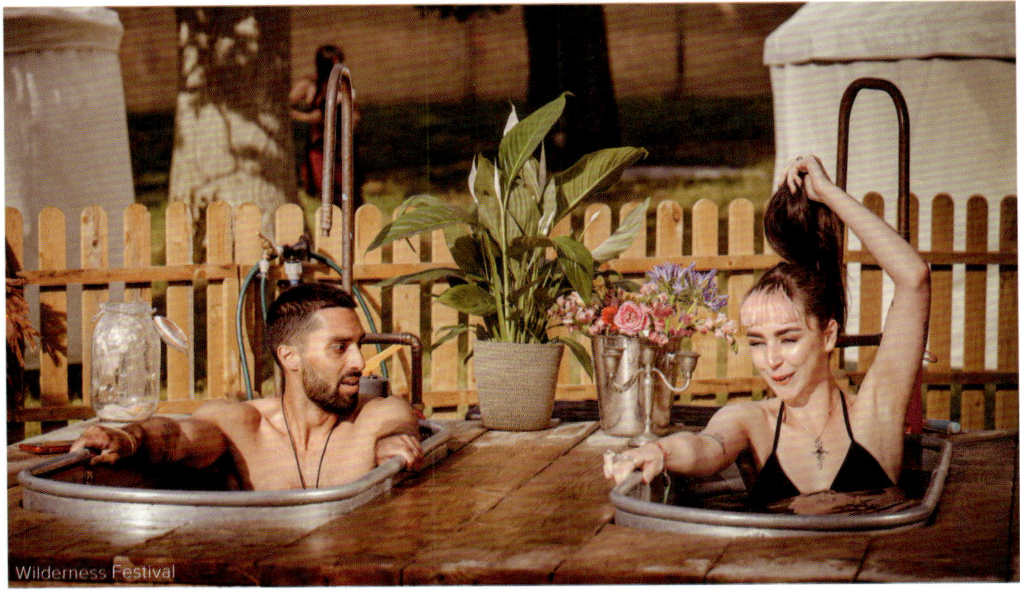
Wilderness Festival

sessions to NHS workers, and those who are prescribed sauna through their GP. Myth Mondays cater to women, non-binary and intersex bathers; there's also a Trans sauna, Queer Poetry sauna, Mum's sauna as well as other less frequent events, such as 'For Brothers That Talk' aimed at black men.

SAUNA AID

Sauna Aid was set up as a humanitarian initiative by the International Sauna Association (ISA), a non-profit organisation made up of more than 20 sauna-bathing nations. Its mission is to send portable saunas to people facing natural and man-made disasters, by collaborating with international organisations and NGOs. Ukraine is the current focus, and to date Sauna Aid has deployed five mobile saunas to the war-torn country.

The idea is not as strange as it sounds; in Ukraine, the sauna, or *laznia*, is known as the 'second mother'. It's not seen as a luxury, but rather as an everyday space where people of all ages, social classes and backgrounds come together for some physical and mental respite.

Estonian charity Saunas For Ukraine is also sending saunas to Ukraine, to troops on the frontline. Again, this idea is not as strange as it sounds, because Baltic, Russian and Finnish troops always build themselves saunas as washhouses and places of respite, wherever they go.

'One of the greatest sins is the unlived life'

Aman Cara, John O'Donaghue

Jumping in an untamed ocean, sweating on a hot bench next to a stranger and leaving the trappings of comfort far behind may sound daunting - terrifying even - but it's a sure fire route to better health and wellbeing. Just ask any of the people featured in these pages. Give it a go, and follow this guide. Here you can plot adventures to extraordinary, exciting places where unexpected connections and unpredictable nature are matched by compassion, warmth and good humour.

On my nine-month UK sauna marathon, a country I didn't know or recognise came into view. A happier, healthier, kinder place. And it's largely thanks to all those sauna operators who light fires and open doors and bring a moment of relief to us all. This book would not have been possible without their hard work, generosity, passion and resilience, and I thank them all.

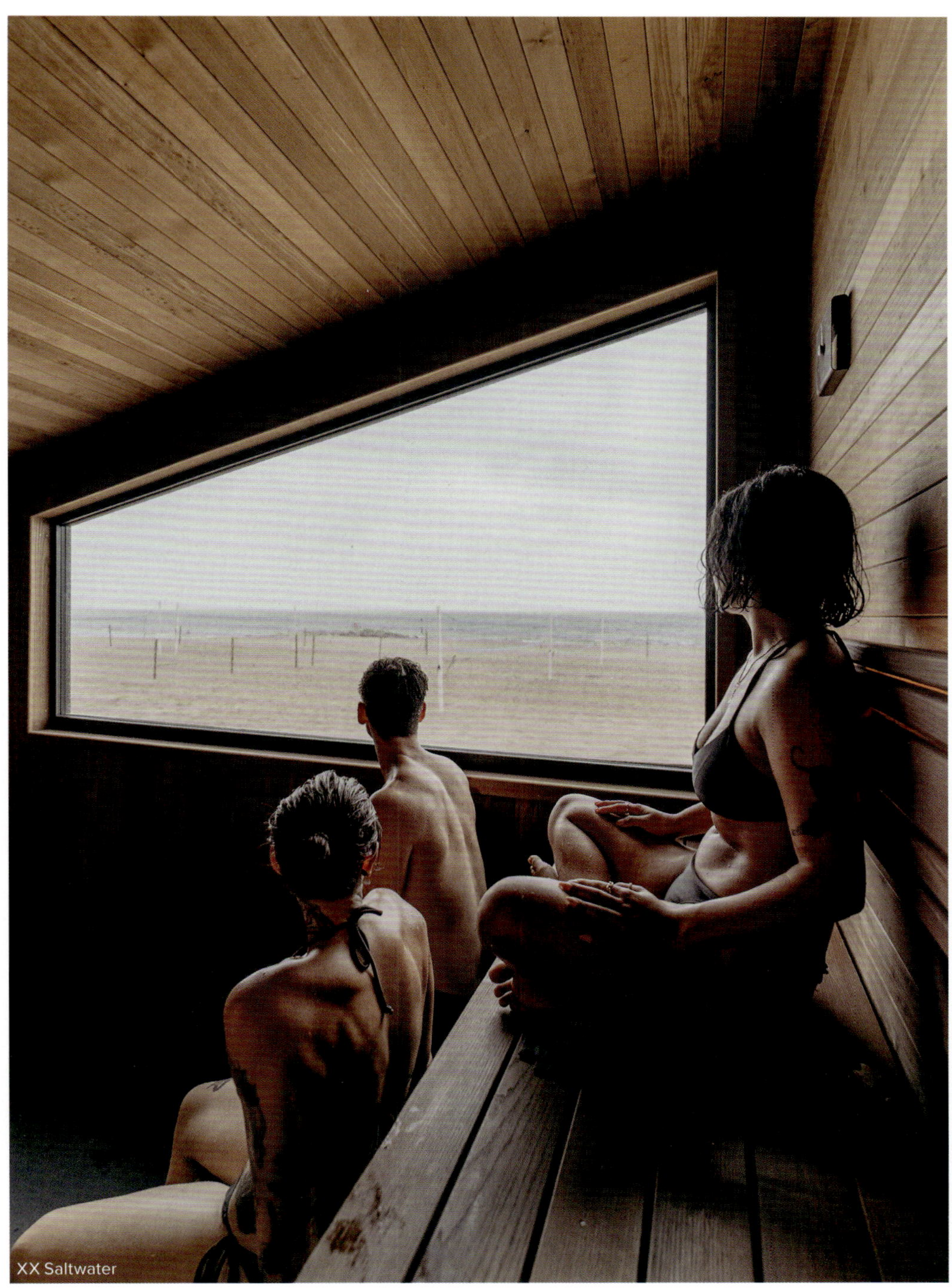
XX Saltwater

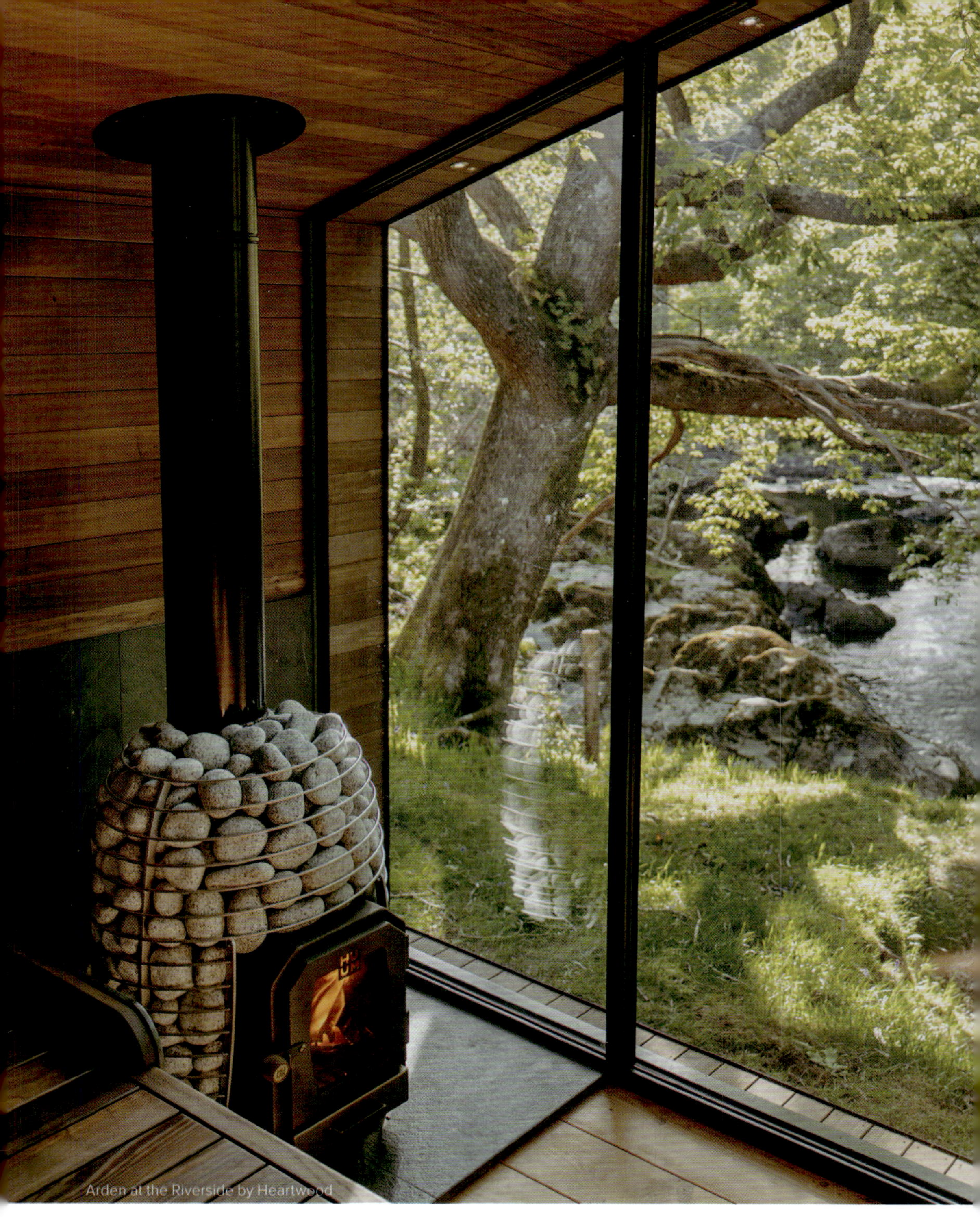
Arden at the Riverside by Heartwood

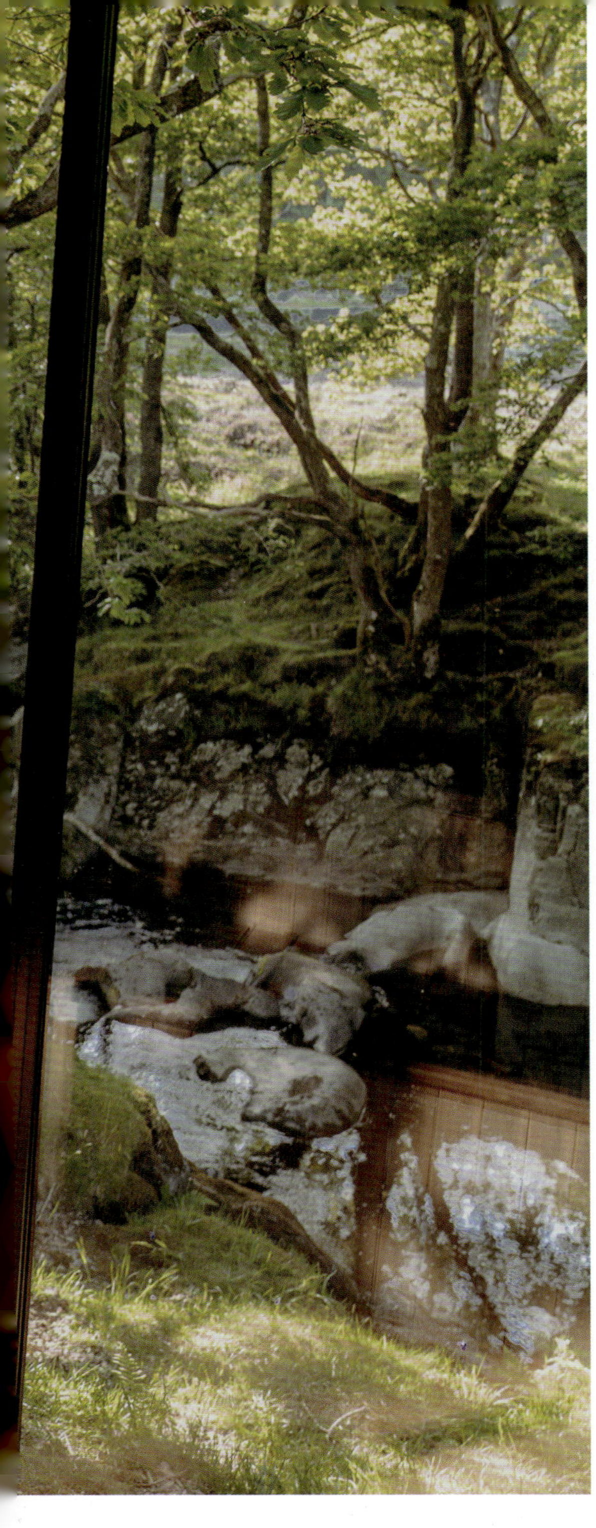

SAUNA MAKERS DIRECTORY:

aspensaunas.com

barrelsaunauk.co.uk

dorsetsaunas.co.uk

finnmarksauna.com

heartwoodsaunas.com

iglucraft.com

kernowsprings.co.uk

ludgatebloom.com

oodhouse.com

outofthevalley.co.uk

pixxla.com

portasauna.co.uk

redkiteyurts.com

revilldesign.com

saunabox.co.uk

saunacraft.co.uk

saunaverse.co.uk

scandinaviansauna.dk

skotlanti.co.uk

wildhut.com

Tent Saunas:

Arctinar.com

Mobiba.ie

Morzh.eu

savotta.fi

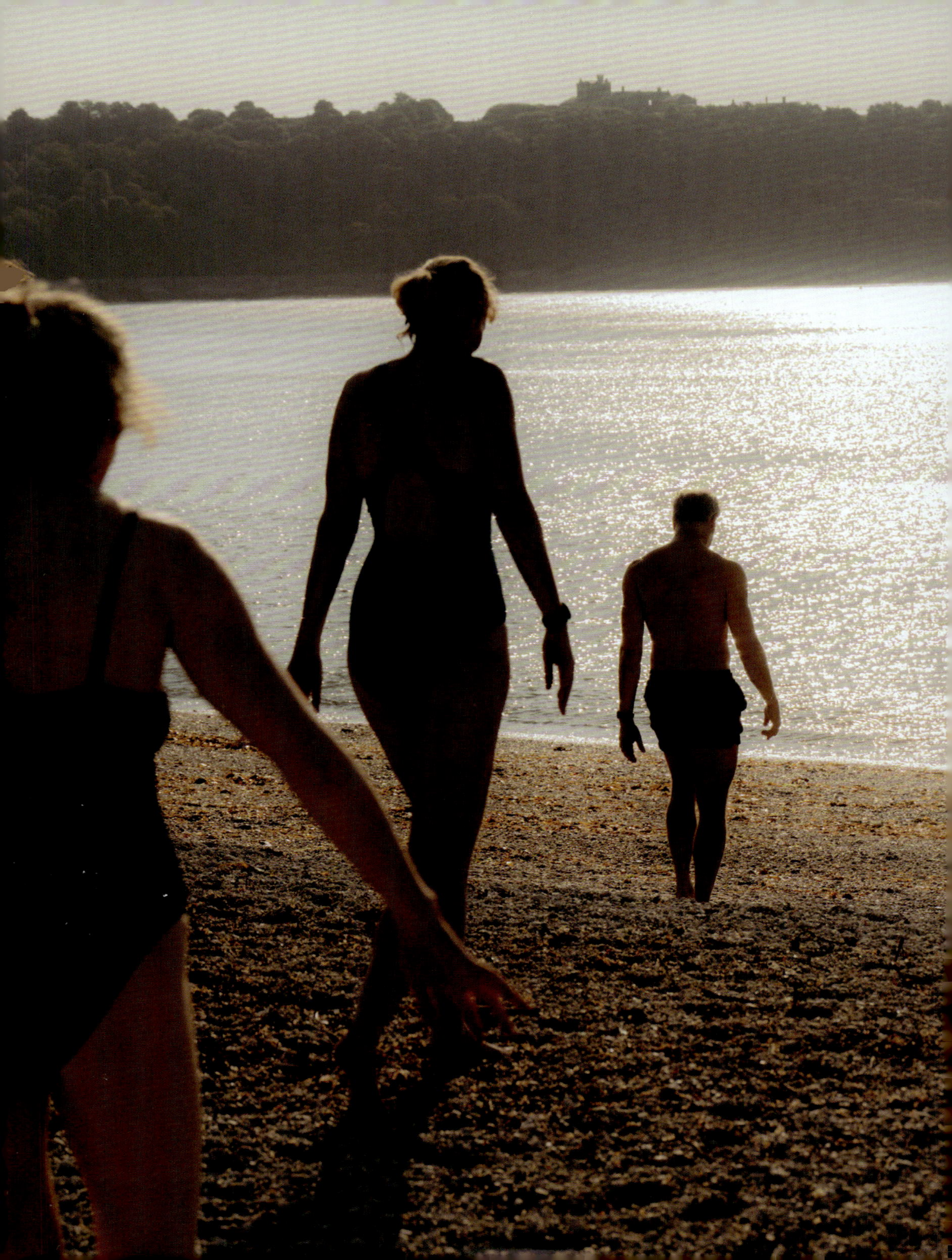

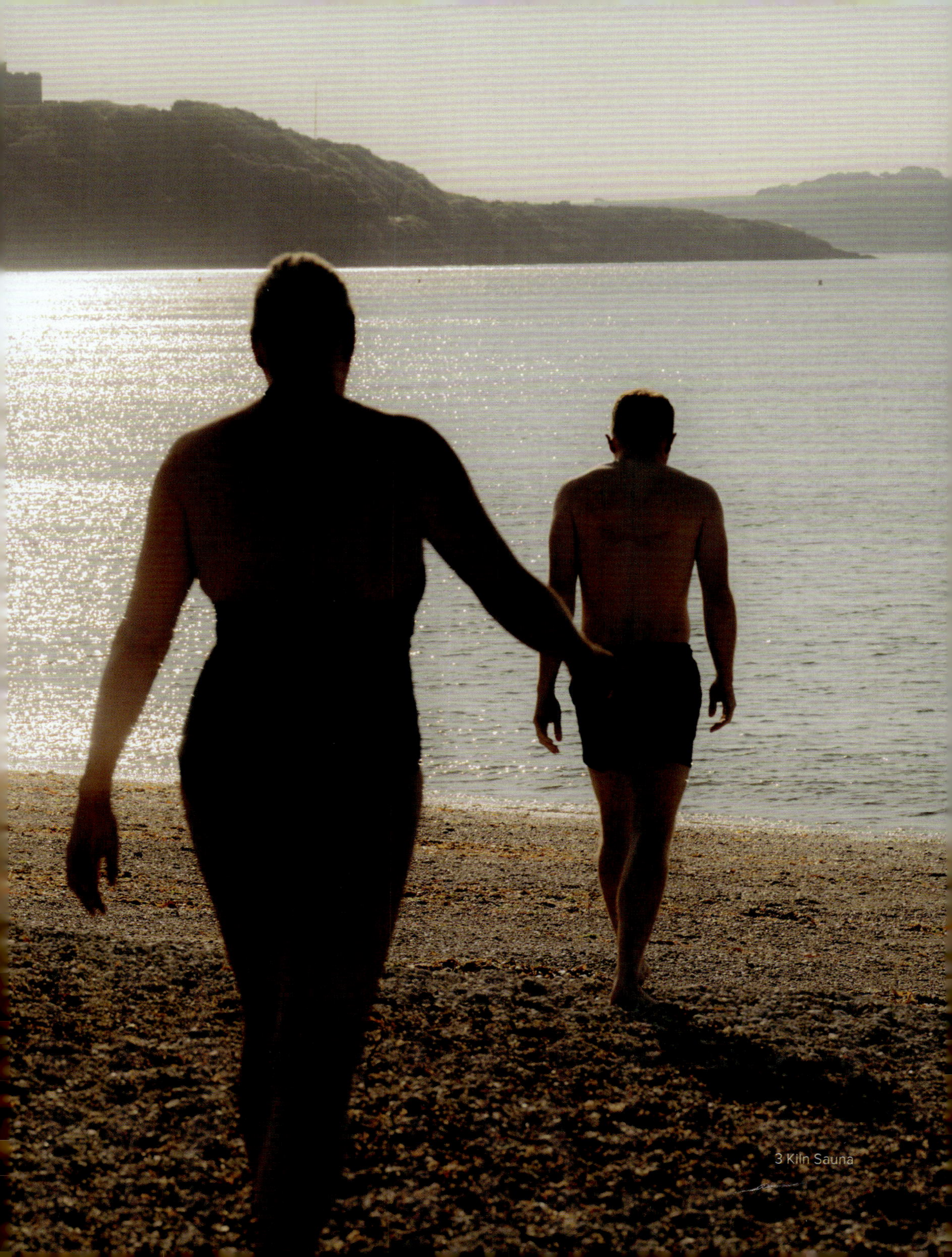

3 Kiln Sauna

WILD SAUNA
The best outdoor saunas in Britain

WORDS:
Emma O'Kelly

PHOTOS:
Those credited

EDITING:
Kate Michell

DESIGN AND LAYOUT:
Emma Stebbings

DISTRIBUTED BY:
Central Books Ltd
Freshwater Road,
Dagenham, RM8 1RX, UK
Tel +44 (0)20 8525 8800
orders@centralbooks.com

WITH THANKS TO:
The British Sauna Society supports best sauna practice in the UK
Britishsaunasociety.org.uk

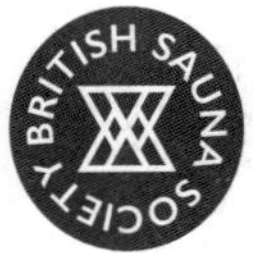

PUBLISHED BY:
Wild Things Publishing Ltd
Freshford, Bath, BA2 7WG, UK
www.wildthingspublishing.com

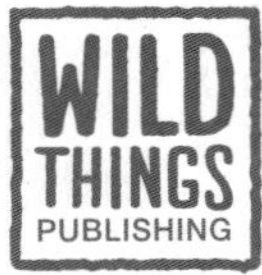

hello@wildthingspublishing.com

ACKNOWLEDGEMENTS

Thanks to my editor friend Jo Lal, who knew the UK was ready for this guide before anyone else did. How right she was. The UK sauna scene is mushrooming so quickly I couldn't keep my arms round it. Alfie, Janet and Lois, your driving skills and insights were top-notch, and thanks for being great company on those long sauna road trips; thanks to Mark for being top sauna partner in crime, and thanks to my father-in-law Richard Dehn for his forensic research, passionate write-ups and for whipping that vast, unwieldy sauna spreadsheet into shape. Thanks too to Daniel, Kate, Emma and everyone at Wild Things who transformed words and pictures into this book.

PHOTO CREDITS

Cover image: Haar Sauna, Shetland, Ritchie Williams. Back cover: Finn Lough, Enniskillen, João Guimarães. Inside front: Kiln Sauna, Cornwall, Jenna Foxton. Inside back: Wildwater, Pembrokeshire, Scott Chalmers & Richard Lynch. Page numbers: 3 Revill Design, 4 Watershed Sauna, 9 Claire Waddell, 10 Sam Cripps, 13 Ritchie Williams, 15 Marc Nichol, 15 Scott Chalmers & Richard Lynch, 17 Finn Beales madebyfinn.com, 18 Dillon Osborne, 19 Saunadelic, 20 Holly Farrier, 21 @jothornephotography, 3 Mikkel Aaland, 23 ITAGO MEDIA LTD, 24 Mikkel aaland, 27 Sam Scales, 28 Nichola Smith, 31 ablinq.co, 33 Marc Millar, 33 Bill Measom, 35 Beth Steddon, 35 Jez Tozer, 35 Paul Winch-Furness, 37 Marc Miller, 37 Olivia-Grace Smith, 39 Des Iles, 40 Louise Mather, 43 Des Iles, 43 J Foxton, 44 Ian Wood / Wood & Co, 49 Robyn Leonia, 49 Robyn Leonia, 51Sam Cripps, 51 Olivia-Grace Smith, 51 Michael Rummey, 51 Dominic Burgess, 52 Sam Scadgell, 53 Lily Bertrand-Webb, 54 Felix Russel-Saw, 55 Des Iles, 56 Dan Kennedy, 57 Lily Bertrand-Webb, 59 Max Newport, 61 Jay Barnett, 63 Dillon Osborne, 65 Liz Seabrook, 67 Holly Farrier, 68 Nathaniel Reeks, 70 Jack Johns, 73 Samuel Boot, 72-73 WE ARE // THE CLARKES, 73 Carla Worden Risen Wild Photography, 74-75 Jenna Foxton, 76 Kathryn Tyler, 76 Jenna Foxton, 77 Kathryn Tyler, 78, 79 Alexa Poppe, 80 Connor Duffy, 81 Janina Fleckhaus, 82, 83 Connor Duffy, 84-87 Jay Barnett, 88,89 Jez Tozer, 90 Jem Wallis, 91-93 Steve French, 94-95 Jay Barnet, 96 Megan Roberts, 97 Keiran Hammond, 98 Lara Kramer, 99 Marc Nichol, 99 Jay Stone, 100-101 Alice Carfrae, 102-103 Olivia-Grace Smith, 104-105 Louise Roberts, 106 Mark Lamb, 107 Sofia Tyson, 108-109 Alex Sergison, 110-111 Izabela Haase, 111 Beth at Folio Creative, 112 Catherine Candler, 113 George Cory, 114-115 Bill Measom, 115 Nathaniel Reeks, 116-117 Seb JJ Peters, 118-119 Olivia-Grace Smith, 120-122 Felix Russel-Saw, 124-126 Dominic Burgess, 128 Kirstie Allen, 129 Shutterstock Robert Harding Video, 130-131 Cole McLean, 134 Revill Design, 136 Simon Buck, 138-139 Sam Scadgell, 140-141 Ben Watson Media, 142-145 @Wasing1759, 146 Leah Maclean, 147 Mark Lamb, 148-149 Tom Keeling, 150 The Quays, 151-153 Michael Antony, 154-155 Nicky Allen, 156 Peter J Fox Photography, 157 Daria Szotek, 158 Luna Hut, 159-161 Claire Waddell, 162-163 Beth Steddon, 163 @jothornephotography, 164 Mark Lamb, 165 Kathy Thomas, 167-169 @jothornephotography, 170-171 Charlotte Monkhouse, 172-173 Holly Farrier, 174-175 Ceri Stokes, 176 Sophie Milligan, 177 Liz Seabrook, 178-179 Liz Seabrook, 180-181, Nick Howe Photography, 182 Victoria Maddox, 182 Victoria Maddox, 183 Zulfiya Wilds, 183 Zulfiya Wilds, 184-185 ablinq.co, 186-187 Frankie Enticknap, 188-189 Hannah Kasza & Ryan King, 190 Oliver Rzosinski, 191 George Cory, 192-193 Zandri Arnold, 194 Sam Scales, 194-195 Andrew Buckley, 197 Anna Hammond, 197 Simon Buck, 198-201 Dan Kennedy, 202 Hannah Louise, 203 Tom Sutton, 207 Dylan Parry Evans, 208-211 Scott Chalmers & Richard Lynch, 210 Sean Ellison, 212 Simon West, 213 Sea+Steam, 214-215 TySawna, 215 Max Webborn, 216-217 Paul Fenrich, 218-219 Felipe Sabbag, 220-221 Sam Farnsworth, 223 Finn Beales madebyfinn.com, 224-225 Nick Thorpe, 226-227 Emma O'Kelly, 231 Jonny Walton, 232-233 Robin Zahler, 234 InaHarrisPhotography, 235 Cat Wynne, 236-237 Jonny Walton, 238 Dave Hemming, 239 Laura Bond, 240-241 Daniel O'Connor, 242-243 Ian Wood / Wood & Co, 244 One Slow Sunday, 245 João Guimarães, 246 Danny Morton Photography, 247 João Guimarães, 247 One Slow Sunday, 248 Jacek Ramus, 249-251 Dillon Osborne, 252-253 Mark Lamb, 254-255 Liam Wiltshire, 256-257 Nick Davies, 258-261 Alex Barlow, 265 Michael Rummey, 266-267 Dave Bennett, 268 Rosie Barge, 269 Immerse Hebrides, 269 Margaret Soraya, 270-271 Louise Mather, 272-273 James Gillies, 273 Claire Ferguson, 274 M Dickie, 275 Aga Urbanska, 276-277 Theodora Van Duin, 278-279 ITAGO MEDIA LTD, 280-281 Seth Tinsley, 282-283 Michael Rummey, 284 Olivia-Grace Smith, 285 Marc Miller, 285 Anna Deacon, 286-287 Olivia-Grace Smith, 288-289 Kim Grant, 290 Rory MacPhee, 291 Daisy Grant, 292-293 Suzanne Black, 294 R Cairney, 295, 297 Marc Millar, 298-299 Suzanne Black, 300-303 Sam Cripps, 303 Shona Armstrong, 303 Annie Armstrong, 304 Watershed Sauna, 305 Claire Ferguson, 306 Shelley Mackie, 307 Debbie Thornton, 308-311 Ritchie Williams, 313 Olivia-Grace Smith, 317 Liz Seabrook, 317 Paul Winch-Furness, 319 Bill Measom, 320 Beth Squire, 323 Jenna Foxton.